# ANATOMY AND THE ORGANIZATION
# OF KNOWLEDGE, 1500–1850

# THE BODY, GENDER AND CULTURE

*Series Editor:    Lynn Botelho*

# ANATOMY AND THE ORGANIZATION OF KNOWLEDGE, 1500–1850

EDITED BY

Matthew Landers and Brian Muñoz

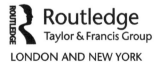

Routledge
Taylor & Francis Group

LONDON AND NEW YORK

First published 2012 by Pickering & Chatto (Publishers) Limited

Published 2016 by Routledge
2 Park Square, Milton Park, Abingdon, Oxfordshire OX14 4RN
711 Third Avenue, New York, NY 10017, USA

First issued in paperback 2015

*Routledge is an imprint of the Taylor & Francis Group, an informa business*

BRITISH LIBRARY CATALOGUING IN PUBLICATION DATA

Anatomy and the organization of knowledge, 1500–1850. – (The body, gender
and culture)
1. Human anatomy – Study and teaching – Europe – History. 2. Human anatomy – Research – Europe – History. 3. Human dissection – Study and teaching
– Europe – History. 4. Human dissection – Research – Europe – History.
I. Series II. Landers, Matthew. III. Munoz, Brian.
611'.0071'04-dc23

ISBN-13: 978-1-138-66462-3 (pbk)
ISBN-13: 978-1-8489-3321-7 (hbk)

Typeset by Pickering & Chatto (Publishers) Limited

# CONTENTS

# LIST OF CONTRIBUTORS

**Kevin L. Cope** is Professor of English and Comparative Literature at Louisiana State University. The author of *Criteria of Certainty* (1990), *John Locke Revisited* (1999), and *In and After the Beginning: Inaugural Moments and Literary Institutions in the Long Eighteenth Century* (2007). He is also the editor of *1650–1850: Ideas, Aesthetics, and Inquiries in the Early Modern Era* and of *ECCB: The Eighteenth-Century Current Bibliography*. During his three decades as a scholar of the long eighteenth century and the history of philosophy and religion, Cope has published over 100 essays and reviews on topics ranging from eighteenth-century cartography to eighteenth-century theories of volcanism to the literature of American fundamentalism and on to the heroic poetry of John Dryden and Alexander Pope. He is currently at work on a book on the 'underground', seismic eighteenth century and is planning a study of joke and jest anthologies of the same period. In 2011, Cope received the Distinguished Research Master Award from Louisiana State University. He has held fellowships from many international research organizations, including the Alexander von Humboldt Stiftung and the University of Aberdeen.

**Nick Davis** is a lecturer in the Department of English at the University of Liverpool. He works mainly on literature–science relations, including cosmology, popular culture and the image of the popular, narratology and early modernity, including transitions to the modern. He is preparing monographs in the privatization of collective experience in early modern literature, and on the treatment of causation in English drama *c.* 1600; and, with Maryam Farahani, an edition of Ibn Tufail's *Hay Ibn Yaqzan*, an account of mentality's development in separation from a social environment.

**Touba Ghadessi** is Assistant Professor of Art History at Wheaton College in Massachusetts. Her book-length study focuses on the ways in which human monstrousness and physical deformity have been historically represented, categorized and interpreted in the various Italian and French courts of the late Renaissance. Ghadessi has been awarded several grants and fellowships; the most recent one was a Whiting Fellowship which allowed her to attend seminars on the history of the body in Paris at the École des hautes études en sciences sociales and also to travel to Mantua, Ferrara, Florence, Rome and Orvieto. Ghadessi has been invited to Wellesley College and the University of Massachusetts at Amherst, where she was a keynote speaker at the Annual Mark Roskill Symposium. She has presented her work at the College Art Association, the Renaissance Society of America, the Social Science History Association and the Western Society for French Historians.

**Jérôme Goffette** is Maître de conférences at Université Lyon 1 in France, where he works in philosophy of medicine. He is the author of *Naissance de l'anthropotechnie* (2006). He is the editor of the collection *L'imaginaire médical dans le fantastique et la science-fiction* (2011). His main research topics are human enhancement, philosophy of the body, philosophy of the imaginary. He works in the research laboratory S2HEP, University Lyon 1 / ENS.

**Craig Ashley Hanson** is Associate Professor of Art History at Calvin College. The author of *The English Virtuoso: Art, Medicine, and Antiquarianism in the Age of Empiricism* (2009), Hanson has published articles in the *Burlington Magazine*, *Journal for Eighteenth-Century Studies* and *Eighteenth-Century Fiction*. He completed his PhD from the University of Chicago in 2003. He has taught as a visiting professor at Emory University and has benefited from programmes at the American School of Classical Studies in Athens, The Wellcome Trust Centre for the History of Medicine and the Attingham Trust for the Study of Historic Houses and Collections. He serves as second vice-president of the Historians of British Art and as newsletter editor for the Historians of Eighteenth-Century Art & Architecture. In the latter capacity, he is the founding editor of *Enfilade*, a daily blog that receives over 7,000 hits each month.

**Hisao Ishizuka** is Associate Professor in the Department of English at Senshu University, Japan. He has published articles in the journals *History of Science* and *Literature and Medicine*, and most recently contributed to *Liberating Medicine, 1720–1835* (2009) and *Neurology and Modernity* (2010). He is co-editor of *Shintai Ibunkaron [Body, Medicine and Culture]* (2002). He is currently writing on fibre theory in Enlightenment medicine, William Blake and medical sciences, and the medico-cultural experience of dyspepsia in nineteenth-century Britain.

**Matthew Landers** is an Assistant Professor of Humanities at the University of Puerto Rico, Mayagüez, where he teaches courses in eighteenth-century British literature and the Enlightenment. He is currently working on a manuscript that examines the relationship between anatomy, philosophy and literature in Europe during the seventeenth and eighteenth centuries. In addition, he has just started work on a new project that reconstructs the development of the word 'culture' in the eighteenth century. He regularly collaborates in the creation of interdisciplinary courses that combine the concerns of the humanities with those of the biological and physical sciences.

**Filippo Pierpaolo Marino** received his bachelor's degree at Alma Mater Studiorum, University of Bologna in 'Visual Arts, Music, Performing Arts and Fashion Studies'. In 2007 he earned his master's degree at the Academy of Fine Arts (Bologna) in 'Planning and Set up of Exhibition Areas', presenting a dissertation on the complicity between art and medicine. He conducted an interview with the scientific journalist Pietro Greco for the Museum of Modern Art in Bologna – *Mambo* (forthcoming). He collaborates on projects with international artists such as Lucy and Jorge Orta, Enzo Cucchi and Sissi. He is currently working at the Academy of Fine Arts in Bologna. His critical investigation, as well as his artistic research, is often tied to the relationship between art and other expressive forms, both in the humanities and scientific fields.

**Brian Muñoz** (co-editor) is a doctor of philosophy from the University of Malaga, Spain (2002) and from the University of Paris X Nanterre, France (2007). He worked as an assistant professor at the University of Lyon I Claude Bernard until 2004. He was a professor at the University of Puerto Rico from 2007 to 2012. Currently he is a collaborative researcher with S2HEP (Science et société, Historicité, Education et Pratiques, University of Lyon and Ecole Normale Supérieur de Lyon). His research areas are contemporary and modern philosophy. His work with S2HEP deals with body and health transformations, especially in neuroethics. He has published several peer-reviewed essays and has arranged numerous conferences in an international context.

**Sarah Parker** has a PhD in comparative literature from the University of North Carolina at Chapel Hill. Her dissertation, 'Contrary Signs: Categorizing Illness in Early Modern Medicine', provides new insights into the relationship between early modern medical uses of the first person and the works of Renaissance writers. Sarah is the recipient of the Evelyn S. Nation Fellowship at the Huntington Library, the Samuel H. Kress Fellowship at the Ackland Art Museum, and she was a visiting scholar at the History and Philosophy of Science Program at Notre Dame in 2012.

**Jonathan Simon** is Maître de conférences at Université Lyon 1 in France, where he teaches history of pharmacy and history and philosophy of science. He is author of *Chemistry, Pharmacy and Revolution in France, 1777–1809* (2005) and *Chemistry, the Impure Science* (2008). He has also published several articles on the history of serotherapy and the history of anatomy. He works in the research laboratory S2HEP in Lyon.

**Mauro Spicci** received his PhD in English Studies in January, 2008. From 2004 to 2008 he worked as an assistant professor in the history of British drama at the Università degli Studi di Milano, Italy, where he also worked as a lecturer in English culture at the faculty of Mediazione Linguistica e Culturale. He has taken part in several national and international conferences. He has published several articles on body metaphors in Shakespeare's plays, the relations between medicine, drama and literature in early-modern England, the link between medical anatomy and Elizabethan allegorical poetry, bodily fragmentation in contemporary drama, and the iconography of Shakespearean characters/actors. His monographic work entitled *The Purple Island (1633) di Phineas Fletcher: un'anatomia. Corpo e ibridazioni discorsive nell'Inghilterra elisabettiana* was published by Ed.it in 2009. He is currently working of an edition of Robert Underwood's *A New Anatomie* (1605), which will be published by the end of 2011.

**Ionut Untea** has studied Christian orthodox theology and political philosophy in Romania (University of Bucharest) and France (Université Lyon 3, Université Sorbonne Nouvelle, Ecole des Hautes Etudes en Sciences Sociales – EHESS, Ecole Pratique des Hautes Etudes- EPHE). He presented papers on Thomas Hobbes, Carl Schmitt, American politics, Passive and Active Resistance, Individual liberty, Toleration, etc. in different academic events organized in Paris, Lyon, Oxford, Cambridge, London, Nottingham, Glasgow, Rome, Venice, Bucharest, Istanbul, Cracow, etc. He is the founder of *Ars Identitatis, Cultural Research Association* (January 2011). He is the author of a number of academic papers, among which 'Excommunication, exile et discrimination chez Thomas Hobbes', in the revue *La Licorne* (Presses Universitaires de Rennes) and 'Carl Schmitt's Interwar Perspective on Political Unity in Europe', in Mark Hewitson and Matthew D'Auria (eds), *Europe before the European Community, 1917–1957* (forthcoming).

**Amy Witherbee** is an assistant professor at the University of Arkansas. She has published recently in the *Eighteenth Century: Theory and Interpretation* and *New Literary History* and is completing a manuscript that looks at time, mathematics and orientalism in Britain in the long eighteenth century.

**Charles T. Wolfe** is a research fellow at the Centre for History of Science, University of Ghent, and an associate member of the Unit for History and Philosophy of Science, University of Sydney. His work focuses on the interrelation between early modern philosophy and the history and philosophy of the life sciences – primarily medicine, 'biology' and natural history – centring on themes such as the man-machine, mechanism and organism, vitalism and materialism; and figures such as Locke, La Mettrie and Diderot. He has published in journals such as *Early Science and Medicine, Perspectives on Science* and *Dix-huitième* *siècle*; his edited volumes include: *Monsters and Philosophy* (2005), a special issue of *Science in Context* on *Vitalism without Metaphysics?* (2008); *The Body as Object and Instrument of Knowledge. Embodied Empiricism in Early Modern Science* (with Ofer Gal, 2010); *The Concept of Organism* (with Philippe Huneman, special issue of *History and Philosophy of the Life Sciences*, 2010), *Vitalism and the Scientific Image* (with Sebastian Normandin, forthcoming). His current project is a monograph on the conceptual foundations of vitalism.

# LIST OF FIGURES

# INTRODUCTION

## Matthew Landers

In 1699, Edward Tyson published the influential work, *Orang-Outang, sive Homo Sylvestris*, which established for the first time a theoretical argument for the comparative study of anatomy among different species. Tyson based his investigation on the 'great Agreement'[1] that natural historians had observed between men and chimpanzees, but which could be studied more systematically in Tyson's time, because of advances in the practice of dissection and anatomy. Drawing from observations made during a dissection of an ape that he performed in the preceding year, Tyson set out to compare the anatomies of chimpanzees and humans, commenting:

> formerly dissecting a *Lion* and a *Cat* at the same time, I wondred to find so very great Resemblance of all the Parts, both in the one and the other; that the *Anatomy* of the one might serve for the other, allowing for the magnitude of the Parts, with very little other alteration: And not only for this, but for several other *Animals*, that belong to the same Family ... But I shall take care to draw up in a shorter view, wherein our *Pygmie* [chimpanzee] more resembled a *Man*, than an *Ape* and *Monkey*, and wherein it differ'd.[2]

Tyson's work thus attempts to address implications that arise from recognition of the 'resemblance of all the parts' between man and chimpanzee – a recognition made possible only through relatively innovative comparative studies.

Comparative anatomists use two terms to characterize structural similarities between different species: analogous and homologous. Analogous similarities are those that develop in the physical structures of different species independently. One of the more traditional examples of analogy is the dorsal fin of sharks and dolphins. The shape and function of these structures are said to converge, meaning that shared environmental forces tend to produce similar (or analogous) physical traits. Such similarities are not homologous, however, because sharks and dolphins do not share a recent common descent. By definition, homologous structures occur only in species that share a common ancestor. Certain structural resemblances between man and chimpanzee are prime examples of homology; and though Tyson appears to sense the difference between analogical and homological structures, he does not go so far as to claim that the resemblances between man and ape suggest that they share a common ancestor.[3] That controversial argument would not be made until 1871.

In 1964, French philosopher and sociologist, Lucien Goldmann, appropriated the term homology to describe the way in which artistic (and I would include intellectual) structures emanate from 'aspects of social life', such that 'one might speak of one and the same structure manifesting itself on two different planes'.[4] Goldmann employs this idea to ground his claim that the novel and the social contexts that it seemingly records are actually homologous structures. In other words, Goldmann views the early novel as a reification of the conscious attitudes/beliefs of a social group. Such manifestations are not mere imitations, Goldmann argues, but the 'culmination of tendencies peculiar to the consciousness of a particular group, a consciousness that must be conceived as a dynamic reality'. Goldmann argues that these attitudes and beliefs become the 'form of the content', or the mental structures that 'organize ... the imaginary universe created by the writer'.[5]

As with the anatomy of related species, Goldmann's use of homology argues for the existence of inherited similarities, by intellectual rather than biological descent. Homologous structures spring from a single font. Biological homologies exist as resemblances that are passed on by the inheritance of structural adaptations. Intellectual homologies exist as resemblances that are passed on by the succession of structuring ideas.

The term homology is fundamental to the claim running through this collection: namely, that the intellectual structure of anatomy came to exist as a dynamic *form* during early modern and Enlightenment periods; and more importantly, that this form manifested itself in various intellectual, political, economic and artistic structures throughout the cultural centres of Europe. In large part, it is the re-emergence of materialist philosophy during the seventeenth century and the idea of *systems* that makes such a claim possible. As many of the essays in this collection will show, arguments about the conformity of nature to universal, physical laws made conjecturing about the corresponding organization of *everything* in the physical universe rather enticing for natural philosophers. In a sense, anatomical explorations of the human body provide a key text. If one can understand the physical laws that govern motion and rest in the body system, one can extrapolate to a 'system of the world'.

The essays included in this collection demonstrate just how strongly anatomical science shaped intellectual and cultural production between the sixteenth and nineteenth centuries. We hope to show that the spread of anatomical approaches during this period speaks to the emergence of a dynamic reality – a structuring attitude towards the world that springs from understandings of the body and the logic of its 'fabrick'.

The collection is divided into three sections: The Body as a Map; The Collective Body; and Bodies Visualized. Essays in the first section explore the central claim that the systematic study of Anatomy during the early-modern period provided Europe with new perspectives about the potential arrangements of knowledge. The first essay, 'Early Modern Anatomy as a Model of Organization', explores the emergence of an anatomical model during the sixteenth and seventeenth centuries. I begin by examining the organization of Andreas Vesalius's *De fabrica* (1543), with the intent of showing that his text, working with different objectives than the texts of his predecessors, establishes a new system of digressive logic, as Vesalius attempts to mimic the non-linear fabric of the body. I argue that it is this form of physical logic that gives rise to an anatomical genre, resulting in an explosion of related medical, literary and philosophical anatomies during the seventeenth century.

Amy Witherbee's essay, '"Who Will Not Force a Mad Man to be Let Blood?": Circulation and Trade in the Early Eighteenth Century', discusses the development of the idea of economic circulation in the eighteenth century. Witherbee explains how late seventeenth-century attempts to create an enclosed, national marketplace in England were linked to William Harvey's theory about the body's closed circulatory system. According to Witherbee, 'the theory that the heart forces blood through the body in a cyclical-motion circulatory system suggested how money, like blood, could be re-circulated, increasing wealth and production through continuous repetition rather than through an increased supply of bullion into the system' (p. 25, below). Taking Harvey's revolutionary explanation of the heart's capacity to pump large volumes of blood as a central reference, the author explains how economic theorists like William Paterson likewise imagined the economy as a closed body-system were wealth could be circulated and re-circulated.

In the third essay of this section, '"After an Unwonted Manner:" Anatomy and Poetical Organization in Early-Modern England', Mauro Spicci discusses Robert Underwood's poem, *New Anatomie* (1610), and Phineas Fletcher's *The Purple Island* (1633), with special attention given to Fletcher's use of the body as a kind of unexplored geography. Spicci's essay begins with the claim that the study of anatomy 'discloses the world of the self', transforming men into 'colonizers of themselves' (p. 60, below). Writing the body thus becomes an act of discovery and conquest; the body yields itself to the poet as 'a universal map', revealing the 'condition of all humanity'. Discourses intersect and converge in the body, allowing the poet to accumulate a wide range of voices, from the medicinal to the political to the philosophical. As Spicci comments, for the poet, 'the human body does not speak one single specific language, but stands at the point of convergence of many different interrelated and mutually interfering discourses'. In short, the body, viewed in the poetic environment, creates opportunities for exploration, discovery and mastery of the human condition.

In her essay, 'Subtle Bodies: The Limits of Categories in Girolamo Cardano's *De subtilitate*', Sarah Parker examines the persistent connection between anatomy and philosophy in early modern Europe. Her essay skilfully contextualizes the importance of Aristotlian and Galenic theory in the works of Mondino and Vesalius and the controversies that arose from the publication of *De fabrica*; but the real weight of Parker's analysis lies in her examination of Cardano's difficult concept, '*subtilitas*'. Although subtlety embraces all that is difficult to explain in the fabric of the human system, Parker argues that it is best glimpsed in Cardano's organizational plan itself, which attempts to compensate for the immense complexity (the hidden interconnectedness) of the body's parts by making digression part of the scheme. As Parker states, 'Cardano's work is guided by the potentially digressive relationships that *subtilitas* reveals', suggesting that the body itself challenges traditional organizational models of scientific inquiry.

Kevin L. Cope's essay, 'Earth's Intelligent Body: Subterranean Systems and the Circulation of Knowledge, or, The Radius Subtending Circumnavigation', expands on the various ways in which anatomy was applied to non-medical topics during the eighteenth century. Taking Thomas Robinson's work, *The Anatomy of the Earth* (1694), as his example, Cope describes how Robinson treats the structure and operations of the earth in nearly the same manner that an anatomist would approach the body. According to Cope,

> Robinson relies in a remarkably straightforward way on the analogy of earth to the human body to establish the relations between levels of anatomy and the various processes that they support. He associates whole classes of telluric phenomena with whole physical systems, thereby creating wide bandwidths for his various efforts at scientific explanation. (p. 42, below)

Along the way, Cope attempts to clarify the procedures of an anatomical methodology, using Robinson as a kind of touchstone. The author insists that Robinson's account of the earth is 'truly anatomical in the sense that he accounts for everything requisite to a given system, in the same way that a physiologists's account of the human body shows how the muscles and bones may support the human frame without recourse to angels, demons or miracles' (p. 50, below).

The second section of this collection, The Collective Body, is a study on the influence of anatomy from the vantage of philosophy and political theory. Nick Davis's essay, 'Mirroring, Anatomy, Transparency: The Collective Body and the Co-opted Individual in Spenser, Hobbes and Bunyan', examines *The Faerie Queen* (1590), *Leviathan* (1651) and *The Holy War* (1682). Famously, each of these texts builds an image of the body that symbolizes the main terms of the argument. Davis's goal is to show how the 'constructedness of the symbolic body image' and its subsequent textual anatomization, 'forms a crucial part of the texts' mediations between the presumptively collective and the prescriptively individual'. 'Considered together', Davis argues, these texts 'offer a lens on the large-scale cultural transition, characteristic of early modernity, from predominantly collectivist to predominantly individualist conceptions of selfhood.'

In 'From Human to Political Body and Soul: Materialism and Mortalism in the Political Theory of Thomas Hobbes', Ionut Untea discusses the importance of Hobbes's understanding of the material body in the formation of his political theory. The essay examines Hobbes's notion of Leviathan, the artificial body of government, asserting that it is related more closely to his beliefs about the material body and physical motion than previously thought. Untea writes that Hobbes drew 'a close parallel between the natural [body of man] and the artificial bodies [of government]', which 'enabled him to build a coherent political theory of the state as an autonomous "artificial man"'. The author maintains that Hobbes believed Leviathan would be subject to the same 'laws of causality' that govern all 'physiological reactions'. Thus because Leviathan is an artificial body composed of natural bodies, as the frontispiece so famously reveals, physical laws that govern the natural body necessarily will influence the course of the commonwealth as well. Untea concludes that the correspondences Hobbes conceived between the body and the body politic – including the communication of 'disease' – led him to formulate a preventative approach to governance, clearly declaring his preference for 'authoritarian regimes'.

In 'Visualizing the Fibre-Woven Body: Nehemiah Grew's Plant Anatomy and the Emergence of the Fibre Body', Hisao Ishizuka discusses the development of Nehemiah Grew's fibre theory and its impact on Enlightenment medicine and models of human society. In reconstructing the idea of a fibre body, Ishizuka reveals the role that fibre theory played in forming a culture of sensibility during the eighteenth century, and eventually concludes that fibres were more important in laying the foundation for the idea of sensibility in the eighteenth century than nerves, because of unique characteristics that fibres were believed to have had, such as '"tone," "tension," "elasticity," "vibration," "oscillation", and many others that frequently propped up in eighteenth-century medical and cultural discourses' (p. 127, below). In the interwoven, textile-like quality of Grew's fibre body, Ishizuka identifies an alternative to the atom, which is to say a solution to 'the radical instability of matter' and the 'chaotic social order' that it suggests.

In the last essay of this section, 'Forms of Materialist Embodiment', Charles T. Wolfe presents a case for the existence of a strictly materialist definition of embodiment during the Enlightenment. Wolfe draws a line between strictly atomistic materialism (which he argues may not really exist) and what he terms embodied materialism. From the standpoint of figures like Fontenelle and La Mettrie, the latter implies that we are 'neurologically determined ... rather than physically determined by the states of the universe as a whole'. The essay goes on to consider the extent to which embodied determinism is reductive of a sense of 'self' and subjectivity, asking: 'Is there such a thing as subjectivity for the materialist? If there is, it will be essentially synonymous with embodiment.' Against traditional interpretations of materialism in the seventeenth and eighteenth centuries, Wolfe argues that embodied materialism explains the mind in terms of 'something bodily rather than the basic physical facts about the universe'.

The third section of the collection, Bodies Visualized, surveys the importance of anatomy from the level of culture and cultural production. Touba Ghadessi's essay, 'Visualizing Monsters: Anatomy as a Regulatory System', employs a novel approach, choosing to consider the impact of anatomical anomalies, rather than paradigms, on cultural and societal norms. According to Ghadessi, anatomical anomalies, or 'monsters', provided an interesting counterpoint to the systematic treatises of Vesalius and others, which gathered and arranged knowledge of the human body around anatomical structures that were deemed to be normal, or functioning according to a created teleological 'end'. On the other hand, Ghadessi argues, the 'systematization of anatomical particulars [monstrosities] provided early modern philosophers, scholars, doctors, scientists and courtiers with a grounded method for the validation of monstrous bodies as new bodies of knowledge', which, in turn, made monstrosities into a kind of scientific (and at times a theological) commodity. Ghadessi concludes that eventually the inclusion of monsters in the systematic study of anatomy 'not only provided an alternate way of understanding human bodies, but they also expanded what constituted cultural conformity'.

Craig Ashley Hanson's essay, 'Anatomy, Newtonian Physiology and Learned Culture: The *Myotomia Reformata* and its Context within Georgian Scholarship', discusses the visual representation of bodies in the anatomical atlases of William Cowper, the last of which was edited by Dr Richard Mead. Attending to the professional advantages of embracing Newtonian methodologies (or at least the rhetoric and social circles of Newtonianism), the essay considers how Cowper's Myotomia reformata, the first edition of which appeared in 1694, was reworked under Mead's direction for publication in 1724. Hanson addresses how Newtonian theory shaped this much-expanded second edition through the inclusion of a new introduction with explanations and illustrations of movement in increasingly mathematical and geometric terms, while concluding that the book might best be understood within the wider context of Georgian antiquarian publishing. Lastly, Hanson comments on the possible impact that Newtonian-based depictions of the body might have had on Georgian art, including the work and theory of such important figures as Hogarth.

In 'Art and Medicine: Creative Complicity between Artistic Representation and Research', Filippo Pierpaolo Marino explores the important contributions of artists, Gaetano Giulio Zumbo, Ercole Lelli, Giovanni Manzolini and Anna

Morandi, in both the medicinal and artistic disciplines of eighteenth-century Europe. Considered together with the 'terrible realism' created by anatomically informed depictions, Marino highlights the facility of wax models as pedagogical tools, capturing and presenting highly accurate levels of detail. This function would have been of great interest to academies, the author comments, given the insufficient availability of cadavers for anatomical dissection. The essay also discusses a number of innovations made possible by modellers, including the ability to visually deconstruct the body into 'vital systems' by generating a series of progressive dissections – each capturing a single step in the journey from exterior to interior – which would have allowed viewers to see and understand bodies in a 'progressive resolution, gradually moving from the superficial systems ... to the most internal ones, and finally arriving at the skeletal structure'. Marino asserts that the ability of such models to create three-dimensional representations (really four-dimensional, given the inclusion of sequence) 'became an essential tool in reproducing a complete mapping of the body'.

The final essay in our collection represents a slight departure, both in its timeframe and in its emphasis. Jérôme Goffette and Jonathan Simon's essay, 'The Internal Environment: Claude Bernard's Concept and its Representation in *Fantastic Voyage*', examines the formulation of an idea of the '*milieu intérieur*' in the writings of Claude Bernard. The authors assert that Bernard attempted to shift the perspective of anatomy from a macro to a micro scale, asking his colleagues to imagine the *milieu intérieur* from the perspective of 'a living cell': 'the physiologist's view of the internal environment should be like our view of the world around us'. This shift in paradigm allowed Bernard to argue that life is 'not a question of the world being contained in every constitutive part, but rather that each element of the living world lives in its own specific world'. The authors proceed to discuss how this shift changed the way that the body was imagined in works of fiction and (later) in film depictions of the body as a new, fantastic world. Special attention is given to Richard Fleischer's 1966 film *Fantastic Voyage*, which marks, the authors argue, 'a turning point in the representation of the human body in film following the conceptual path prefigured in the writings of Claude Bernard' (p. 194, below).

It would be impossible to argue that each of the essays in this collection proves the existence of a 'strict homology' between anatomy and the subject being explored. It is the hope of the editors that the essays contained herein lead scholars of art, economics, literature, sociology and politics to reconsider the intellectual and cultural place of Anatomy between the years 1500 and 1850. Use of the word 'analogy' has been attractive in the past, because it implies a direct influence; however, we believe that evidence is mounting to suggest that anatomy played a larger role in giving shape to the early modern and modern world than ever suspected.

# 1 EARLY MODERN DISSECTION AS A MODEL OF ORGANIZATION

## Matthew Landers

Anatomical texts find a particularly receptive audience in Europe towards the end of the early modern period. K. F. Russell notes in his seminal work, *British Anatomy: 1525–1800*, that England produced only nine books on anatomy between 1500 and 1600; however, that number rose to fifty between 1600 and 1650, eventually climbing to '230 in the second half of the century'.[1] Such an explosion of interest stems in part from Henry VIII's approval of human dissection for the advancement of medical knowledge in 1540.[2] England, which had remained far behind the rest of Europe with regard to the development of the anatomical sciences, appeared ready to stake its own claim. It was not until William Harvey's publication of *Exercitatio anatomica de motu cordis et sanguinis in animalibus* (1628), however, that England had its first groundbreaking contribution to anatomical knowledge. Russell comments, *De motu* 'at once placed Harvey in the forefront of anatomists and physiologists and put British anatomy on the scientific map'.[3]

Harvey's first-hand knowledge of human anatomy played a crucial role in the discovery of the circulatory system. He was a student of Fabricius ab Aquapendente, who lectured at the celebrated medical school in Padua. Padua was at the time the uncontested centre of anatomical science, due in part to the reputation of its most famous anatomist, Andreas Vesalius, who published the revolutionary text, *De humani corporis fabrica*, in 1543. Harvey was exposed to the Vesalian model of anatomical demonstration through Aquapendente (himself a student of Vesalius), thereby establishing a clear line of influence between Padua and England (via Harvey). This influence would continue to grow during the latter half of the sixteenth century, spawning a number of Vesalian texts and inspiring new approaches to the logical organization of information.

In this essay I will examine the importance of Vesalius's *De humani corporis fabrica* as a genre-defining example of the anatomical mode. Using *De fabrica* as a theoretical framework, I will discuss Vesalius's impact on English anatomists Thomas Geminus and Helkiah Crook. Central to the argument of this essay is the assertion that the medical anatomies of Vesalius and his followers experiment with new modes of textual arrangement, which they establish on the systematic organization of the human body itself. Lastly, from these examples I hope to construct a definition of anatomy (as a genre), from which an explanation for the emergence of the 'literary anatomy' in the seventeenth century, typified by Robert Burton's *The Anatomy of Melancholy* (1621), will emerge.

## Vesalius and the Anatomical Mode

Vesalius's contribution to the discipline of anatomy, and science in general, has been the subject of countless books and essays. Most histories of modern medicine begin with an account of the publication of *De fabrica*. The reasons for Vesalius's reputation can be traced to his willingness to break with certain elements of traditional medicinal theory, and the subsequent development of new pedagogical approaches for instructing physicians in the university, which he anchored in visual demonstrations of human dissections (both public and private).

Ancient and medieval practitioners of medicine held that anatomical knowledge had only an ancillary value. Physicians were expected to be familiar with basic internal structures for the purposes of diagnosis and treatment; yet the idea of having a systematic understanding of the interior of the body was considered both excessive and unnecessary.[4] Traditional medical theory rejected the idea that perfect knowledge of internal structures was even attainable, citing the tendency of the body to change structurally once it begins to decay. Galen and his followers, as a result, approached the practice of human dissection with uncertainty, doubting whether the therapeutic benefit of such an extreme approach outweighed the social drawbacks.[5] The principle motive behind the practice of medicine is, after all, the treatment of disease; and if dissection produces no real therapeutic advantage, the negative social and religious associations raise too powerful an argument against its use.

In the *Praefatio* to *De fabrica*, consequently, Vesalius addresses the potential benefits of anatomical demonstrations before making a case for their inclusion in medical curricula. He begins by highlighting the kinds of errors that are perpetuated by separating traditional medical knowledge from anatomical practice. Vesalius argues that by dividing the duties of the physician from those of the barber-surgeon traditional medicinal theory creates an 'evil fragmentation of the healing art'.[6] Successful treatment of disease, he maintains, depends on the physician's ability to achieve a balance of medical knowledge, between what he calls doctrine, the use of medicines, and surgery [*ratio, medicaminum usus*, and *manus opera*]:[7]

> Previously this study [anatomy] was uniquely pursued by physicians, who strained
> every nerve in the process of mastering it; but when they handed over the task of

surgery to others they lost the art of dissection, and this meant that the whole of anatomy went forthwith into a sad decline. For so long as the physicians declared that the treatment only of internal afflictions was their province, they considered that knowledge of the viscera was all that they required, and they neglected the fabric of the bones and muscles, and of the nerves, veins, and arteries that permeate the bones and muscles, as if it were none of their business.[8]

In response to this perceived neglect, Vesalius employs *De fabrica* as an argument against the pedagogical routines of anatomical demonstration – the *quodlibetarian* model – that had persisted since antiquity. '[T]hat detestable ritual' involved the reading of an authoritative anatomical text (such as Galen's *De usu partium corporis humani*) and the simultaneous dissection and demonstration of the internal structures of the cadaver, before a crowd of curious onlookers. Individuals with specialized expertise carried out the various responsibilities of the demonstration. The recognized authority of the proceedings was the physician, who, as the *lector*, read *ex cathedra* from a Latin text. The *ostensor*, perhaps a professor or medical student, used a *radius* to demonstrate a particular part of the body; and lastly, the *sector*, most often an uneducated barber, made the actual incision.[9] Because physicians never actually participated in these dissections, except in a perfunctory manner, Vesalius condemned the practice, complaining, 'a butcher in shambles could teach a practitioner more than the spectators are shown amidst all this racket'.[10]

For the reformer, Vesalius, *quodlibetarian* demonstrations had little or no pedagogical value. He maintained that physicians relied more on the authority of writers like Galen for their anatomical knowledge than on observation. Vesalius, on the contrary, was adamant about the importance of direct knowledge. He goes to great lengths to reveal errors in Galen, whom Vesalius claims never performed dissections on a human body, but relied on the structure of apes for his anatomical knowledge.[11] The emphasis Vesalius puts on visual demonstration works to de-centre the text of the *quodlibetarian* model in favour of first-hand experience. *De fabrica* is thus, primarily, an effort to reconstruct medical knowledge around the authority of personal observation, as opposed to textual precedent.

## Print as an Organizational Tool

*De fabrica* is a work deeply concerned with its own print identity. Vesalius is said to have overseen most aspects of its production, including the creation and arrangement of 171 woodcut illustrations, which supplement the text. *De fabrica* is novel precisely because of the vigour of Vesalius's reforming energy, which aimed at creating innovative organizational structures that collaborated with new print technologies. Vesalius recognized that one of the problems with earlier anatomical texts, including those of Berengario da Carpi and Mondino di Liuzzi, was the difficulty faced by a student or professor trying to identify internal structures during a dissection, based solely on textual descriptions.[12] The *quodlibetarian* model only made the dilemma worse by creating a gulf between the dissector and physician.

Because illustrations were nearly impossible to reproduce for handwritten manuscripts, most anatomical textbooks of the Middle Ages and early Renaissance lacked visual depictions of anatomy. The limited illustrations that did adorn certain volumes were borrowed from earlier works (and often redrawn for each copy), thereby perpetuating a tendency towards the transmission of error and inaccuracy. In an attempt to remedy this problem, Vesalius – taking advantage of contemporary print technologies – commissioned an unprecedented number of woodcuts to complement his text, cross-referencing illustrations with anatomical descriptions in a systematic fashion. He worked closely with the artists of Titian's workshop to produce accurate representations of the internal structures of the body (many for the first time), providing the best available images of human anatomy in his time. Collaboration between anatomist and artist was uncommon during the early history of book culture. Vesalius was among the first medical authors to appreciate the full potential of new print techniques, which promised to enhance the ability of a text to express and communicate accurate information.

In explaining the organizational scheme of *De fabrica*, Vesalius uses the Latin word *ratio*, or system, to signify the scope of the information that he wished to circumscribe. Though *De fabrica* is a book concerned primarily with the internal composition of the human body, Vesalius tries to situate anatomy within a larger intellectual sphere, arguing that

> the most calamitous result of this unfortunate division of the means of treatment amongst a variety of artisans has been that it has inflicted a deplorable and most disastrous shipwreck upon the study of anatomy. Anatomy is an important part of natural philosophy; to it, since it embraces the study of man and must properly be regarded as the prime foundation of the whole art of medicine and the source of everything that constitutes it, Hippocrates and Plato attributed such importance that they did not hesitate to ascribe to it first place among the component parts of medicine.[13]

Vesalius considered the loss of anatomical expertise crippling to any system of medicine:[14] a system of medicine must be 'whole' if it is to achieve its goal of curing the sick. The attempt to define such a system involves, for Vesalius, a complete description of the healing arts, not just anatomy. Removing the study of anatomy from the 'system' creates an opportunity for misdiagnosis and maltreatment.

Vesalius's specific use of the word 'system' seems to imply that 'knowledge' and the body are homological structures. Bodies of knowledge can be organized systematically if one can only discern the interconnections between disparate parts. Systems exist, at least theoretically, by means of the internal relation (*ratio*) of information. Vesalius regards knowledge of anatomy as part of a larger system of natural philosophy, envisioning anatomy itself as a system within a system, just as man is a microcosm within a macrocosm. In short, the study of the interior of the body has its place because it sheds light on the relation of man to the universe within the context of a broader system of philosophy.

Nancy Siraisi observes rightly that *De fabrica* borrows this obvious teleological trajectory from Galen's *De usu partis corpori humani*, which maintains that every part of the body has a divinely elected purpose. Vesalius alters the terms and associations of Galen's scheme, but his notion of systems (and systems within systems) suggests that knowledge is unified.[15] As mentioned above, Vesalius is attempting to fashion a system of human anatomy as well as to situate that system within a larger system of natural philosophy. The text of *De fabrica* thus embodies the intellectual act of system creation (identifying and accurately describing the relationships that bind knowledge into a unified whole). Because the amount of information brought within this system was enormous, however, and because no typographical paradigm for such complex arrangements existed, Vesalius found it necessary to experiment with new methods of textual organization.

Prior to the publication of *De fabrica*, the textual arrangement of books relied more on the established conventions of the *scriptorium* than on the generic demands of specific content. From a structural standpoint, anatomical texts were hardly discernable from any other kind of book – a situation that results from the fact that incunabula of the fifteenth century tended to mimic the scriptographical layout of medieval manuscripts.[16]

## The Print Identity of Anatomy

By the mid-fifteenth century, anatomists had been using Mondino's *Anothomia* for at least a hundred years. Mondino finished his manuscript in 1315, although the first printed edition, by Antonius Carcanus, appeared in 1478. Carcanus's edition of *Anothomia* is rather ordinary, even for the period. The layout is characteristic of early incunabula, lacking even a title page. In fact, the only decorative choice that Carcanus seems to have made is the one to print the text in two columns. Carcanus's use of a traditional gothic font is even more conventional, giving Mondino's text the austere look deemed appropriate for the genre. The result is a book that appears overcrowded and encumbered.

Various editions of Mondino's *Anothomia* emerged over the following few decades, although little changed in the presentation of the text. If anything, some editions took several steps back towards medieval practices. With the rise of humanism, however, came new possibilities in print. Antiqua or roman type became fashionable among humanists of the fifteenth century, in part because it evoked ancient authority, but also because it was easier to read. However, medical texts, like the 14⁹⁴⁄₅ edition of *Anothomia*, published in Venice, continued to make use of gothic type. The printer, Hieronymus de Durantibus, even chose to present Mondino's *Anothomia* in a single, block column. This unfortunate arrangement continued to dominate the layout of editions through the late 1530s, with only occasional additions, such as a title-page on the 1507 edition (Pavia) and marginal notation in the 1519 edition (Genève).[17] The typographical conservatism of fifteenth- and sixteenth-century printers epitomized the ongoing conflict between humanism and errant scholasticism of the Middle Ages. When Vesalius's *De fabrica* appeared in 1543, consequently, it represented more than a simple challenge to Galenic authority. *De fabrica* launched a revolution against traditionalism in print culture and against typological habits that limited the freedom of an author to experiment with new organizational schemes.

Elizabeth Eisenstein identifies this early period of printing as a moment for which the attempt to 'modernize' and 'rationalize' the procedures of organizing textual information represents the emergence of an *'esprit de système'*.[18] *De fabrica* demonstrates the actual working-out of such a 'spirit', taking full advantage of sixteenth-century technical innovations, in order to gather and view data in a highly organized, rational form. *De fabrica* is, therefore, largely an editorial project: the concern for structure is governed primarily by a desire to correct Galenic tradition. Vesalius understood, however, that such an undertaking was possible only through the accumulation and systematic organization of *all* existing knowledge, with reference always to first-hand experience of human dissection.

Fittingly, Vesalius's organizational scheme mirrors the methodology of his subject. As an anatomist, he divides his textual material into endless sections. Unlike Mondino's *Anothomia*, *De fabrica* represents a negotiation between text and image. Vesalius's intent was that *De fabrica* be used as a visual aid; and because of this he insisted that it include observable references for the dissector. First among these 'cues' is the structure of the text itself. Vesalius divides his work into seven books, each corresponding to a system of the body: skeletal, muscular, venous, nervous, digestive (nutritional) and reproductive, cardiopulmonary and cerebro-sensory. Each of the seven books is further separated into *capituli*, which serve to subdivide each system into its constitutive parts, by function. Vesalius's use of chapters as divisions is not particularly innovative. In fact, this arrangement is reminiscent of ancient Greek and Roman encyclopaedias, which compiled a diversity of subjects 'within the bounds of a single work'.[19] Nonetheless, the idea of dividing a subject systematically, or in relation to its function within a larger scheme, is relatively novel.

As one might suspect, the process of making cuts or sectioning a narrative can lead to a diminished sense of cohesion. In other words, the real difficulty involved in making divisions in a narrative is the need to imagine each section both as an abstract particular and (at the same time) as an integrated component of the whole. Although Mondino divided *Anothomia* into forty-four sections, each corresponding to a major organ, or set of organs, Vesalius takes this systematic impulse even further. Over the course of *De fabrica*'s seven books Vesalius divides the text into 188 chapters. Amazingly – and perhaps appropriately – the first two books, discussing the skeletal and muscular systems, account for 102 of these sections. It is evident from the headings, moreover, that Vesalius divides his text according to the needs of an anatomist, rather than those of an editor.

The text of *De fabrica* functions as a narrative that follows the chronology of dissection from the inside out, beginning with the skeleton. Each chapter represents an individual section, or cut, of the *sector* – and, therefore, a cut deeper into (or out of) the body, or subject of the text. *De fabrica*'s narrative is not strictly linear, since the action being plotted is at times cross-spatial, just as the organs of any given system often are distributed unevenly throughout the body. This high level of spatial abstraction makes textual cross-referencing necessary. As a result, the structure of *De fabrica*'s text is a product of the opposition between its chronological and achronological narrative elements. The text is aware of its own non-linear organization, freely referencing and cross-referencing within its own body.

Vesalius solves many of the problems of this kind of oppositional description by creating links between text and image. Traditional anatomical works lacked the physicality of *De fabrica*'s 'integral arrangement',[20] relying more on textual description, which, more often than not, hid error, instead of shedding new light on the function and relationship of internal structures. Illustrations gave Vesalius the freedom to compile descriptions from traditional texts, while using visual analogies to provide evidence both for and against the claims of authoritative works. This new approach added an unknown dimension to conceptualizations of the human system and, by extension, the idea of systems in general. Elizabeth Eisenstein observes that such innovations in print technology generated a kind of 'combinatory activity' between scholars and artisans, which 'changed relationships between men of learning as well as between systems of ideas'.[21] Vesalius's alignment of textual description with the empirical evidence of illustration – thereby reducing the occurrence of error – epitomizes the *esprit de système* which gave 'a newfound coherence to preexisting material'[22] and set a new standard for thinking about and representing perceivable reality.

## Vesalius's Influence in England

Historians often find it difficult to trace the influence of a text across geographic borders. Yet *De fabrica* was distinctively visible in England. A plagiarized version of the *Epitome* to the work appeared in England only two years after the original publication of *De fabrica*. In his bibliographic history of British anatomy, K. F. Russell writes:

> In 1545 Thomas Geminus issued a plagiarized version of them [Vesalius's plates] under the title of *Compendiosa totius anatome delineatio* in which the name of the original author is casually mentioned in the dedication. It proved popular at once and Geminus had it translated into English in 1553 and again in 1559.[23]

Harvey Cushing speculates that Geminus – an Italian – may have worked among the engravers commissioned by Vesalius, giving him access to the plates.[24] Whatever the case may be, Geminus's version of the *Epitome* bears little resemblance to Vesalius's original, beyond the scaled-down reproductions of the plates. Cushing points out that the text is likely compiled from Thomas Vicary's *Anatomie of the Bodie of Man* (1548). He credits Dr Sanford Larkey with the discovery that Geminus's version followed traditional textual arrangements of the anatomy, beginning with a cut through the viscera, instead of starting with the skeletal system, as *De fabrica* does.[25] Vesalius's name appears in the dedication of Geminus's text, however, thereby solidifying the reputation of the Italian anatomist almost immediately.

While both Russell and Cushing appear, like most medical historians, to prioritize the emergence and influence of Vesalius's anatomical plates, the eventual arrival of the text of *De fabrica* in England and (more importantly) its system of arrangement deserves some attention. One can assume quite safely that versions of the original edition of *De fabrica* appeared in England during the late sixteenth century. Evidence for such a claim comes from the manner in which certain English anatomical texts mimic Vesalian methods of organization. Russell regards Helkiah Crooke's *Mikrokosmografia: A Description of the Body of Man* as the first example of a 'comprehensive text-book in the Vesalian manner'.[26] Published in 1615, *Mikrokosmografia* exceeds other contemporary examples in the sheer scope of its subjects. Like before, Crooke's text is adapted mostly from other writers – the title-page credits Gaspar Bauhinus and Andreas Laurentius – yet, the organization structure of *Mikrokosmografia* matches Vesalius's attention to systematic detail. Crooke borrows and adapts Vesalius's illustrations, including his prolific letter-index of body parts. Now, however, smaller versions of the images flow within the body of the text, doing away with the need to flip back and forth throughout the work.[27] With regard to sectioning, Crooke arranges the text of *Mikrokosmografia* into thirteen books, with 294 chapters. To these chapters he adds 178 '*Questions*', which, for all purposes, form additional chapters that address the controversies of the various books. Taken together, Crooke divides the text of *Mikrokosmografia* 485 times.

The frequency of Crooke's divisions is no accident. Sections, or 'parts', take on philosophic importance in the argument for *Mikrokosmografia*. As with Vesalius, the issue for Crooke is one of systematic arrangement, though at first the organizing principle of the text is not always apparent. Book 1 is compendious in the breadth of its topics. Crooke moves between subjects as dissimilar as astrology, geology, Epicurean philosophy and Christian theology, before finally offering a definition of human anatomy in the fifteenth chapter.[28] Reminiscent of Vesalius's argument in the preface of *De fabrica*, each of Crooke's subjects represents a single partition within a larger philosophical discussion, for which the body of man appears to be an analogue – a microcosm of universal knowledge, as the title suggests.

The importance of Crooke's *Mikrokosmografia* has yet to be fully recognized even by medical historians.[29] In part this is due to the eccentric qualities of the text, which grow with Crooke's attempts to relate every major intellectual subject to human anatomy. Recent scholarship has seemingly rediscovered *Mikrokosmografia*, if only for the purpose of discussing Crooke's challenge to Aristotle's 'one-sex model'[30] – thereby linking the text to gender-based criticism for nearly a decade. Other scholars have pointed to the scandalous content of books 4 and 5, which describe and depict the female form in detail (and more inappropriately, in English). Of course, the content of these books was considered 'quasi-pornographic' at the time, earning Crooke a censure from the College of Physicians.[31]

More importantly, Crooke's contribution to seventeenth-century anatomy remains largely unexamined. C. D. O'Malley, in perhaps the only biography of Crooke, comments:

> The *Microcosmographia* was certainly the largest and fullest anatomical work produced in England up to its day and for a considerable time to follow, but it is to be doubted that the fullness of detail was really essential for the surgeons.[32]

Perhaps it is the 'fullness of detail' that turns modern readers away from Crooke's text. O'Malley certainly implies that readers tend to look for content that is 'essential' for the use of the text, while it is quite clear that Crooke ventures far beyond necessity. The exhaustiveness of *Mikrokosmografia* reveals a great deal about Crooke's scheme and about the logic that guides him.

Crooke's intentions for *Mikrokosmografia* become apparent in chapters 15 and 16 of book 1. Here, in a lengthy but important passage, he defines anatomy, drawing an important distinction between alternate meanings of the word:

> Now there is amongst Physitians, a double acceptation of Anatomy; either it signifieth the action which is done with the hande; or the habite of the minde, that is, the most perfect action of the intellect. The first is called practicall Anatomy, the latter Theoretical or contemplative: the first is gained by experience, the second by reason and discourse: the first wee attaine only by Section and Inspection, the second by the living voice of a Teacher, or by their learned writings: the first we call Historical Anatomy, the second Scientificall: the first is altogether necessary for the practise of anatomy, the second is only profitable; but yet this profit is oftentimes more ben-

eficiall then the use it selfe of Anatomy: the first looketh into the structure of the partes, the second into the causes of the structure, and the actions and uses therefrom proceeding. According to the first signification we may define anatomy thus: *An Artificiall Section of the outward and inward partes ...* If Anatomy be taken in the latter signification, it is defined a *science or Art, which searcheth out the Nature of every part, and the causes of the same Nature.*[33]

Crooke thus begins by drawing a distinction between practical and theoretical anatomy. Practical anatomy corresponds to common understandings of human dissection: namely, physical sectioning of the body into parts, and the subsequent inspection of those parts. According to Crooke, however, practical anatomy is not, by definition, systematic or even organized. He uses the word 'Artificiall' to distinguish between dissections that are undertaken without a plan – such as the accidental discovery and inspection of a corpse – and dissections that are deliberate and, in some measure organized by art or science for the advancement of knowledge.[34] The latter category of anatomies he calls '*Scientificall*', indicating the primary organizing function of reason, the very '*Science or Art*' by which all demonstrations of knowledge (anatomical or otherwise) are framed.[35]

Crooke claims that both modalities can be considered anatomies because the 'subject of both ... is a Part'.[36] Thus the idea of a 'Part' is key to Crooke's definition of anatomy and to his methodology. Anatomy's primary function, as both a practical and intellectual exercise, centres on the nature of a part, both as a singular concept and in relation to the whole. Crooke comments:

> a Part is one of those things which the Logicians doe call τα πρὸς τι ti that is, *have reference or respect to another*: so a part is said to bee a part of the *integrum and whole* ... Now whereas the part must helpe to compound the whole, it is necessary it should adheare or cleave unto it by a connexion of quantity; wherefore in the whole body, a Part hath a true existence, and is *indeed* ioyned thereto, but *in reason* devided therefrom ... *A part is a body cohearing or cleaving to the whole, and ioyned to it in common life, framed for his use and function.* From hence we may gather that two things are required to accomplish the nature of a Part: First, that it should cleave unto a whole, and next, that it should have some end or use.[37]

The overly philosophical character of Crooke's explanation is bewildering at first. Put into simpler terms, he argues that individual parts of the body bear an intrinsic relation to the structure of the 'whole'. In fact, it is this teleological relation that defines parts *qua* parts.

Still, how does one go about arranging a narration of parts? To some extent, Crooke recognizes (with Vesalius) that the demands of trying to textualize the body generate an aesthetic structure – what I call its systematic form. According to Crooke, the organization of a scientific anatomy emanates from the integrating functions of reason, which seek out the 'universall or generall Theorems or Maximes, and common Notions' that define the body as an *integrum*.[38] In other words, it is the intellectual activity of integration that categorizes Crooke's 'Scientificall' or 'contemplative' anatomy.

As a matter of practice, however, Crooke argues that reason recognizes the 'connexions' between parts only after it first understands parts as such. Put differently, that which we perceive to be 'joined' in the visible *'integrum'* must first *'in reason* [be] divided therefrom'. Systematic organization depends, then, on the abstract dismantling of a subject, in search of certain coherences of 'Structure', 'Action' and 'Use'.[39] Crooke's explanation helps to flush out a rather elusive notion of system in the early modern period and offers a clear definition of the anatomy, first as a mode, and second as a genre.

## The Aesthetics of Anatomy

The application of Vesalian methodology in England explains, to some extent, the explosion in the number of literary 'anatomies' written throughout the seventeenth century. To many it became clear relatively early that the systematic structure of the anatomy provided opportunities for examining a variety of topics. As a result, many authors adopted anatomy as a means of giving narration to the particulars of nearly every imaginable subject.

This is not to say that every text that deems itself an 'anatomy of' is in the anatomical mode. Numerous texts aspired to imitate the anatomy without satisfying the conditions of such an endeavour. I would argue, as above, that the criteria for anatomies are three-fold: first, the abstract division of a subject into parts; second, the use of systematic organization as an integrating form to bring diverse parts together; and third, the resulting comprehensive treatment of a subject within the boundaries of the organizational structure. Comprehensiveness is, as such, only a by-product of the anatomical mode. Greater than the desire to include 'everything' is the recognition that the constituent parts of 'everything' must bear a recognizable relation to each other, in terms of *structure, action* and *use*. Without this primary recognition, the anatomy becomes, at best, a hotchpotch of meaningless data, and at worst the work of a madman.

It seems fitting then that one of the finest examples of the literary anatomy treats the topic of madness and melancholy. Robert Burton's *Anatomy of Melancholy* is, according to Crooke's definition, a 'Scientificall', or what we might call a systematic anatomy. The *Anatomy of Melancholy* has little to do with practical dissection or the demonstration of bodily structures; rather, Burton embarks on a narrative journey, for which the primary focus is the abstract division of the constituent elements of melancholy (as a concept) and the systematic reorganization of these parts by the intellect. Having an understanding of the structure of the *Anatomy* is thus key to recognizing Burton's literary plan; however, only one scholar, Ruth A. Fox, has treated Burton's organizational structure to a book-length study.

Fox's efforts (in *The Tangled Chain* (1976)) seem directed mainly at demonstrating the logical unity of the *Anatomy* – an inclination that leads her to regard the work as 'a single vision or "totality" of truth'.[40] Fox argues that the tripartite structure of the book's partitions and their corresponding synopses imitate 'the forms of scholastic treatises', which give it 'the marks of a *summa*' and 'make the claim of totality for Burton'.[41]

Fox shies away from claiming that Burton constructs a perfect order in the *Anatomy*. She argues instead that the synopses outlining each partition exist as 'statements about the functional contexts and logical relationships in the book'.[42] In particular, Fox suggests that the synopses establish connections between the 'logical' narrative structure of the work and Burton's numerous digressions. Accordingly, Burton's numerous narrative digressions must be viewed as logical parts of the whole, with the synopses supporting the structure: 'the digressions in Partitions I and II are outlined in the synopses, and the Third Partition ... is to be seen at the outset as part of the *Anatomy*'s single organization'.[43] By looking at the synopses as graphic demonstrations of the book's logical structure, Fox contends that careful readers anticipate Burton's digressions, thereby robbing them of their irrational relation to the text. According to Fox, the synopses pre-situate digressions within the overall sense of the work schematically.

Notwithstanding a degree of truth in Fox's observations, one still wonders: why call the work an anatomy if the similarities between Burton's methodology and those of the scholastics are so strong? Fox's comments suggest that the structure of the anatomy is practically equivalent to that of the scholastic treatise. In making this argument, however, Fox fails to address the anatomy *as a genre* or as a scientific method of organization. There are, without doubt, cosmetic similarities between the anatomy and the scholastic treatise; yet, Fox does not consider the generic differences with any kind of rigor.

Without becoming overly cumbersome (a difficult task in itself when talking about Burton), I would like to examine a few issues raised by Fox on the structure of the *Anatomy*. Much of her argument hinges on the status of digression within the logical construction of the narration. Fox accounts for digression by citing the formal layout of the synopses, which visually incorporate each digression as a unit of the partition, in such a way that the synopses disclose the 'apparatus' of the argument to the reader beforehand.[44] By way of explanation, Fox offers the use of visual synopses in the second Partition (II.2) as an example. If one looks closely at the synopses, however, it becomes evident that rudimentary illustrations of the chronological order of the argument do not always make the logic clearer for the reader. Rather, the synopses function more like an index, giving the reader a representational idea of the structure of the partitions, without fully revealing the connections between sections. When seen in context with the preceding section, or *Member* (titled, 'the rectification of passions and perturbations – from his friends'), Burton's digression has little to do with the ongoing line of argument.

Fox borrows Panofsky's definition of the term 'Gothic' to account for detours in logic, describing partitions as individual 'rooms' within the framework of the scholastic treatise, which allow for 'internal change without undermining the external fabric' of the logic.[45] Burton seems far less certain about the status of his digression, however, apologizing to his audience:

> I have thought fit, in this following section, a little to digress (if at least it be to digress in this subject), to collect and glean a few remedies and comfortable speeches out of our best orators, philosophers, divines, and Fathers of the Church, tending to this purpose.[46]

Clearly Burton's narrative detours bear a relation to the main argument; however, these connections are not logical – if one means syllogistic – but, rather, systematic in structure. Digressions lead the audience to related material, but not such material that by its inclusion one satisfies the requirements of a premise in logic. The intention of the author is to be comprehensive in his presentation of information, not logical. Systematic organization is *demonstrative*, not persuasive.

With regard to narrative detours then, the author is forced to call them digressions because they tend to confound the reader's ability to perceive associations in the logic. Simply noting a break in the logic beforehand – Burton calling attention in the synopsis to an obvious departure from the subject – does not really help to integrate digressions into the body of the argument, except representationally. Furthermore, the act of drawing brackets around a series of premises does not make them rationally coherent. One suspects, given Burton's insistence on the satirical nature of the *Anatomy*, that the inclusion of obvious failures in logic are in fact necessary.

The existence of digressions marks one difference between the anatomy and scholastic treatise, as modalities. Humphrey Ridley, in his *Anatomy of the Brain* (1695), remarks that digression is so unavoidable in narratives of the structure of the body – the organs of the body being so unevenly and illogically distributed – that digression simply becomes part of 'order of the [anatomical] method'.[47] Whereas treatises exist as expansions on, or extensions of the logical processes of the mind-searching-for-the-*summa*, anatomy affirms the importance of understanding *parts*. The treatise is concerned only with the verifiability of the whole, the anatomy with the demonstrability of the section in relation to the whole. As such, displaying the function of the part – knowledge that remains hidden to the casual observer – becomes, in the hands of the anatomist, more important (or at least more artful) than proving the existence of the whole. The tasks of the scholastic and anatomist are related, insofar as they both cover the same ground: the existence of connections. In terms of method, or modality, however, scholasticism uses logic to build the *summa*; the anatomist uses dissection, or digression to cut the whole into its basic parts. The *summa* grows layer-upon-layer; the anatomy, like that of Vesalius, can be epitomized into more basic partitions. Organizing these divisions has more to do with identifying connections between structures, as Crooke argues, in terms of their action and use, and less to do with the logical coherence of premises. To put it in plainer terms, the 'logic' of the systematic form is primarily 'physical', or related to function. It matters very little to the anatomist if parts are distributed in a non-linear fashion throughout the body, as long as the parts bear a common functional (systemic) relation.

How then does one speak about systematic organization as an anatomical mode, if the primary impulse of the anatomist is division? Perhaps the best analogy one can offer is a similarity between the operation of narration and the function of the anatomist. Narration resembles anatomy insofar as it attempts to demonstrate the diversity of parts, in terms of chronology, action, character, etc., without a primary concern for logical constraints. In order to write an 'epitome' of an individual life or action (as, for instance, in the many biographical novels of the eighteenth century) the author must resort to cutting information (time, location, voice) into parts. In the case of an author like Laurence Sterne, the sectioning of time, location and voice can be extreme – almost unintelligible. However, the relations that exist between the parts of an account are functional in advancing the narratological goals of the author.

Returning to Burton, one recognizes that the organization of the *Anatomy of Melancholy* has a kind of extended physicality to it – or what Walter J. Ong might call 'place' or 'space' logics[48] – resulting from the extreme, non-linear distribution of the parts of the narrative and from the functional relations that these partitions maintain with each other. *The Anatomy of Melancholy* resembles Vesalian anatomies insofar as Burton's organization of the topic relies on a physical logic of function, avoiding the difficulties raised by linear syllogistic thinking. Just as the anatomist narrates the structure of the body in a non-linear fashion, digressing frequently as he encounters organs and structures, drawing attention to function and association, Burton progresses in a manner suited to the dissection and demonstration of his topic: melancholy. Strictly speaking, this arrangement is not logical, in a syllogistic sense. Rather, each section, member and partition of the text exhibits a kind of non-linear coherence, or (to use Crooke's term)[49] a 'cleaving' between narrative parts. In other words, Burton's *Anatomy* maintains a cohesion, despite its achronological, illogical structure, precisely because each section or cut in the narrative bears a relation to the overall function of the work: to cure melancholy. Partitions and digressions simply become a way of linking narrative parts that otherwise demonstrate no logical connection.

But here one must concede that Burton pushes the anatomical impulse beyond the limits of utility. The centrifugal force of Burton's methodology generates endless divisions, examinations, digressions and trials of the subject matter

– so much that the reader eventually gives up on reading the text as a unified system or aesthetic whole. *The Anatomy of Melancholy*, more than any other literary text, demands to be read/examined in pieces. Digressions become aesthetic entities, which can be (and perhaps should be) separated from the whole and read for their own value – just as individual sections of a medical text are consulted according to need. Divisions, according to Burton's methodology, represent individual *curative units* – each aimed at treating melancholy through diversion, distraction and amusement. One can allege then that the 'brain-sickness' of the narrator finds its way into the organizational scheme – and we, the audience, must stand back and wonder at Democritus Junior's passionate dissection and uncontrollable laughter.

As such, satire remains an integral part of Burton's scheme; his project appears to be driven by an effort to lampoon scientific attempts at systemization. He settles on the anatomy as a mode, because of its insistence on the philosophical value of the 'part'. In this way, Burton tweaks the anatomical genre to suit his purposes, in effect creating a mock-anatomy. Democritus Junior becomes a dissector of ideas rather than animals or humans. In the process of reading, one senses Burton's concern that things are getting out of hand. The reader finds, as Democritus Junior's explanations of causes, symptoms, kinds and cures of melancholy grow; as Burton extends the digressiveness of his work to include topics ranging from cosmology to love; as the text of the *Anatomy* expands with each published edition, the seemingly infinite material of Democritus Junior's dissection points to the imminent absurdity of the project. Burton's *Anatomy* can never achieve its systematic ends because, unlike anatomies of the body, the process of accumulating and arranging an infinite body of knowledge is, by definition, interminable and unsustainable.

The aim of this essay has been to suggest (in a limited fashion) how deeply anatomical methodologies altered the way that Europeans went about organizing the world around them. In exposing some of the characteristics of the anatomical mode, I have tried to propose a loose set of rules that shed light on the sudden emergence of a very popular genre during the seventeenth and eighteenth centuries. Lastly, I have attempted to describe how anatomical texts generated an aesthetic form that departed from traditional methods of scholastic examination and explanation, in favour of the new, digressive modality of anatomical demonstration, which, itself, is implied by the 'physical logic' that emerges from the systemic relation of parts in the body.

# 2 'WHO WILL NOT FORCE A MAD MAN TO BE LET BLOOD?': CIRCULATION AND TRADE IN THE EARLY EIGHTEENTH CENTURY

## Amy Witherbee

In his 1690 preface to *Political Arithmetick*, William Petty explained:

> The Method I take to do this, is not yet very usual; for instead of using only compara-tive and superlative Words, and intellectual Arguments, I have taken the course (as a Specimen of the Political Arithmetick I have long aimed at) to express my self in Terms of Number, Weight, or Measure; to use only Arguments of Sense, and to con-sider only such Causes, as have visible Foundations in Nature.[1]

Petty had been trained in medicine and was among the first generation to teach Harvey's theory of circulation at Oxford. As his preface indicates, Petty was fascinated by mathematics' apparent capacity to give experiential, even sen-sual, validity to ideas that are fundamentally abstract. Convinced by Harvey's argument, Petty saw the potential of applying a new sort of reasoning to other subjects of philosophical concern, including politics, sovereignty and wealth. And even those who were less interested in mathematical reasoning appreciated the implications of Harvey's mathematically-inflected concept of circulation for the nation's financing challenges.

Described in the 1628 publication of *De motu cordis* and taught by Harvey as part of the natural philosophy course of study at Cambridge, the theory that the heart forces blood through the body in a cyclical-motion circulatory system suggested how money, like blood, could be recirculated, increasing wealth and production through continuous repetition rather than through an increased supply of bullion into the system. This became a recurrent theme in financial pamphlets. In part the circulation metaphor allowed authors like Killigrew to associate activity, the proliferation of events, with a life-giving motion. Those who chose to save their bullion rather than invest or spend it became hoarders, and their coin was said to 'lie dead' to the detriment of the marketplace and the nation. Circulation was therefore a powerful rhetorical figure; but, I will argue, it also served a crucial function in shaping the political, financial and social subjects of political economics to fit a mathematical framework. This essay looks at the mathematical perspective inherent in both the anatomical and economic models of circulation from the seventeenth-century banking debate and, using Brian Rotman's work, unearths an intimate historical relationship between the virtual worlds of mathematical reasoning and systems that circulate.

## Circulation and Early Banking

In a pamphlet arguing for the establishment of a national bank and paper currency in 1663, William Killigrew exclaimed, 'Ought not a government be oblig'd to make Laws for the Publick Good? ... Who will not force a Mad Man to be let Blood, and take wholsome Medications? Is not the Nation in a Distraction about their money and Credit?'[2] Killigrew's colourful rhetoric plays off an earlier passage in which the author insists that there is surely enough bullion in England to 'Circulate our Trade' in spite of his contemporaries' fears to the contrary.[3] Like so many of those contemporaries and countless economic commentators since, Killigrew found in the human circulatory system a convenient model for describing and managing financial wealth at a national level. Circulation after all could serve as a metaphor for how repetition, rather than older models of loss and gain, could create wealth even as it reinforced the picture of the English nation as an organic political body. In the contentious world of seventeenth-century politics, the argument for a nationally-sponsored bank needed to be made with care. Killigrew's 1663 pamphlet was part of a debate that lasted through most of the century about how to solve the intertwined problems of the English government's over-strained finances and British complaints about the shortage of coin available for domestic and international trade.

Studies like Larry Neal's *The Rise of Financial Capitalism* (1990), Joyce Oldham Appleby's *Economic Thought and Ideology in Seventeenth-Century England* (1978) and P. G. M. Dickson's *The Financial Revolution in England* (1967) document how state debts and international bullion shortages in the late seventeenth century prompted dramatic shifts in how Britons thought about and attempted to manage wealth. As Neal's study shows, the issues of bullion shortages and state debt were largely a product of Britain's growing interaction with international markets. Trade with Asian and Middle Eastern regions and colonial efforts elsewhere might produce wealth in the form of goods, but many Britons feared that coin was being drained from the realm in the process. The East India Company became a particular target of such fears, spurring defences in the form of early economic tracts by interested parties like Thomas Munn. While the debate continued, however, British traders and merchants found their own solutions to coin shortages in complex credit practices that were already in use both in Asian and Middle Eastern markets and on the Continent. The most vocal British proponents of national banking made reference to the banks of Rotterdam and Amsterdam with their exchangeable notes of credit. By the middle of the seventeenth century a lively discussion was underway about the potential benefits of founding national banks in Britain.[4]

Advocates argued that national banks would increase credit available to merchants and landowners, ease the strain on bullion supplies, keep interest rates low and establish a ready supply of funding for the British military efforts that, more often than not, were also in the service of expanding trade. Largely based on the existing use of 'lombards' (early pawn shops) and goldsmiths, capital assets took the form of coin, stored merchandise or land holdings against which the proposed bank would issue some form of credit note to the depositor. In their particulars, many of the British banking plans included provisions for issuing paper currency in the form of freely exchangeable credit notes (Killigrew specified marbled paper but thought metal or wood would do just as well). These notes were secured by coin or goods that might not yet have been collected by the bank and that might not be available to the debtor for an extended period of time.

The question was how to convince potential investors to deposit their goods or coin with the bank and to leave it there over long durations. Advocates hoped that investors in private business would be encouraged by the stability of the bank, the interest income and the exchangeability of its credit notes to make those long-term loans to the bank. The exchangeable credit notes would simultaneously allow the creditor to make more of his or her purchases, thus increasing demand for goods and tax proceeds for the state. The state in turn benefited from these tax proceeds in terms of present revenues, but also could use its estimated future revenue to borrow from the bank for present needs. As such, the state's annual interest payments to the bank, combined with whatever capital base or wealthy guarantors a particular scheme's proposer thought necessary, served as the foundation for the bank and the public's faith in that institution.

As seventeenth-century bank proposals developed from fairly small private arrangements among a select group of merchants or landowners into national finance schemes, the question of credibility became an increasingly difficult issue. At such a scale, national finance operates something like a sophisticated game of musical chairs, for which the music is never meant to stop. The players trust that most of their competitors will not sit down and so remove too many of the secure places in the game. At the same time, the players count on something else: namely, that no external force will suddenly change the balance or rules of the game. In the game of national finance this was a particularly dangerous assumption. Britain's need for more currency and greater access to credit arose precisely *because* its early modern markets were changed, quickly and dramatically, by interaction with more sophisticated commercial networks in South East

Asia and the Middle East and with the rich supply of goods from colonial spaces throughout the Caribbean and Atlantic.

Those who advocated for national banks, credit currencies and the other long-term financing schemes that marked Britain's seventeenth-century financial revolution needed a form of argument that would not only convince the public that this new economy could work, but also that its 'rules' would be followed in a predictable manner. Robert Mitchell convincingly argues that by the end of the eighteenth century the social, political and financial strain created by this dynamic would give rise to an emerging discourse of sympathy. In the formative years of British banking, however, political economists sought out a discourse that could mimic the tangibility of gold and silver coins. Their central arguments, therefore, took the form of mathematics, and their mathematics depended upon an image of circulation that William Harvey had used successfully to convince his contemporaries of the pumping mechanism of the heart a few decades before.

## Harvey's Realignment of the Organs

Harvey's dedication to Charles I in the 1628 publication of *De motu cordis* reinforced both the importance of the heart in natural philosophy and anatomy and the importance of the king to the political body:

> The heart of animals is the foundation of their life, the sovereign of everything within them, the sun of their microcosm, that upon which all growth depends, from which all power proceeds. The King, in like manner, is the foundation of his kingdom, the sun of the world around him, the heart of the republic, the fountain whence all power, all grace doth flow.[5]

As is usual with dedications, Harvey's was meant to invite support from an important patron, but in reiterating the analogy between king and heart, Harvey had another agenda. One of the most significant obstacles to having his work accepted was its conflict with Galen's widely accepted theory on the production, constitution and distribution of blood in the body. According to prevailing theories the liver worked with the gallbladder and the spleen to turn the nutrients of food and drink into blood. The heart then drew blood from the veins (rather than forcing it out through arteries) and worked in concert with the lungs to add vital spirits. The visible signs of pulse and respiration were thus conceived to have the same function of providing life-carrying spirits to the human body.[6]

This theory of the organs had two necessary effects with which Harvey was concerned. In trying to frame the partnership between heart and lungs, Galen and his followers had imagined that the right and left ventricles of the heart served different purposes. The right ventricle was said to nourish the lungs while the left drew materials from the lungs and right sinus of the heart to create spirituous blood, which was sent into the aorta to receive fuliginous vapours and then through the pulmonary vein to the lungs. The complications of trying to make this theory consistent with anatomical findings led to a host of explanations for how 'spirits' related to the more visible blood. There was, however, general agreement on Galen's claim that the heart provided some lesser-known quality to the nutritive blood produced from the liver. This claim made sense within the context of a worldview that recognized all creation as a hierarchical reflection of the divine and the human body as a privileged microcosm of that order. As the human form was closer to the true divine order than that of other animals, so too was the heart associated with the more noble spirituous properties of the blood as opposed to the meaner nutritious blood. Both the bodily organs and their functions were entwined with a much larger discourse of natural philosophy.[7]

When Harvey first sought to convince his contemporaries that respiration and pulse had different functions and that the heart moved blood through its systole rather than its diastole action (pumped rather than sucked), he needed to re-characterize the functions of the heart, lungs and liver and the flow of blood within them. Harvey's theory of circulation gave the heart, 'the fountain whence all power, all grace doth flow', a significantly different import.[8] To be sure, anatomists including Harvey still believed that the heart added to the blood some form of 'heat or spirit or whatever else it needs to be refreshened', but now the primary function of that noble organ was simply motion: 'It must therefore be concluded that the blood in the animal body moves around in a circle continuously, and that the action or function of the heart is to accomplish this pumping. This is the only reason for the motion and beat of the heart.'[9] In shifting the roles of the noble organs, De motu cordis dilutes the question of divine agency in Galenic theories of the body and moves the body one step closer to a closed system in which the emphasis is neither on production nor order, but on repetition and continuous distribution.

Embedded within the field of natural philosophy rather than medicine, Harvey was well aware of the stakes involved in redefining the workings of the human body. Roger French's study traces Harvey's careful attention to the forms and progression of argument customary to his field and to the author's digression from those forms. Long touted as an example of the triumph of empirical science in the modern age, Harvey's theory of circulation succeeded in part because its author found a way around the limitations of both traditional philosophical approaches and empirical evidence through his use of mathematics. Traditionally, an anatomist's lecture within the field of natural philosophy would begin with the lecturer offering a *historia*, that segment of a public anatomy demonstration in which the lecturer provides description with visual observation of the organs. French argues that Harvey's frequent recourse to visual evidence in *De motu cordis* would have been familiar to his contemporaries as part of the *histo-*

*ria*. Philosophical anatomy would then be invoked to describe the actions and functions of the organs and how those related to the macrocosmic structure of the world.[10] Harvey's challenge was to frame the elements of his *historia* in such a way as to produce a body acceptable to the larger field of knowledge encompassed within natural philosophy. His first move in this regard was to expand that field of knowledge through the use of Aristotle's texts on animals.

As French explains, Harvey modelled his comparative work on the human heart and those in other animals on the work of Fabricius of Aquapedente. Fabricius had sought 'to find rules that govern the variation seen in the same organ in different animals. His method is to construct inductive syllogisms to discover significant relationships between related organs in animals (for example between the stomach, teeth and horns of ruminants).'[11] Unlike Galenic approaches which were more concerned with action and cause as they relate to providence, the Aristotelian approach that Fabricius favoured looked for what French terms 'the nature-of-the-thing', a causal knowledge that can be applied to all hearts, horns or livers as they function within animate creatures.[12]

Harvey's reliance on Fabricius's Aristotelian approach is clear throughout *De motu cordis*. The second, third and fourth chapters (those immediately following the author's explanation of his motives for writing) are devoted to observations of the functioning heart in animals. Working with animals allowed Harvey to perform vivisections and thus to observe the heart in motion, even if only in its final motions. Under the premise that the 'nature' of an organ is the same from one species to the next, Harvey then translated his observations of animals to the human body.

This premise was a step towards a more mathematical form of reasoning, allowing the scholar to abstract the organs from larger contexts and place them all within a translatable system. But not everyone was happy with Harvey's Aristotelian premise. Harvey's theories initially came under attack from Galenic scholars, who essentially rejected the new Aristotelian approach by arguing that what we see in lower life forms is not valid evidence of the role of human organs, given the human body's position in the order of nature. On the other hand, the sceptics who rejected such cosmological approaches to science also attacked Harvey's theory, arguing that even with animal vivisections, Harvey did not have enough empirical evidence to support his claim of the blood's cyclical flow from the heart. As French writes:

> It was not only that a Harveian account of the action of the heart destroyed the traditional concoction associated with the passage of the blood through the septum but much more that Harvey's account of circulation was (to a sceptic) a *system* that tried to give confident knowledge about things hidden to the senses, particularly the invisible arteries-to-veins transit.[13]

From our standpoint in the twenty-first century it can be difficult to understand the concerns behind this latter attack. We have no trouble accepting the body as a system in which many processes remain, at least for now, invisible to our observations. But part of the reason for our ease with this notion is our comfort with the idea of systems. Faced with the task of convincing both sceptics and traditionalists, Harvey offered one other form of argument that was new to natural philosophy but crucial to the development of systemic thinking: he resorted to mathematics. What seems to have persuaded scholars in England and on the Continent most strongly of the validity of Harvey's theory of circulation was his now-famous calculation of how much blood was in the human body at any given moment:

> As a reasonable conjecture suppose a fourth, fifth, sixth, or even an eighth part is passed into the arteries. Then we may suppose in man that a single heart beat would force out either a half ounce, three drams, or even one dram of blood, which because of the valvular block could not flow back that way into the heart.
> The heart makes more than a thousand beats in a half hour, in some two, three, or even four thousand. Multiplying by the drams, there will be in half an hour either 3,000 drams, 2,000 drams, five hundred ounces, or some other such proportionate amount of blood forced into the arteries by the heart, but always a greater quantity than is present in the whole body.[14]

Concluding that the amount of blood flowing through the heart cannot be produced solely by the food and drink digested daily, Harvey reasons that blood is not continually produced in large quantities but circulated and reused. Blood is no longer an ingredient produced from external materials and excreted in some other form; it is now an essential part of the body and engages simultaneously with all other parts through its flow. The heart takes its place as a form of pump or engine which manages that flow while the entire question of production fades to the background. The body of *De motu cordis* is imagined and idealized as a closed, self-sufficient system.

Harvey's contemporaries found his mathematics convincing largely because they were able and willing to share Harvey's 'vision' of a self-enclosed body that could not be seen but could be represented imaginatively. This idealized, self-referential system is in fact an essential feature of mathematical reasoning. In his study of mathematical thought, Brian Rotman argues that mathematics can be understood as a series of predictions for which the mathematician convinces him or herself that no other result is possible. The mathematician creates an idealized world in which semiotics are asked to stand in for the events, people and factors that he has deemed significant and in which the problem can be acted out. The process requires that the mathematician imagine three distinct 'selves' that will respectively enact, direct and witness the virtual unfolding of the problem in the idealized world of mathematical semiotics. Each of the three 'selves' involved in mathematical reasoning and persuasion is associated with the overlapping semiotic fields that Rotman terms the Code, meta-Code and Virtual Code.[15] These semiotic fields, rather than referring to some sort of transcendent truth or preconceived concept, constitute the true material of mathematics. Mathematical signs, including numbers themselves, create an enclosed semiotic, purely self-referential world through which the mathematician (using his subject and agent) might enact and perpetuate his thought experiments.[16]

Rotman theorizes that within the world of mathematical semiotics the Code and Virtual Code create and act out, respectively, a Subject who issues commands for the conscious-less agent to perform ('let b = 3' or 'add 5 to 10'). These are the semiotics we associate with mathematics in its most rigorous form, 'real' math. They are meaningless, however, without the presence of a third 'self', what Rotman simply refers to as the 'Person'.[17] The Person is the only subjectivity of the group that belongs to a historically and geographically-bound cultural context. We generally consider the spoken language that he or she employs to introduce, clarify, justify, validate or normalize the process of mathematical reasoning to us to be a mere gloss on the more important work of the subject and agent. But the Person serves the crucial function of serving as the consciousness who must be convinced. As a self-enclosed, agreed-upon system of thought-writing, mathematical semiotics can only speak about itself. However, in convincing the Person that the likeness between Subject and Agent is sufficient (that, therefore, the likeness between idealized world and unidealized world is sufficient) mathematics claims to speak about a world beyond itself:

> the Person (Dreamer awake) observes the Subject (Dreamer) imagining a proxy – the Agent (Imago) – of him- or herself, and, on the basis of the likeness between Subject and Agent, comes to be persuaded that what the Agent experiences is what the Subject *would* experience were he or she to carry out the unidealized versions of the activities in question.[18]

Using the expression '2+3 = 3+2' as an example, Rotman demonstrates that even in the simplest calculations this complex imaginative world necessarily comes into play.[19]

Mathematics in Rotman's model is a translation of the most extreme kind. More than a translation from one language to another, it is the translation of a subjectivity into a virtual world with its own tightly-controlled set of signs, relations and practices. Mathematics 'speaks' (to the extent it can be said to do so) only about itself, such that the real challenge to a mathematical problem is not the internal manipulation of signs but the effort to convince the Person that what he or she imagines is a close enough likeness to the unidealized world to reveal some 'truth'. As Rotman writes, 'what is salient about mathematical assertions is not their supposed truth about some world that precedes them, but instead the inconceivability of persuasively creating a world in which they are denied'.[20] Mathematics, then, can be understood 'in terms of the performing of thought experiments or waking dreams'.[21] In such a practice the empiricist emphasis on sensory experience is displaced onto an imagined experience in the self-contained, idealized world of mathematical semiotics.

Rotman's discussion enables us to see more clearly how and why Harvey shifted from both the traditional forms of philosophical argument and emerging empirical approaches to the less familiar field of mathematics. With his simple calculation of drams of blood Harvey asked his audience to share in the creation of an idealized body whose living systems could become 'visible' (if only to the mathematical imago and subject) in its normal motions. Mathematics offers a parallel universe in which the scientist can mimic, via his imago, the experiential nature of empiricism without the unfortunate limitations of the human senses. Rotman's model also reveals why Harvey was forced to close off his idealized body from the 'outside' world. One must be able to articulate the unidealized problem (in this case the functioning of the heart) as a closed system in order to produce a convincing replica in the idealized realm of a mathematical problem. Harvey's discovery might well be less an example of scientific empiricism triumphing over scholasticism than it is a moment in the rise of a very non-empirical form of persuasion built in the imaginations of mathematicians.

## Circulation and the National Body

The application of Harvey's mathematical reasoning to the emerging field of political economics is obvious. William Paterson, whose 1694 proposal served as the foundation for the Bank of England, proclaimed in that year with great confidence that

> The want of a bank, or publick Fund, for the convenience and security of great Payments, and the better to facilitate the circulation of Money ... hath in our time, among other Inconveniencies, occasion'd much unnecessary Credit, to the loss of several Millions, by which Trade hath been exceedingly discourag'd and obstructed.[22]

This fact, it seems, was the only thing that could be claimed with confidence, as Paterson's treatise goes on to survey several decades' worth of contentious debates about the establishment of a national bank. Within that debate, explained Paterson, many have been concerned that a bank would give too much power to the monarch on the one hand, or too much to a few major lenders on the other. Other proposers (Killigrew among them) wrongfully attempted to coerce the nation to accept a non-bullion form of currency through legislation; 'they would anticipate Ages, and attract, or rather imagine, inestimable Value form innumerable Years to come; all which was to be crammed down Mens throats as a Punishment of their Infidelity'.[23]

Paterson's plan offered what seemed to be a reasonable solution. We must accept, he argued, that gold and silver are the customary measure of financial value and thus base the bank's security solely on bullion. The royal charter would be issued to a committee of private men who would provide the funds for the original loan and management of the Bank in accordance with a set of established regulations. Paterson recommended an immediate loan in the amount of 1,200,000 pounds to the British government at an interest rate of 8 per cent per year to produce a 96,000 pound profit (though Paterson rounds this up to 100,000 pounds in his own calculations).[24] All of the business of the Bank would be founded on this single ongoing loan to the government such that the Bank would be secured by both the wisdom and self-interest of the chartered members and the stability of the nation. Paterson confidently estimated the increase in circulating money and trade resulting from the establishment of the Bank:

> It is an infallible sign that Money abounds and is plentiful, when the Interest thereof is low; for Interest or Forbearance is the Price of Money, as it is such; and if Money be plentiful, People will thereby be enabled and induced to Trade and Purchase, and by the plenty of Money other things must in proportion bear the better Price. And if the Proprietors of the *Bank* can circulate their Fundation of *Twelve hundred Thousand Pounds*, without having more than *Two* or *Three Hundred Thousand Pounds* lying dead at one time with another, this Bank will be in effect as *Nine Hundred Thousand Pounds*, or a *Million* of fresh Money brought into the Nation[25]

In Paterson's continued list of economic benefits to the nation it is easy to overlook the holes in his argument. By securing his Bank with a loan to the government, Paterson displaced the uncertainty of both currency and trade values to the nation.

As J. G. A. Pocock and, more recently, Patrick Brantlinger, Catherine Ingrassia and other 'new economic' critics have argued, state financing schemes yoked the personal financial concerns of a mass of individual investors to the stability and growth of governments. This arrangement reinforced the conceptual boundaries of the nation; in fact, part of the reason that Paterson's argument worked was that it conveniently ignored the effects of people and events outside the imagined space of the national marketplace. Gone are the seventeenth-century anxieties that the foreign trade (and the East India trade, in particular) were draining bullion from the English nation. Gone, too, is any mention of how events in Europe and around the world might affect interest rates, trade opportunities, tax revenues or the ability of the English government to make its debt payments.

Tony Aspromourgos observes in his history of classical economics that the sort of vibrant political-economic theorizing we see in the seventeenth century arose precisely because commerce became too complex and integrated to be comprehended through existing frameworks; 'in a real sense there was an international "economy" (integrated and interdependent economic relations) *before* there were national economies, such that seventeenth century London was more economically integrated with Amsterdam than it was with large parts of England'.[26] In light of Aspromourgos's argument, Paterson's effort to close off the English system of finance conceptually makes sense, *especially* because this could not be accomplished in actuality. The need to create a closed system is inherent in the sort of mathematical argument that Paterson uses, whether the boundaries are synonymous with the nation or not.

However, Paterson's numbers are remarkable in another sense as well. Seventeenth-century banking proposals used mathematics as a persuasive technique in an era for which understandings of what constitutes 'fact' or 'data' was shifting.[27] Political economics challenged the public to accept an abstract, systemic manner of thought that, like Harvey's circulatory system, was anchored neither by traditional philosophical forms of knowledge about the polis nor by experiential, sensory data. To no small extent, this challenge nurtured the fixation on the sorts of material that could serve as currency.[28] What political economists offered instead of the tangible forms of currency at the centre of their debates was the virtual 'sensory' experience of mathematical argument.

Paterson's relatively simple calculations thus invoked an imaginary, idealized world that he needed to make convincing as a stand-in for the complex and constantly shifting accumulation of diverse commercial events that made up his audience's daily trade practices. Inspired by the sort of mathematical persuasion that Harvey had used earlier in the century and supported by the anatomist's compelling image of a self-sustaining body, political-economic thinkers like Paterson finally convinced their audiences to gamble money on their quintessentially modern field of knowledge. Harvey's theory of circulation had articulated a far more enclosed body, one that functioned through systems that operated with greater self-sufficiency than had been imagined in prior centuries. In adopting that body as a crucial reference point for their own emerging field of knowledge, political economists invited us all to share in the creation of a similarly self-referential, imaginary world with which the twenty-first century continues to grapple.

# 3 EARTH'S INTELLIGENT BODY: SUBTERRANEAN SYSTEMS AND THE CIRCULATION OF KNOWLEDGE, OR, THE RADIUS SUBTENDING CIRCUMNAVIGATION

## Kevin L. Cope

Anyone who has built, repaired or renovated a home, hut or hovel anywhere in North America has probably come across the famous logo of the largest paint and finish supplier west of the prime meridian, the Sherwin-Williams Company. In what an environmental law blog from the Berkeley and UCLA law schools describe as a 'breathtakingly anti-green' hallmark,[1] this renowned vendor of colour coatings takes as its emblem a bucket of brilliant red paint spilling all over the terraqueous globe. This paint-dispensing bucket seems to hang on a point in space as its contents incarnadine roughly three-fifths of the earth, with the initial splashdown occurring at a point near the ecological utopia of the Galapagos islands. Three words emblazon the Sherwin-Williams logo: 'cover the world'. Oddly enough, that goal is not accomplished within the logo. Those who yearn for a revival of old-world culture will delight to discover that, contrary to cartographical custom, both western Europe and western Africa have been tipped ninety degrees off the standard north-up orientation so as to hang upside-down at the bottom of the escutcheon, there to remind viewers of the prehistoric African origins of humanity and to celebrate the Italian ports from which began the exploration of the Sherwin-Williams 'world'. Although surface tension adheres the paint to the globe a few degrees beyond the girdle of the tipped, formerly blue-green sphere, the bottom half of the planet remains open to daylight. Meanwhile, prodigious paint drops as large as the Sahara fall off the globe and into unknown spaces.

With its sentimental sparing of the continents from which exploration originated, the Sherwin-Williams logo makes a point about the complexities of the great age of investigative travel that commenced with Columbus and then flourished in the long era of modernization. Exploration, discovery, investigation and analysis transpired in linear and superficial ways, with 'linear' and 'superficial' carrying their best rather than their pejorative meanings. Sailing, tramping or otherwise moving across the surface of the earth or its seas, itinerant adventurers and scientists traversed the earth along paths or waterways that could be easily delineated on maps. In print culture, the exploits of these travellers took the equally linear, pleasingly superficial form of step-by-step narratives or instalment-by-instalment technical reports that were recorded on the printed superficies of books, broadsides and occasionally ballads. Both the rough hewn mariners and the enthusiastic 'virtuosi' of the period knew that they were travelling around the irregular outer surface of a three-dimensional, slightly oblate sphere. They recognized that their journeys led to countless discoveries with regard to human cultures and to those parts of nature that abided on or near the surface of the planet, but revealed comparatively little about the immense space from which the aforementioned Sherwin-Williams bucket would later dispense its paint or about the depths of a convex planet that could be 'covered' only on its thin mantle. Modern exploration was circumferential to so high a degree that it eventually raised questions about the radius: about what abided within the earth as well as what soared to the zenith.

Similar challenges with respect to depth perception pop up in the modernized practice of anatomy that peaked in Richard Burton's *Anatomy of Melancholy*. The 'anatomy' tradition guided the works of thousands of collectors, indexers and organizers, whether the divertingly baroque Thomas Browne, with his collections and commentaries on everything from morals to mausoleums; whether the joke-collecting if pseudonymous Joe Miller; whether publishers such as Nathaniel Crouch who made a good living assembling information collections that were never completed and that kept reappearing in updated editions; or whether over-wrought medical men such as Samuel Tissot and John Armstrong who hoped that organized arrays of medical anecdotes might somehow penetrate to the root causes of masturbation. As a genre, the anatomy, whether medical, literary or otherwise, is committed in the first instance to collecting data that has been gleaned from properly superficial observation. At the same time, and by contrast, the anatomy is also committed to discovering deep causes and uncovering underlying explanations. This bivalent commitment to the study of surfaces as well as to the delivery of in-depth explanations cerates an assortment of procedural paradoxes, the study of which would fill a dozen books. This somewhat shorter study will follow the genially superficial lead of the great anatomists by presenting a case study of one particular area of inquiry in which those paradoxes are most salient, the geological history of earth. This pilot project will offer an outline of anatomy and its subtleties that will invite further study of this subject.

*

However unresolved the questions about the origins and import of the 'anatomy' genre may be, by the late seventeenth century its medical associations were here to stay. An author might write an anatomy of broad topic such as the world or of a psychological problem such as melancholy or of a refined matter such as etiquette, yet the background suggestion of plain old physiology resonated in every utterance of this most physical of words. When combined with the ambition to review and classify a very large range of information, ideas or phenomena, the anatomy, with its inveterate physicality, tends to move towards allegory, for its medium and its message – its tenor and its vehicle – tend to diverge. Allegory postulates a distance of some sort – physical, conceptual, ideological, semiotic – between its intended meaning and the words or images that deliver that content. In its heritage physical but in its application highly intellectual and abstract, anatomy as a genre postulates a rift between the material that it reviews and the structure and meaning that it discovers. Anatomy, whether as a method or as a particular body of information about a particular topic, negotiates between the wide range of knowledge that it conveys, discovers or imparts and the system that it proposes for the arrangement of material. Any particular anatomy thus postulates a rift between content and procedure. Anatomy as a general *method* is not anatomy as a body of knowledge, say the anatomy of frogs. Neither the anatomical method nor the anatomy of the particular frog necessarily lead to an exact anatomy of science, religion, the world or anything else. The author of an anatomy is committed to at least a degree of metaphorical or analogical or otherwise accommodated discourse whether addressing either content or methodology.

The semantic distance inherent in an anatomy – the space between what is 'in' an anatomy, what an anatomy means, how an anatomist works and what an anatomist says or produces – was further complicated by the emergence, during the late seventeenth century, of a spate of topics that were all characterized by immensity. A complete anatomy of any topic is a challenge. Even the anatomy of a frog could lead to a thousand diversions, from the history of amphibians to the proper seasoning of edible bugs. Big topics were harder still. Followers of Sir Isaac Newton, for example, seldom if ever offered anatomies of the universe. That task would have been daunting. Conversely, the emphatically local character of anatomy – its habit of diagramming, organizing and classifying the components of a particular, finite body – fit poorly with the idea of an infinite cosmos as propounded by Cambridge's leading gravitationalist. Even topics in the middle range of complexity such as government, which is certainly bigger than a breadbox and yet smaller than the universe, became more difficult to anatomize as explorers discovered new and diverse tribes and as colonies multiplied across cultures and continents.

One middling to large topic that stimulated relentless interest among anatomists throughout the long eighteenth century was that of the earth itself. For one, earth provided the substratum supporting all the other diversity in the world. It was a good place for an anatomist to start. More profoundly, the earth, in its immensity and newly-reckoned depth, resisted comprehension, its diameter being too big for most minds, ships or caravans to girdle. Neither the immensity nor the variety of the earth, whether manifested in its geological bowels or on its floral and faunal surface, were completely without order. On the contrary, the long-eighteenth-century eye tended to see either design or taxonomy everywhere. However profuse or numerous nature might be, it always suggested a scientifically explicable system.

Among the keenest long-eighteenth-century eyes were those of the country parson Thomas Robinson, who, we learn from a sparse entry in *The Dictionary of National Biography*, supplemented his pastoral duties by enjoying ale and sponsoring sporting events while collecting minerals and other natural novelties. Modest Robinson epitomized the spectacular Augustan confidence in the explanatory powers of the intellectually entrepreneurial individual. Ensconced in his rectory in a tiny Cumberland village, he issued a series of not altogether voluminous books explaining single-handedly the entire geological and natural history of the earth. His first work, *The Anatomy of the Earth*, opens with an enactment of that whole suite of contrasts and paradoxes that define the modern, non-physiological anatomy. Reflecting on the volatile conditions at play during the first days of creation, Robinson develops an analogy between the growing but still juvenile body of earth and more stable, standard notions of human anatomy:

> In this [primordial chaotic] state they [particles of primeval matter] continued, bound up and hanper'd with a vast thick Fogg or Mist of a waterish substance, extending it self as far as the Moon's Vortex, until the *Spirit of God moved* upon *the Face of the Waters* ... and, by the vital Heats and Insulations, did digest it into an orderly World: by whose infusing into it, and every part of it, a vital Spirit, it became a great Animal; having Skin, Flesh, Blood, Bones, Nevers &
>
> **Chap. II .** Of the Skin of this Animal; the production of Living creatures, &c.
>
> The Outer Coat and Surface of the Earth is its *Skin*; which (being concocted and digested by the influence of the Sun's Beams, and having a *Plastick Power* infused in it by the *Spirit of Nature* became productive not only of Grass, Trees, and other Vegetables, as the Skins of other Animals naturally grow hairy; but, when it was in its full strength and vigour, it brought forth all kinds of Birds, Beasts, and Serpents, as naturally as it now brings forth divers kinds of Insects, or, as the Skins of other Animals bring forth Lice.[2]

Salient in Robinson's account is the drive to reconcile the Mosaic narrative of creation, in which the early universe transits from one inchoate to a later, better, more orderly format, with anatomy, which seems not to require a narrative, being static in its description of immobilized organisms. Robinson pushes early geological history into a story line that culminates in a set of analogies that lack any obvious temporal, narrative extension. He explains how a 'Plastick Power' converted chaos into a whole classification system full of diverse organisms, but then he drops the story, contenting himself with showing the panoply of creatures rather than, say, explaining how the lion preys on the gazelle or what might be the mating customs of the walrus. The result is a forward-moving history that culminates in an immobilized process. This frozen or perhaps suspended story looks somewhat allegorical insofar as it conceals or even ignores as much as it discloses. For one, it glosses over the obvious breakdowns in the analogies. If plants are the hair of the earth, it seems reasonable enough to declare animals to be its lice, yet that analogy distorts as much as it reveals, striking readers as downright weird. Surely normal observers would see major differences between the actions, uses and dispositions of pleasing animals and those of pestilent parasites. The analogy seems not to work yet seems to emerge from the logic of the story line. The fact that Robinson is writing an 'anatomy' amplifies the expectation that some sort of storyline will make the anatomy look complete – that the anatomical narrative will somehow contain or account for the entirety of nature as well as the process that led to it even as it shows, indeed revels in the fantastic diversity of our planet.

To return to the Sherwin-Williams logo with which this essay opened, we can speculate that a non-mathematical, clumsily allegorical, natural-language representation of a highly complex process such as either the creation of the earth or the covering of the planet with paint can remain stable and accurate over only a small segment of its full range of possible meanings. It is easy enough to understand the punning message of the 'cover the world' logo, which asserts that a paint manufacturer controls the entire worldwide paint market. It is perverse, pedantic and even impossible to insist on an explanation of the manufacture of a paint bucket that is greater in size than the continent of Asia or to ask where so vast a quantity of paint, which seems to exceed the mass of the earth, was distilled. Similarly, Thomas Robinson's opening dramatization of creation, a set of not altogether felicitous comparisons between our planet and our bodies, manages to characterize the fertility, variety and productivity of the earth in a fairly complete way, but at the cost of requiring readers to overlook an assortment of oversights or absurdities. 'Anatomy' as practised by the geologically minded Robinson thus highlights a more fundamental tension, in the genre, between anatomy as process – say, the doing of dissections or the making of discoveries – and anatomy as description and classification. Carrying out the extended comparison between planet and body requires overlooking some content issues (and vice versa). This tension between process and product reached its greatest potential in the writings of rambling authors such as Richard Burton and

Thomas Browne, who are always balancing collecting, gathering and occasionally interpreting against describing and classifying.

What we discover in Thomas Robinson is an awareness that anatomy operates not only at differing levels of resolution but also at differing levels of interactivity. As the physiologist must decide whether to start with the gross anatomy of the body or with the parts of the pancreas or perhaps at the cellular level, so the anatomizing geologist must decide whether to cavort about the surface of the globe or to plunge into its depths or to peruse individual rock formations. As the medical anatomist must recognize that bones interact with muscle and devolve from blood, so the anatomist of the earth must consider the relation of geological scaffolding to the processes that either produce or depend on structure. The ingenious Robinson relies in a remarkably straightforward way on the analogy of earth to the human body to establish the relations between levels of anatomy and the various processes that they support. He associates whole classes of telluric phenomena with whole physical systems, thereby creating wide bandwidths for his various efforts at scientific explanation. Rocks, as a class, correspond in gross to all skeletal matters, which are also congregated into a class, with no distinctions being made between the knee bone and the thigh bone.

> Under the Flesh [i.e., the surface of the earth] lye the Bones, that is, Stones, Metals and Minerals: All which the Miners have reduced to seven *Genera* or Kinds, containing under them as many subordinate *Species* as there are either of Vegetables or Sensitives upon the Earth's surface.[3]

Robinson recognizes that bones and rocks both include in their numbers many subspecies, but he relies on forceful analogy to smooth these differences and thereby to establish that *there is an anatomy*, that there are indeed larger categories that, with a fully ontological force, connect otherwise differing phenomena. A femur and a tibia and a chunk of granite differ at the level of the various subspecies to which they belong, but their service in the cause of supporting the operation – the process – of the human or the geological bodies also demonstrates that they are not fully independent entities, that anatomy is something more than a mental recreation.

In Robinson's approach, both classified objects and the classification system itself slip into a secondary position. Both depend on an assortment of physical and literary processes that hold together the analogies on which the seemingly ontological practice of anatomy depends. Processes offer Robinson a kind of liquid mental mucilage that flows slowly enough to hold materials into a classification scheme while it also lubricates the processes that it celebrates, whether those of life or those sustaining geological activity. The complicated structure of the earth, which features apparently useless gaps and interstices that might puzzle those who affirm the divine design of nature, thus sustains processes fundamental both to the operation of the planet and to life itself.

> In the Earth there is a constant Circulation of Water, as in the Animals of Blood; every particular Metal and Mineral having its proper Feeder, which, by thus circulating it, preserves its Life, and carries in it the Spirit and Flavour of that kind to which it belongs: as may be readily distinguish'd, sometimes by Tast [*sic*]; sometimes by Colour; but most commonly by its Effects and Operations. Hence proceeds the great Variety of *Medicinal Waters*.[4]

Underlying Robinson's affirmation that underground seepage is something more than a random trickle – that it is a formalized 'Circulation' – is an amazing affirmation that *everything* can be anatomized, that even a seeming miasma of cracks and crevices can be classified as core and critical to a complex system. Indeed, Robinson's view suggests a commitment to the evolution of design. If new cracks corrupt earth's components they will ultimately contribute to the subterranean circulation. Still more striking is the analogical correlation of compartmentalized anatomies. In the concluding sentence of this passage, the segregated if analogically coordinated circulation of underground water and circulation of human blood converge as a trickle-up effect sprays 'Medicinal Waters' that enter and cure bodies. Presumably, the cavities through which the underground water is circulating are also wet, suggesting that seepage creates an explicable, allegorically significant interface between systems and structures even in the inanimate underground.

What is perhaps most spectacular about Thomas Robinson's project to create an 'anatomy of the earth' is its overall counter-systematic flow: its running affirmation that irregularity is more conducive than is regularity to design, process and, in sum, anatomy. Regularity and predictability stymie the instabilities that make for a system. With that, they create the kind of complex, interactive arrays of phenomena that anatomists prize. Thomas Burnet, for one, had argued that prelapsarian perfection required a smooth planet, a notion that Robinson, in his sequel study, *New Observations*, thinks compromises the systematic variety and interactive complexity of creation.

> Dr. Burnet, in his Theory of the Earth, conceits and endeavours to perswade the World, that the Primeval Earth was Spherically or Mathematically round, without Seas, Mountains or any inequalities upon its Surface.
> Which Hypothesis (or rather ingenious Conceit) seems in the first place to be inconsistent with the Original State of this Material Globe; which being design'd for a place of Habitation for several Kinds of Animals of a mixt and compounded Constitution, whose vital flame is nourish'd and maintain'd by a continual respiration of a soft vaporous Air; which must not only be frequently fann'd with the brisk gales and blasts of a cleansing Wind, but also moistned and sweetned with showers frequently falling through it; all which have the Original cause from the constant flux and reflux of the Sea, and those inequalities upon the surface **fo** [*sic*] the Earth: Without which

these would neither have been an Atmosphere, Wind, Raid, or Are; but the Superficies of the Earth would have been [by the sun] Baked and Incrusted into the hardness
of Brick and Tyle.

This hypothesis seems also inconsistent with the different Nature of those Animals with which the Almighty Creator has been pleas'd to stock it; some of which
being only produc'd in a Warm and Fertile Soil, others only in a Cold and Sterile:
So some Animals delight only to delight only to breath a warm and soft Air, others a
more bleak and piercing: Thus Strawberries and Gilliflowers will not thrive upon the
tops of cold and barren Mountains; nor Mountain Vegetables in the most fertile Soil,
or best prepar'd warm Beds ... it cann't [*sic*] be imagined that all this variety of Matter
would settle in a Figure Spherically and Mathematically round.[5]

To drive his point home, Robinson devotes another ten pages to citing examples
of 'inequalities' in nature, whether differences in height, composition or form,
that allow an uneven earth to promote variety worthy of an infinite creator. This
passage demonstrates Robinson's skill in maintaining several parallel anatomies
as he simultaneously reviews and at least cursorily comments on relations among
members of the animal, plant and mineral kingdoms. What is novel as well as
ingenious in Robinson is that he implies the possibility of a higher level of anatomy – 'meta-anatomy' would not be altogether incorrect as a descriptive term
for it – in which these various systems also interact. Robinson asks for more
than a convenient taxonomy of flora or a Baedeker to gemstones. He aspires to
explain how the variety of minerals and the apparent miscellaneousness of their
distribution interact with similar complexities among living creatures, amidst the
weather, with respect to human custom and with regard to a host of other con-
stellations. Robinson moves far beyond the traditional 'argument from design'
in which, say, the worm exists to feed the songbird and the songbird to feed
the hawk, to ask why it is that certain species of wigglers feed certain species of
birds, why both birds and bugs can be classified in any number of ways, including
with respect to weather and physical habitat as well as to genetics or morphology, and how it is that all these systems not only interact but continually suggest
some grand overarching anatomy known only by God and maybe by a lucky few
in Robinson's tiny Ousby congregation. So strong is his drive to discover order
specifically within irregularity that Robinson routinely postulates the existence
of complex systems without a shred of evidence. Knowing only that the earth
rotates once a day, for example, Robinson infers that the centre of the earth must
contain a vast variety of molten ores, the mutual incommensurability of which
leads to a volatile circulation of magma: a circulation that, although it might
seem random, yields, through friction, the steady turning of our planet and all
the salutary benefits that this rotation brings to us.

Robinson presents himself as a more thorough version of his rival, Dr Burnet: as a student of the earth who possesses the patience not only to present the
macroscopic story of earth's genesis and evolution but also to explicate the book

of creation line by line, disclosing not only the system of the whole but also identifying an array of interlocking subsystems. Robinson is eager to go beyond the
standard taxonomic tree, to represent nature not as one schematic drawing with
assorted creatures occupying the boxes in the organizational chart but as an array
of systems that together support an enlarged universal order. In this, he again
resembles allegorical, moralizing authors such as Ralph Austen, whose *Spiritual
Use of an Orchard* (1653) also combines scientific, botanical classification with
spiritual hermeneutics. Filling in his picture of a world that is proceeding into
taxonomic order, Robinson writes another sequel work, *A Vindication of the
Philosophical and Theological Paraphrase of the Mosaick System of the Creation*,
the method of which is a line-by-line and sometimes word-by-word glossing of
the first few chapters of the Book of Genesis and the goal of which is the demonstration of the congruency of revelation with Robinson's geological theories.
Implicitly analogizing himself to Moses and with that raising questions about not
only the authority of a writer on big topics but about the process for acquiring
that authority, Robinson affirms that his 'design at present shall be only to give
a short Account how *Moses* came to be qualify'd for so great an Undertaking as
to write a *Description* of the World's *Creation*'.[6] He proceeds to explain that the
children of Israel were accustomed to thinking in a figural and 'hieroglyphic' way.
Moses needed a combination of geological, narratological and inventorying skills
in order to explain the genesis of the world to an audience more familiar with
desert rocks and folklore than with philosophical subtleties. Moving from verse
to verse, Robinson postulates a harmony between the bits and pieces of the geological record and the grand (and complicated) narrative of creation that emerges
from it. He distinguishes himself from writers, such as Thomas Burnet, who privi-
lege the big picture over the minute details – over the 'petrify'd *Shells*' and 'other
*Marine* Insects, which we meet with inclosed in hard Rocks, upon the tops of
high Mountains': fossils that, far from challenging the biblical account of ancient
times, not only can but must create a highly interesting and profusely detailed
story. 'The Majesty of the Scripture-Style', Robinson opines, 'consists in the *Metaphor* and *Figure*'.[7] That style, in turn, parallels the subject matter that Moses and
other Scriptural authors embrace. Robinson is one of the few exegetes willing to
address the actual content of what he explicates. He inclines less to talk about the
origins of 'the world' or similar abstractions than to elucidate the scratches on
rocks and what they might add to a 'hieroglyphic' interpretation of natural history. Thus Robinson never hesitates to descend from his speculations about the
whole maelstrom of creation to investigate such local curiosities as some alleged
knocking, drumming and even groaning coming from a well in Bantry, apparent
percussive messaging that the locals regarded as 'Mineral Spirits' attempting to
steer miners towards a mother lode but that Robinson treats as yet another anecdote for his simultaneously Mosaic – and mosaic – rendering of creation.[8]

Discussed above, the universalizing energy of anatomy – its drive to explain or at least to describe objects or events or beings in their entirety and its occasional ambition to organize the whole body of knowledge – led to selectivity in explanation like that seen in the Sherwin-Williams company logo, where paint covers the world but where information about the setup of this colossal paint job is scarce. The inverse is also true: claims either to explain or to taxonomize either everything or everything about a specific topic lead anatomists into digressions and extensions of their assignments. Anatomizing navigation will inevitably lead to divagations on the wood used to manufacture rudders and, with that, into considerations of the loams that nurture the trees of northern Europe; anatomy of the human body will surely lead into reflections on the urinary system or on nutrition or on any of a thousand other topics. Combined with the narrative drive among anatomists – with their tendency to convert sheer classification or bald description into extended accounts or stories about the action as well as about the structure of the anatomized object – this digressive tendency leads even a topic-focused anatomist like Robinson far afield from his designated subject matter. The fact that the earth is covered predominantly by oceans, for example, drags Robinson into a protracted discussion of tides. In that discussion, Robinson rejects the standard notion that the moon pulls the tides from the seas, opining that it would be equally 'reasonable to conclude that one Man is the Cause of another's Running, who runs the same Race with him Shoulder by Shoulder, and foot by foot' and instead crediting the tides to the differential drag on opposing hemispheres with differently sized oceans.[9] Robinson is thus intellectually pulled, like the Sherwin-Williams paint bucket, off and away from the planet that he considers and ever further afield from classification, taxonomy or anything fundamental to anatomy. What anatomist Robinson produces is an oscillation between the very particular and the universal. His intended subject matter occasionally comes into view during transits between the two. Robinson, for example, develops an early version of a unified field theory in which he seeks in the earth a common cause for meteorological, geological and oceanic phenomena, from weather to tides to volcanic eruptions.

> When the Damp ... upon some Class of the Superintended Strata, it either splits them, making Cracks and Chasms in the Exterior parts of the Earth for some Miles in length, which at the instant of the Shock openeth, and in the Interval between the Shocks closeth again: [Of this Kind was the Crack or Chasm which open'd and swallow'd the Tents of Korah, *Dathan*, and *Abiram*; and no doubt, but the Shock struck a Terror into the whole Camp].
>
> Or if the grand *Flatus* be very Strong and Vehement, it either elevates the whole Class above the Superficies of the Earth, forming a Mountain; or else it sinks down into the Vault, and the vacant place is immediately fill'd with Water [not from Dr. Woodward's Abyss] but from the Veins of the Earth which break into it.[10]

Robinson's argumentation is characterized by alternation. He vacillates between vast operations within the earth and an assortment of digressive comparisons, whether his hermeneutic response to a tremor reported in the Bible or his glancing blow at rival geologist Dr John Woodward. This inability to stay on the topic or to maintain a continuous level of resolution or generality may account for the irony attributed to many anatomies (again, Browne and Burton come to mind), where the frequent juxtaposition of vast observations and particular anecdotes suggest a kind of hyper-intellectualized mock-heroism. For Robinson, a country parson, irony and wit are only after-images of his struggle to account for everything pertinent to the earth only to discover that pertinence tends to dissipate into everything.

Affective bipolarity, whether expressed in the contrast of the sublime and the ridiculous that characterizes the mock-heroic or in the blend of truth and sarcasm that generates irony or in the mix of stead judgement and burning outrage that animates satire, is an essential part of any anatomical project. Anatomy claims to cover the whole of a part: to give a complete account of a topic that is only a small excerpt from nature. Its claims of comprehension fit awkwardly with the particularity of its subject matter. The many modulations of this contrast between the diffusely immense and the identifiably small play themselves out, among other ways, in liberal approaches to the management of space and time. Robinson, for example, takes a nearly fundamentalist approach to the Book of Genesis, explicating its every line and its every event as if there were no distance at all between sign and signified. Yet he expansively grants large and loosely defined intervals to the days of the generative act. Moving from day to day within Genesis, he suggests that earth was

> created perhaps some Thousand Years after the Creation of the *Coelum Imperium*; for notwithstanding that Omnipotent Power might have created the whole World at one stroke, by an Imperious *Fiat*; yet it would not have been agreeable with the Infinite Wisdom, which consists in Deliberation and Counsel.[11]

One can only giggle at this characterization of God as a something of a cross between Oliver Goldsmith's Vicar of Wakefield delivering pious aphorisms and Royal Society virtuoso John Ray gathering natural-historical anecdotes. Robinson seems to expect that God will take the same deliberate, step-by-step pace that allows anatomists to bridge the gulf between the thousand details that a particular body of knowledge and the great volumes that, per Sherwin-Williams paint, 'cover the world'. Indeed, Robinson himself is key to the long process that converted the anatomy on a particular topic – the *Anatomie of Protestancie* or *The Anatomie of Absurditie* – to his anatomy of *the World*. This tendency towards enlargement animates every aspect of Robinson's investigations. Robinson, for example, takes a similar approach to a spatial, geometric and statics problem, the question of the stability as well as of tall and slender volcanoes such as Vesuvius or Ætna. A person who regards these burning mountains as things-in-themselves susceptible of small-scale anatomical treatment will quickly wonder why these hollow hills resist collapse, especially given that they seem to discharge their contents and thereby to empty their foundations and their cores while also growing tall, thin and turbulent. Robinson solves the problem by extending it over space as well as time. He suggests that the volcanoes we view stand atop far more massive configurations that extend deep into the earth, down to an immense reserve of magma shared by 'Spiracles' around the world.[12] That spatial extension simultaneously solves the genre problem, suggesting that the process of anatomy writing can go on, through detail after detail, until reaching the very centre of the earth, and the publishing or sequel problem, in that so vast a phenomenon will require a vast series of studies over a vast period of time. Arriving at the universal pool of magma that joins all earth's volcanoes in a single pool of combustible material is a multi-step process that culminates in an emblem of the unity of knowledge: an image of a vast pool of energetic material that explains not only one volcano, not only all volcanoes, but the mechanics of an entire planet.

Robinson's ingenious attempt to account for the stability of visible volcanic vents by anchoring them in a common pool of global 'gunpowder' (as he calls it) points up that, despite its haphazard methods and sprawling dimensions, the anatomy serves a regulatory, pressure-relieving purpose. One message of the anatomy is that there is always some deeper, more fundamental phenomenon underlying the apparent topic and that finer levels of resolution always lead to more mechanisms, more structures and more explanations. Perhaps perversely, an anatomy is always about something other than its proclaimed topic. If the work offers an anatomy of beekeeping, chances are that it will diverge into architecture (via the construction of beehives) or dietetics (via the uses of honey) or agriculture (via a review of hymenopteran pollination habits). Like the essay genre as practised by Michel Montaigne and later Sir Francis Bacon, the anatomy continually opens up the possibility that something else is involved with whatever is being explained or that a multiplicity of possible explanations will all point to the stability of nature – to, say, the very low probability that volcanism signals the imminent explosion of the planet. Robinson, for example, piles up rival or other possible theories regarding the internal operations of the earth. He records the opinions of those who believe that desiccation may lead to the heating and eruption of the earth; he wonders whether the interior of the earth is a vast cauldron of conflicting chemical processes; and he reviews the exegetical theory that the 'Fountains of the great Deep' mentioned in the Scriptures as the cause of Noah's flood might have been submarine volcanoes.[13] None of these theories coincide with one another. One is based on dryness, another on wetness; one is based on chemical abundance, the other on mineral aridity; one draws on Scriptural texts while the others draw on evidence-aided speculation. All these theories suggest some limit to the earth's potential action, whether through the cooling action of the waters atop the undersea vents or the limit of solar power with respect to drying mountainous rocks. All of these potential explanations also suggest that volcanism falls within the range of both human science and ordinary mechanics. The act of giving explanations – even multiple, contradictory theories – tends to tame and domesticate the seemingly awesome objects of geological inquiry. That which can be debated and explained is very likely not that which is supernatural. Postponing conclusions until geological theories can be weighed and checked and until the anatomy can be completed is a way of postponing disaster, of affirming that the apocalypse can wait. Composing an anatomy, surely not the quickest of assignments, is a way of calming fear and buffering anticipated disasters.

*

One challenge that anatomists implicitly face is whether they have reached the top of their own hierarchy of explanations. Is the anatomy offered by Thomas Robinson, being an anatomy of the entire earth, the anatomy to end all anatomies, or is there some higher level of discourse, some anatomy of anatomies, in which it is but one entry? In considering an out-of-the-way character like Robinson and, doubtless, while questioning whether the 500-inhabitant village of Ousby where Robinson plied his twin trades of clergyman and geologist could produce enough evidence to explain the entire world from core to volcano-top, recourse could be made to a metaphor that always underlies the anatomy, to wit, the body. What Robinson presents to us, as he proposes a vast underground cauldron that links together an array of volcanic outlets, is the geological equivalent of a combined circulatory and nervous system. The flowing and mingling of volcanic fluids ensures the routine, regulated and minimally destructive release of energies and pressures which, in his character as a pastor, Robinson reflexively attributes to the fall of man, with all its odious consequences. For Robinson, the earth is at least analogous to a living and sensitive body. It is a complete system that regulates, distributes and refreshes an assortment of fluids, minerals and resources that contribute to the maintenance of life. Conventional to the core, Robinson certainly is no pantheist, but he includes in his rendering of telluric creation an array of feedback loops that suggest the interaction of mind and body and that cap what could be an infinite regress (or progress) in the production of anatomies. For Robinson, the beauty of the anatomy is that it does more than explain this or that phenomenon. It goes beyond telling readers why a volcano erupts and leaving it at that. Rather, the anatomical approach traces the continual interaction of the various parts and processes that sustain the operations of and in the earth. Working step by step, the anatomy as a genre encourages readers and researchers to follow what happens after the explanation of a thing or event. After a volcano explodes, where does the steam, the bitumen and the energy go? Is there some system for reprocessing the waste of dramatic underground action? Thus the anatomy, like the brain monitoring its body, is always bending back towards both its topic and towards the outflow and outcome of whatever it studies. The anatomy is a perpetually running feedback loop that never loses sight of the origin or the destination of the components in its topic. When the topic is the earth, the anatomy follows igneous action from the interplay of subterranean materials through the eruption and then on to the gradual redeposit of those materials in the depths of the earth, where, recharged, they re-enter the volcanic process. Despite its bold universalism, the anatomy as a genre, Robinson's work teaches us, keeps everything within such compact loops. Sulphur ejected from Ætna stays in the volcanic cycle; it does not end up either on the surface of Venus or on the head of a matchstick, but rather circulates within its assigned zone.

Robinson attempts to explain everything that matters with reference to the self-contained, seemingly comprehensive yet geometrically limited ball of the earth. He offers an exposition of planetary processes that accounts for at least a miscellaneous assortment of biblical pronouncements without invoking extra-planetary forces or supernatural influences. For Robinson it is not necessary to look to God for the energy required to power volcanoes or to develop extraneous mechanisms for the delivery of water during Noah's flood. His effort is truly ana-tomical in the sense that he accounts for everything requisite to a given system, in the same way that a physiologist's account of the human body shows how the mus-cles and bones may support the human frame without recourse to angels, demons or miracles. Robinson thus epitomizes a cadre of geological writers who were eager to account for seismic processes by postulating the existence of complicated infrastructure within our home planet. Michael Escholt, for example, argued that the earth contained an abundance of interconnected capillaries and tubes that allowed for water, steam, vapours, electricity, and, in sum, just about any imagi-nable fluid or gas to transfer energy from one venue to another,[14] while Erasmus Warren wonders where in the earth the water for the great flood might have been stored.[15] Earthquakes that were felt in both England and in continental countries in 1692 and 1750 gave rise to dozens of pamphlets, reports and even sermons that asked whether the steam pressure that allegedly both caused and resulted from these shakings might be transmitted through vast cataracts or tubes running through the earth, passing from nation to nation at high velocity via underground canals. Speculation about underground plumbing that looks for all the world like earth's circulatory system takes the theological edge off the actions of the earth. It blunts the old saw that earthquakes or other major geological events represent judgements of God against an erring people, a common enough interpretation, for example, of the earthquakes in Jamaica in 1692, which allegedly resulted from the arrant wickedness of the mirthful Jamaican people.[16] All physical systems have their weak points and pathologies, and so it is that an earth that operates through its circulatory system will, sooner or later, experience a rupture or blockage somewhere, whether or not the people taunt their God.

This study opened with the thought that the anatomy, as a genre and as a method, was committed to negotiating the space between, on the one hand, miscellaneous data collection and superficial observations and, on the other hand, the discovery of deep explanations that, being in need of explication, might well lead to further instalments in the open-ended anatomizing process. Writers such as Thomas Robinson show us how the anatomy emphasizes the negotiating process. Many of the facts, anecdotes and evidences that comprise the tissues of the anatomy lack significance outside the anatomy itself. The interest in lumps of sulphur or phosphorus or pumice derives less from their intrinsic properties than from their participation in the process that the anatomy is trying at once to assemble and, to a degree, to replay for the sake of science-based entertainment. The geological anatomy as practised by Robinson and others thus takes on a life of its own. The anatomy emerges as a machine for the production of stories about stories, about the way in which interesting phenomena fit into more interesting processes that, in turn, lead to even more stimulating speculations.

# 4 'AFTER AN UNWONTED MANNER': ANATOMY AND POETICAL ORGANIZATION IN EARLY MODERN ENGLAND

Mauro Spicci

## Anatomy as a Textual Genre

Originally quoted in its Latin form (*anathomia*), the term 'anatomy' made its first appearance in English medical language in the first half of the sixteenth century, when the rediscovery of the anatomical knowledge of the ancients started to go hand-in-hand with active experimentation. In sixteenth-century England the term 'anatomy' denoted primarily a branch of natural philosophy. This is suggested by the printer and bookseller Robert Copland, who combines anatomy with surgery stating, 'the scyence of the Nathomy is needful and necessarye to the Cyrurgyen'.[1] In many cases the term 'anatomy' also denoted the kind of medical knowledge that could be obtained through anatomical dissections. This emerges from the words of the satirist Stephen Gosson, who uses the term to designate the arrangement of the parts of the body that can be shown *by* anatomy ('The anatomy of man is set out by experience').[2] The word 'anatomy' also indicated proper anatomical texts: i.e. dissection manuals or treatises dealing with animal or human anatomy. Such 'anatomies' were called 'printed', 'paper' or 'fugitive' anatomies, depending on their length and format.

When the term appeared as 'natomy', 'notomy' or 'atomy', however, it acquired a more specific meaning, referring either to a corpse ready for dissection or, figuratively, to a withered and skeletal figure. Such a variation, which probably originated from the fact the Greek prefix '*ana-*' was confounded with the indefinite 'a/an', became very popular in non-medical writings.

It is not unusual to find the word 'anatomy' on the frontispiece of English vernacular texts. Not surprisingly only some of them were dissecting treatises, such as Thomas Vicary's *The Anatomie of Man's Bodie* (1543), hailed as the first English-language 'popular dissecting manual';[3] the anonymous *The Anathomy of the Inwarde Partes of Man Lyuyelye Set Fourthe and Diligently* (1545); and the anonymous *Anatomy of a Hande in the Manner of a Dyall* (1554). Nevertheless what is really surprising is that in the sixteenth and seventeenth centuries non-medical printed anatomies greatly outnumbered their medical counterparts. One is forced to reformulate the concept that anatomies were only (or prevailingly) an extension of medicine, or that their circulation was limited to the medical field.[4]

The tradition of non-medical printed anatomy started in 1576 with the publication of *A Philosophicall Discourse, entitled, The Anatomy of the Minde* by Thomas Rogers, and *A New Anatomie of Whole Man* by John Woolton, archbishop of Exeter. The former is a moral treatise that adopts Saint Paul's body–Church allegory to dissemble the collective body of 'Christians, which ... by notable examples of others ... maye knowe them selves',[5] while the latter intends to 'describe mans excellencie before his fall, miserable ruine, together with the causes and consequences thereof'.[6] Both texts were reprinted many times after 1576, permitting one to suppose that the demand for this new branch of anatomy – i.e. moral anatomy or anatomy 'of the mind' – stemmed from more than mere curiosity.

After 1576 moral anatomy became a proper textual genre. In 1596, for instance, the pastor John More published *A Livelie Anatomie of Death*, in which the author's moralistic aim is combined with the medieval tradition of the *Nosce te ipsum*, such that the anatomical dissection became a sort of 'lesson in human mortality'.[7] The same didactic and universal tone can be traced in *The Anatomie of Sinne* (1603) by Joseph Hall, archbishop of Norwich, whose 'anatomy' is a proto-encyclopaedic treatise on human vices and their corresponding virtues, as well as in George Strode's *The Anatomie of Mortalitie* (1618), and Ephraim Huit's *The Anatomie of Conscience* (1626). All of these moral anatomies testify that in the seventeenth century the alliance between anatomy and moral reflection was greatly productive.

In the light of this premise it is no wonder that a large part of English early modern printed anatomies had a palpable literary quality. The first literary anatomy came to light two years after Rogers and Woolton had inaugurated the tradition of moral anatomy. In 1578, John Lyly published *Euphues. The Anatomy of Wit*, a text in which the typical Renaissance taste for *divertissement* is matched with the anatomical tendency to 'dissect or open the corruptions and weaknesses of wit'.[8] Lyly's was the first of a series of works in which anatomy acted as a productive nucleus of literary tropes and metaphors. Such was the case, for instance, for Philip Stubbes's *The Anatomy of Abuses* (1583), and Thomas Nashe's *The Anatomie of Absurditie* (1589), whose bitter disruptiveness suggests a further productive connection between the practice of bodily dissection and satire.

While it is true that in the literary field anatomy fully loses its narrow medical connotation, it is likewise true that what remains unaltered of its original meaning is its potential as a cognitive process of discovery. This seems to suggest that what lies at the core of the early modern concept of anatomy is the idea that the body can be analysed, discussed and transformed into a cognitive paradigm, which then can be applied creatively to a variety of different discursive contexts.

## The 'Fantastic Voyage' of Early Modern Anatomy: *A New Anatomie* (1610) by Robert Underwood

The first reference to an anatomical dissection in Britain can be found in Edward Edwardes's manual *De Indiciis et Praecognitionibus* (1532). Between 1532 and 1633, the latter being the year of publication of Phineas Fletcher's extraordinary anatomical poem *The Purple Island*, more than seventy 'anatomies' were printed in Britain. Among them, many use anatomy as a demystifying instrument combining moralistic reflection, universal didacticism, and a strong religious and satirical streak. Despite being heterogeneous in their content, all English early modern anatomies promise a new form of knowledge built on the primary role of vision in the process of knowing. In moralistic or political reflection anatomy demystifies ancient rhetorical constructions, revealing their sustaining ideological scaffoldings, while in the literary field the anatomical method polishes ancient metaphors (like the 'body politic') and gives new strength to old figurative traditions (such as the body/house association). In all these cases, however, anatomy discloses new, unusual and fascinating perceptive landscapes, where the categories of the ordinary and the known are presented, according to Robert Underwood's definition, 'after an unwonted manner'.[9]

Placed within this context, where literature and science establish fruitful exchanges, Underwood's *New Anatomie* (1605) is the first of a series of English early modern texts that transformed the human body into the perceptive setting for an actual 'fantastic voyage', where the adjective 'fantastic' implies the idea of a journey of discovery in which the man, with his own body, is at one and the same time a protagonist, an object and a victim.

Underwood's poem is a proper literary anatomy for many reasons. First, as shown by its epigraph, Underwood's poem acts on and offers a precise 'description' of the human body. It is also pervaded by a strong anatomical fury, which can be seen in the hyperarticulation of its sustaining metaphorical constructions (i.e. Spenser's original association between house and body and the even older one between the body and a political community). It offers an unusual form of knowledge that combines wit and didactic purpose (the subtitle describes the poem as 'No lesse pleasant to the Reader, / Then profitable to the / Regarder'). It also proposes a kind of knowledge that is essentially visual (in the frontispiece Underwood addresses the reader with the words 'A Man, a Household, and Cittie large, All three in one, described you *may see*'). Lastly, by dispensing a kind of knowledge that is explicitly declared as original, on several occasions the poem insists on the theme of novelty. Thus the adjective 'new' qualifies both the nature of the anatomical knowledge offered by the poem and the original form through which this knowledge is made available.

In the opening lines of his poem, Underwood sketches a narrative frame that relies on the motif of dreaming and preludes to an unusual revelation. This almost supernatural experience is introduced as follows:

> Late in the night, not long agoe
> As I lay in my bed,
> Musing alone of many things,
> Which then came in my hed:
> Were by Revelation,
> By Vision, or by Dreame:
> Or yet as lying in a traunce,
> Or by some other meane,
> I knew not well.[10]

Lingering between dream and hallucination, the poet discloses to the observer's ravished eyes an extraordinary vision, which is made readable by the use of similes. From his privileged optical perspective ('One caught me up to the Aire'),[11] the author first sees what seems to be a well-organized city:

> I did discrie
> A Cittie large, of bignes such,
> As it the World had been:
> A thousand thousand Houses there,
> A man might well have seene.[12]

Then he focuses on specific elements of the urban landscape, which soon acquires an architectural connotation. Once introduced, the body–house association is hit by anatomical fury. This fragments the original analogical nucleus into a myriad of atoms and visual suggestions that follow one another in an infinite – and somehow improbable – process of accumulation: the corporeal building is, for instance, sustained by 'Two *Pillars* framed like an *Arch*',[13] while these are sustained by '*Lases* very strong and white'. Every house has a chimney and two spherical 'turrets' in which the poet can see 'Two *Windowes* ... / Which are so like to eyes, that I, / Do thinke them eyes to be.'[14] The landscape observed by the poet is so estranging, fascinating and luxuriant that it can be associated with an unexplored and Eden-like 'new world', where the harmony of natural shapes and luminous tones ensnares the human eye and testifies to the perfection of their divine creator.

The act of contemplating something, the excessive beauty of which goes beyond the boundaries of the known – yet offers itself spontaneously to the poet-anatomist – leaves the observer's eye in a state of constant desire. The promise of ever-new perceptive experiences implied in the anatomical method leads the eye to search for new visual pleasures. After observing the external surface of the body-houses, the poet realizes:

> If these things thus without
> These Houses, be so wonderfull,
> And glorious; then no doubt,
> Those things, the which we cannot see,
> Which in these Houses are,
> Must nedes exceede these outward things
> And go beyonde them farre.[15]

Much like Vesalius's flayed men, who offer their bodies in a sort of spontane-ous self-sacrifice to the observer, Underwood's bodily structures literally 'unfold' themselves to the eye of the poet-anatomist. These corporeal edifices reveal their secret order and transform an estranging vision into a source of 'new' and precious knowledge. The original metaphor is thus fragmented into a variety of motives and details, which include a kitchen, a complex piping system, a magical cauldron, several purple fountains and a series of thick walls. Then it is possible to see a pillar, followed by a door and a mill, which hides a small room covered with ivory.

The thick web of metaphors, through which the poet rewrites the geography of the body, is fed by the perceptive horizons offered by early modern anatomy, which enlighten the obscure recesses of the human body and impose the neces-sity of finding a new vocabulary to describe it. The architectural analogy (which in the second part of the poem, with the introduction of the image of the city, acquires a clear edifying meaning and underlines the harmony between body and soul) gives voice to the obscure geography of the human body. Actually, the language of metaphor builds a new body, because the language adopted to mould its forms is new.

Nevertheless, if anatomical fragmentation inaugurates a rhetoric of the body whose metaphorical renditions are potentially infinite, we cannot deny that such infinity implies the risk of chaos. In Underwood's poem, figurative anarchy is exorcised by the adoption of an editorial criterion that reproduces the structure of early-modern surgical manuals and gives order to the poetical discourse. In fact, the margins of the page contain a dense apparatus of notes that reflect, sim-plify and summarize the metaphorical structure of the poem. On the one hand, the poetical discourse hyperarticulates the architectural body metaphor; on the other, the figurative scaffolding of the metaphors that nourish the poetical dis-course is made explicit by marginal notes, which act as a sort of countermelody to poetry and give a further level of legibility to the body. Eventually the body comes to be rewritten both by poetry and by the marginal notes.

The new ways of rewriting the human body offered by anatomical science give poetry, as shown by Underwood's poem, an extraordinary series of motives and figurative suggestions. The anatomical body offers itself spontaneously to being rewritten and reformulated through a rhetorical strategy that exploits the method, the complex system of figurative associations and the intertextual discursive references of anatomy.

In the period when Underwood writes his *New Anatomie*, another poet, Phineas Fletcher, draws inspiration from anatomy to elaborate his *The Purple Island* (1633), an ambitious poetical allegory, the product of a complex network of discursive and figurative associations related to early modern anatomy. As textual surfaces mirroring the multiple meanings of anatomy, Underwood and Fletcher's poems reflect the contradictions that are implicit in the evolution of anatomical science: not only does it strip off the flesh from the textual and poetical body, imposing the need to continually rewrite the human body, which is its main object of interest and scrutiny, it also establishes a series of acrobatic alliances with literary genres and motives, producing a kaleidoscopic and estranging bodily icon.

## *The Purple Island* by Phineas Fletcher: The Analysis of the 'Preface'

As a striking example of literary anatomy, Fletcher's *The Purple Island* reflects the revolutionary purport of early modern anatomy with great clarity. This is particularly evident if we consider the texts that appear in its prefatory section. The 'Preface' opens with the author's usual dedicatory epistle: this text, written by an intentionally obscure, yet unambiguous 'P. F.', is addressed to Edward Benlowes, 'Mecenas of the North',[16] who repays Fletcher with the first of the short poems contained in the preface to *The Purple Island*.

The title of Benlowes's poem – 'On the Excellent Moral Poem, entitled the *Isle of Man*'[17] – inscribes Fletcher's allegory within the tradition of 'moral' anatomy, whose origin dates back to Thomas Rogers's *The Anatomie of the Minde* and John Woolton's *A New Anatomie of Mans Bodie* (1576). However, Benlowes's words are peculiar in their insistence upon the autobiographical motif. Benlowes declares that after years of straying and vain erring Fletcher's poem enabled him to discover that 'travelling the world' is pointless unless it is combined with a desire to know one's moral condition:

> How my youth with this vain world hath err'd,
> Applauding theirs as th' onely happy fate,
> Whom to some Empire bloud, choice, chance preferr'd,
> Or who of learned arts could wisely prate;
> Or travelling the world, had well conferr'd
> Mens natures with the mysteries of state![18]

Exhausted by the dangers of imperialistic expansionism, which foments only human selfishness, Benlowes proclaims the need for a counter-tendency decision. Thus he wants to become a master of 'moral anatomy', an art of discovering and taking possession of the territory of one's self:

> Reigne o're the world, not o're this Isle of Man,
> Worse than a slave thou thine own slaves obey'st.
> Study all arts devis'd since time began,
> And not thy Self, thou studiest not, but play'st.[19]

Benlowes's verses suggest a process of self-knowledge that leads the Renaissance man to transform his original condition of slavery ('a slave') into sovereign power over the self, as the term 'reigne' seems to suggest. In the context of Renaissance colonial expansionism, Benlowes's poem ends with an original plea for self-awareness and self-containment:

> Let me (o Lord) but reigne o're mine own heart,
> And master be of this self-knowing art,
> I'le dwell in th'Isle of Man, ne're travell forrain part.[20]

The final goal of Renaissance anatomy (which, as shown by the periphrasis 'self-knowing art', is the process by which man knows himself) is therefore a mastery over the alien territory of the self.

Due to the Renaissance system of correspondences between microcosm and macrocosm, anatomy also offers the chance to combine self-knowledge with some deeper awareness of God's imprint within the universe. This is what the Protestant polemist Daniel Featley hints at in the epistle addressed 'To the Readers', which stands between Fletcher's dedicatory epistle and Benlowes's poem. Featley's epistle opens with the following words:

> He that would learn Theologie, must first studie Autologie. The way to God is by our selves: It is a blinde and dirty way; it hath many windings, and is easie to be lost: This Poem will make them understand that way; and therefore my desire is, that thou maist understand this Poem.[21]

The neologism coined by Featley (*Autologie*) semantically recalls Benlowes's 'self-knowing art', but it also links anatomy and theology in a close relation of synonymy. By virtue of the fact that 'the way to God is by ourselves', Featley's final exhortation to the reader – 'Peruse it as thou shouldst thy self, from the first sheet to the last' – must be taken literally, suggesting that the human body is a text that can reveal God's mystery only if it is dissected anatomically. By progressively dismembering the organic unity of a complex body, anatomy thus allows those who practise it to gain a form of knowledge that optimistically preludes happiness ('I invite ... all readers to be understanders; all understanders to be happie').[22]

The same relationship between anatomy and self-scrutiny stands at the core of 'To the Unknown Mr. P. F. Upon Survay of his Isle of Man', which can be considered the most curious among the poems contained in the preface. The poem was written by Lewis Roberts, a professional merchant and the president of the East India Company between 1639 and 1640. Roberts's only other published work was *The Merchants Mappe of Commerce* (1638), the primary concerns of which were, as the title suggests, commercial rather than literary. 'To The Unknown Mr. P. F. Upon Survay of his Isle of Man' thus represents Roberts's debut in the literary field and as such it can suggest the appeal anatomy had over a professional merchant and traveller like Roberts.

Roberts himself explains the reasons behind his literary debut in the following couplet: 'Yet rarer wonders in this Isle of thine / I view'd this today, then in twice six yeares time.'[23] Fletcher's poem attracts the 'Merchants eye' because it promises the wonderful vision ('I view'd') of a virgin, 'undiscover'd' land, which arouses the same sexual excitement that informed early modern experiences of colonization. According to Roberts, Fletcher deserves greater merits than the greatest of explorers. He comments that Fletcher

> hath descried an unknown World at home
> A World, which to search out, subdue, and till,
> Is the best object of mans wit, strength, skill:
> A World, where all may dangerlesse obtain
> Without long travel, cheapest, greatest gain.[24]

Fletcher's anatomy titillates the desires of Western men ('the best object of mans wit') because it offers the vision of an entirely unexplored world, a dark territory that can be discovered ('search out'), colonized ('subdue') and earned by labour ('till'). But in so doing Fletcher provides his readers with the most estranging of experiences: anatomy discloses the world of the self and transforms men into colonizers of themselves. In other words, what stems from Fletcher's literary anatomy is a sort of 'purified' colonial experience. Under the anatomist's gaze, the body of man appears as an edenic land whose hidden geography can be controlled and subdued ('curb') only through brand new expressive means. *The Purple Island* rewrites the geography of the human body mainly through an extensive use of anatomical allegorism, in order to offer a bodily icon that is the source of a truly *autoptic* vision because it can be perceived by the eye, it is destined to the eye, and it represents the triumph of eye perception. Being described as a 'a place too seldom view'd, yet still in view',[25] Fletcher's body offers itself to the observer's eye as a dialectic entity, which is 'fair',[26] yet 'most unknown'.[27] This eye, however, must be properly educated in order to decode the double nature of the Fletcherian body, which seems fatally to attract both the eye, obliged to rely on analogy in order to lessen 'the cognitive anxiety of discovery',[28] and the language of poetry, which tries to rewrite the body through an obsessive accumulation of figurative details.

## The Anatomical Landscape and the Triumph of the Eye

Not even one reference to hearing, smell, taste or touch can be found in the anatomical cantos of *The Purple Island*. This implies a drastic ocular polarization of the ways in which the body is made an object of poetry. In this regard Fletcher's manipulation of the island metaphor is highly meaningful. By eliminating all the details of the actual voyage of discovery that precedes the direct experience of the human body, Fletcher discloses the metaphor of the island directly to the eyes of the observer, and presents it as something unexpected and hence highly fascinating. Fletcher's island, unlike the remote lands that were the destinations of early modern voyages of discovery, can be reached 'without long travel',[29] as expressed by Lewis Roberts in the preface. But this does not mean that Fletcher's island does not share the trait of geographic remoteness with the typical alien lands of travel literature. Rather than physical distance, however, what characterizes Fletcher's island is a strictly metaphorical distance, which permeates the exotic enchantment produced by the vibrant and luxuriant corporeal landscape shown by the poet. The role of the reader is therefore not dissimilar to that assumed by Elizabethan explorers, for whom the experience of exploration of new lands was primarily and essentially *ocular*. The ecstatic contemplation of the beauty of landscape is not only a triumph of sight, but also the essential preliminary step towards the domestication and conquest of the unknown. This concept is underlined by Wayne Franklin, who suggests, 'at the heart of the discovery narrative stands the ravished observer, fixed in awe, scanning the New World scene, noting its colors and shapes, recording its plenitude and its sensual richness'.[30]

From this viewpoint, the hyper-articulation of the original metaphorical nucleus of the poem – which most of the critics identify as one of the principal faults of Fletcher's poetic project – and the subsequent profusion of visual details of anatomic origin, might well be the poetic equivalent of the same rhetoric of 'wonder, rapture ... haste of enumeration'[31] of Renaissance narratives of discovery.

However, the visible nature of the human body does not mean that it can be immediately read. In fact the wilderness of bodily landscape needs to be inscribed within a set of precise norms that make it possible for the reader to decode its unknown geography. The metaphor of the island serves this purpose perfectly because it is aimed both at multiplying the possible allegorical pathways stemming from the Spenserian body–house association, and at translating bodily geography into natural images that evoke the suspended landscapes of pastoral poetry, the timeless scenarios of utopian literature and the narratives of discovery. In this sense, like Underwood's suspended 'Cittie large' or Shakespeare's island in *The Tempest*, Fletcher's 'little isle'[32] is not a real and realistically defined place; rather, it is a 'playground for fantasy ... not confined within the cage of literal meaning', but constitutionally open to disclose 'the realm of imagination'.[33] However, Fletcher's island is not 'an alien habitat ... an unchartered territory': unlike Prospero's island in Shakespeare's *The Tempest*, which is 'fearful [and] disorienting' for its inhabitants because it has no 'place names'.[34] Fletcher's somatic isle represents the natural playground for the linguistic capacities of its explorers. The landscape of Fletcher's island is in fact so meticulously marked by fixed linguistic signs that the observer is naturally forced to call it 'home'.[35] The accuracy of Fletcher's medical terminology is therefore not simply a benchmark for the author's scientific expertise. It also corresponds to the precise aesthetic aim of representing the body as a territory that shares the language of its colonizers. The accuracy of the anatomical lexicon in *The Purple Island* is thus a Foucaultian 'art of naming', a strategy by which the poet triumphantly colonizes the island, defines the rules and limits of its 'predictability' and lastly exorcises its wilderness, transforming it into an entity that can be linguistically determined, then recognized, and finally controlled.

Encapsulated within the island metaphor and marked by the language through which Renaissance anatomy colonized it, the human body becomes a map, a universal chart that, as suggested by Peter Charles Hoffer, makes order 'out of the sensory chaos of novel locations ... reducing vast spaces to measured relationships ... transform[ing] raw sensations into precise linearity ... [thus becoming an] intellectualized mastery of the natural world'.[36]

Such universalism makes it readable as if it were a geographic chart or, more generally, 'an Index'[37] that is a 'vast abstract theoretical edifice' which '[tries] to explain all the variable and mutable structures of the world'.[38] This is a typical trend of Elizabethan literature, in which, as demonstrated by M. H. Nicolson, the microcosmic tradition acquires a specific cartographic connotation, maybe by virtue of the primary role played by Britain in the process of early modern discovery and conquest. Such a trend is shared, among others, by John Donne, who expresses the nature of the bond between the human microcosm and the universe through the images of the 'index' and of the 'book' in one of his well-known sermons: 'The world is a great volume, and man the Index of that Booke; Even in the Body of man, you may turne to the whole world.'[39] The reader of *The Purple Island* is therefore invited to scrutinize both the physical body of man, which functions as a universal map reflecting the condition of all humanity, and the textual body, which adopts the words and images of poetry to express the divine matrix inscribed in the entire universe:

> Look as a scholar, who doth closely gather
> Many large volumes in a narrow place;
> So that great Wisdome all this All together
> Confin'd into this Islands little space[40]

What first strikes the reader's attention in Fletcher's depiction of the human body is the poet's insistence on its circular quality. The body in *The Purple Island* reflects

> that perfection which is found in Spherical Figure, which God hath also pourtray'd in all his works, which observe the same exactly or come as near as their use will permit; as is seen particularly in the fabrick of Man's Body, his master-piece, whereof all the original parts have somewhat of the Spherical or Cylindrical Figure, which is the production of a Circle.[41]

However, the circle is much more than a recurring metaphor in Fletcher's poem; it is something on which the poet insists obsessively. The observer's eye is continuously attracted by curves, circular shapes and spherical volumes. This is the case of the world itself, which the poet describes as spherical even *before* its actual creation: the creation of the world – hinted at as an 'undigested Ball'[42] or 'earthly ball'[43] – is a pure emanation from the mind of God, the 'first and last',[44] who circularly epitomizes the beginning and the end of the whole process of creation. The world is therefore a spherical island that floats in a geometrically circular universe: this is the same image as used by Frances Quarles, author of one of the poems contained in the preface to *The Purple Island*, who describes the 'vast circumference' of the earthly island as 'yet but a rolling stone'.

Similarly the bodily island reflects the circular shape of the universe, fragmenting it into infinite atoms. The role of the heart in the fabric of the body, for instance, is defined by a series of images linked to that of the sun, which is itself circular. Since the sun is 'the great worlds heart', the heart becomes 'the lesse worlds light'; as 'the lesse world' floats 'in the calm pacifick seas'[45] of the universe, it is in the 'circling profluence'[46] of blood that

> This Citie, like an Isle, might safely float:
> In motion still (a motion fixt, not roving)
> Most like to heav'n in his most constant moving:
> Hence most here plant the seat of sure and active loving.[47]

The shape of the cervical region, which is 'fram'd like heaven, sphericall',[48] suggests its structural harmony as well as the nature of the bond that ties all its components, which coexist in 'sure and acting loving'. Among the cranial bones, for instance, the pericranial bones 'the citie round *embrace*',[49] while the double layer of skin surrounding them 'all the Citie round *enlaces*'.[50] Furthermore in the eye the *corpus vitreum* 'girts the Castle with a close *embrace*',[51] while a tissue as 'slight, and thinne'[52] as gossamer 'round enwraps the fountain Cristalline'.[53] The extensive repetition of verbs like '[to] embrace' and '[to] enlace' shows that the principle of unity regulating the whole body is the purest kind of mutual love, which is physically mirrored by a strong bond between all the parts, whose intersections make it possible for the body to live as a perfectly self-regulating organism.

The mutual combining of all parts also becomes a creative principle: in fact, because of the endless interweaving of its components, the body acquires its three-dimensional shape. What is striking in this regard is that Fletcher persists in exploiting the ideal of circularity even when depicting the *volumes* of the human body, whose three-dimensionality is revealed by the adoption of lexical items referring to arches and domes. In the middle of the cervical region, for example, 'two caverns stand, made like the Moon half spent;'[54] the intersection between the two gives birth to a 'Third cave ... his sides combining / To th'other two, and from them hath his frame.'[55] This cave is sustained by a dome made of 'three fair arches',[56] and overlooks a valley 'where two round hills shit in this plaesant dale'.[57]

Mutual love also becomes a structural principle regulating the functioning of the whole isle. The peritoneum, for instance, is described as a strong wall that 'girts with strong defence'[58] the ventral exapolis; the belly is composed of 'six goodly Cities, built with suburbs round',[59] which are 'joyn'd in league & never failing bands'.[60]

Circularity, whose mechanism was first described in 1628 by William Harvey in his highly influential *De Motu Cordi*, also epitomizes the life-principle of the body: blood, 'circling about, and wat'ring all the plain',[61] brings life to the whole body; its circulation is made possible by Galen's concoction, which 'never from his labour ... retires / No rest he asks, or better change requires: / Both night and day he works, ne're sleeps, nor sleeps desires.'[62]

Regulated by the so-called 'ocularcentrism'[63] of discovery, the rounded shapes of Fletcher's bodily geography reveal an infinite variety of colours and luminous reflections. The colour 'purple' itself, featured in the title of the poem, contains a myriad different nuances: blood vessels, for instance, first described as 'azure chanels',[64] are like rivers that 'with luke-warm waters di'd in porphyr hue, / Sprinkle this crimson Isle with purple-colour'd dew'.[65] The 'skie-like blue' of the blood system is juxtaposed to the 'milky wave'[66] of the nervous one, whose channels are as opalescent as 'lacteall stones which heaven pave'.[67] Moreover, the imperial dignity of the liver, 'the Isles great Steward' is underlined by the hyper-articulation of colour reflections: red is the colour of the liver's garments ('In purple clad himself'); of its palace ('His porphyre house glitters in purple dye'), and of the invigorating liquid oozing from its many fountains.[68]

Though of primary importance, blood red is not the only colour in *The Purple Island*. As previously suggested, many are the sub-tones that mitigate the intensity of the reds. The most pervasive of them is the neutral nuance of white. This is the colour of the skin, whose 'lilie white'[69] is so delicate that it seems almost transparent. Such transparency is not only aesthetically pleasing; it is also functional, because

The inward disposition detecteth:
If white, it argues wet; if purple, fire;
If black, a heavie cheer, and fixt desire;
Youthfull and blithe, if suited in a rosie tire.[70]

The readability of the body enabled by its whitish external surface inspires a voyeuristic play of transparency, which frequently titillates the observer's erotic imagination. It is no wonder that in many stanzas of *The Purple Island* the body is, if not explicitly compared, at least powerfully associated to a female entity, which sexually provokes the onlooker:

As when a virgin her snow-circled breast
Displaying hides, and hiding sweet displaies;
The greater segments cover'd, and the rest
The vail transparent willingly betraies;
Thus takes and gives, thus lends and borrows light:
Lest eyes should surfet with too greedy sight,
Transparent lawns withhold, more to increase delight.[71]

Fletcher's verses reveal the same dialectics of 'possession and feverish sexual excitement' as can be traced in the Elegy XIX by John Donne, where the female body is explicitly compared to a 'new-found land.'[72] The human body is therefore the object of authentic sexual desire, fostered by broken visions ('Thus takes and gives, thus lends and borrows light'), aroused by transparencies ('The vail transparent willingly betrays'), and fed by the hope of its eventual, yet constantly deferred fulfilment. Fletcher's bodily isle ensnares the observer by its far-away, yet tangible vision ('this fair Isle, sited so nearly neare'),[73] an alien ('forraine home'), yet homely land ('a strange, though native coast')[74]: a sexually attracting *terra incognita*, whose colonization requires the same 'complex of anxiety, voyeurism, [and to which] attractions can be traced in many 'texts and images of early contact between European and Native'.[75]

## A Paradigm of Political Stability

The human body has always been described as something whose integrity must be defended against possible intrusions. From this viewpoint it is clear that one of the reasons why Renaissance anatomy was so revolutionary is that it gave full visibility to the human body by overcoming most of the physical and cultural boundaries that made it an 'inviolable' entity. In coherence with the paradigm of impenetrability, the body in *The Purple Island* is 'constructed around one overriding principle: it must be defended'. This explains why the anatomical cantos of the poem are so full of images of and linguistic references to 'battlements, moats, strategically placed mountains'.[76] The bodily island has a threefold political structure:

> By three Metropolies is jointly sway'd;
> Ord'ring in peace and warre their governments
> With loving concord, and with mutuall aid:
> The lowest hath the worst, but largest See;
> The middle lesse, of greater dignitie:
> The highest least, but holds the greatest soveraigntie.[77]

Fletcher's adoption of the rather obsolete term 'metropolies' suggests that the kind of authority that resides in these three regions is not only political (each of them is the seat of a peculiar government), but also religious (originally a 'metropolis' was the seat of a metropolitan bishop). Of these three regions (i.e. the belly; the thorax; the cranium)

> Deep in a vale doth that first province lie,
> With many a citie grac't, and fairly town'd;
> And for a fence from forrain enmitie,
> With five strong-builded walls encompast round;
> Which my rude pencil will in limming stain;
> A work more curious[78]

The constant menace of external attacks weakens their perfect harmony. To reduce the danger of foreign invasions, they are surrounded by 'five strong-builded walls', namely 'the skinne, the fleshie panicle, and the fat … the muscles of the belly-peese or the inner rimme of the belly'.[79] Similarly the city of Hepar stands on a hill, which grants it a position of 'ocular' supremacy over the entire region of the belly. Nevertheless, Hepar itself needs to be defended: this is the reason why it is characterized by

> sure barres, and strongest situation;
> So never fearing foreiners invasion:
> Hence are the walls slight, thinne; built but for sight & fashion.[80]

Moreover, the primary importance of the heart within the body implies an extremely complex system of defence: besides common barriers (skin and muscles), the heart can rely on 'another Guard':[81]

> Built whole of massie stone, cold, drie, and hard:
> Which stretching round about his circling arms,
> Warrants these parts from all exteriour harms;
> Repelling angry force, securing all alar'ms.[82]

Together with the sternum, other organic barriers that protect the heart are the muscles of respiration, which are described as a 'Guard, both for defence, and respiration;'[83] the 'border-citie' of the midriff, which 'like a balk, with his crosse-builded wall, / Disparte the terms of anger, and of loving;'[84] and the pleura, a 'peculiar wall, / The whole precinct, and every part defending':[85]

Sheltered by this complex system of walls and fortifications,
Kerdia seated lies, the centre deem'd
Of this whole Isle, and of this government:
If not the chiefest this, yet needfull'st seem'd,
Therefore obtain'd an equall distant seat,
More fitly hence to shed his life and heat,
And with his yellow streams the fruitfull Island wet.[86]

But disruptive menaces might be external as well as internal; the bodily isle is in constant danger of intestinal perturbations. From the city of Hepar, for example, stem 'three pois'nous liquours',[87] whose streams must be carefully regulated to avoid

The cloudie Isle with hellish dreeriment
Would soon be fill'd, and thousand fearfull rumours:
Fear hides him here, lockt deep in earthy cell;
Dark, dolefull, deadly-dull, a little hell;
Where with him fright, despair, and thousand horrours dwell.[88]

Imbalance is only a theoretical threat. The efficient cooperation among the defence systems of the body reduces the risk of mutiny, so that the island floats 'in the calm pacifick seas.'[89] Fletcher's island is therefore not only a self-sufficient organism. It is also an *exemplum* of political stability, communitarian cohesion, and benefic harmony. As such, it is also a surprising somatic 'utopia', a 'perfect society where social cohesion and the common good are not imperiled by individual appetite'.[90]

The political implications of Fletcher's allegory are striking: while depicting the anatomy of the human body in all its medical details, the poet also offers a political paradigm of cohesion and stability to Britain, itself a real island. The intersection between these two 'insularities' – Britain as a real island, Fletcher's as a metaphorical one – gives a strictly political value to the poet's anatomy.

The contemplation of the perfect self-sufficiency that characterizes the life of the physical body leads Fletcher to condemn those 'Vain men, too fondly wise, who plough the seas, / With dangerous pains another earth to find'.[91] The desire to add 'new worlds to th' old, and scorning ease, / The earths vast limits dayly more unbind'[92] is violently execrated by the poet because it is doubly dangerous. On the one hand, it contradicts the implicit belief that insularism is a synonym of stability and peaceful coexistence; on the other, the discovery and possession of 'farre distant worlds', defined as 'needlesse sweating' by the poet, leads men to self-oblivion ('You never find your selves; so lose ye more by getting.'[93] Therefore

Let others trust the seas, dare death and hell,
Search either Inde, vaunt of their scarres and wounds;
Let others their deare breath (nay silence) sell
To fools, and (swoln, not rich) stretch out their bounds
By spoiling those that live, and in wronging dead;

That they may drink in pearl, and couch their head
In soft, but sleeplesse down; in rich, but restlesse bed.
Oh let them in their gold quaff dropsies down;
Oh let them surfets feast in silver bright:
While sugar hires the taste the brain to drown,
And bribes of sauce corrupt false appetite,
His masters rest, health, heart, life, soul to sell.
Thus plentie, fulnesse, sicknesse, ring their knell:
Death weds and beds them; first in grave, and then in hell.[94]

Fletcher contrasts the disruptiveness of colonial *hybris* with a vision of integrity
that finds its fulfilment in the 'Island fair':[95]

Let me under some Kentish hill
Neare rowling Medway 'mong my shepherd peers,
With fearlesse merrie-make, and piping still,
Securely passe my few and slow-pac'd yeares:
While yet the great Augustus of our nation
Shuts up old Janus in this long cessation,
Strength'ning our pleasing ease, and gives us sure vacation.[96]

The insular metaphor of the body thus sustains an ideal of stability and evasion
('sure vacation') which is both private, because it is rooted in the autobiographical experience of the author, and public, because it is only by defending its own
organic insular self-sufficiency that England will be able to maintain its status
of God's 'Vice-roy'.[97] What emerges from the 'fantastic voyage' into the hidden
geography of the human body accomplished by Fletcher is, therefore, the idea
that in the early modern age the human body is a problematic icon, an improbable organic whole where a complex variety of interrelated discourses – subjective,
scientific, poetic and politic – can coexist and mutually influence one another.

## Conclusion: The Languages of the Body in Early Modern England

Underwood's *A New Anatomie* and Fletcher's *The Purple Island* turn out to be
two striking attempts to give voice to the narrative urgency that emerged as
soon as Renaissance men started to peer into the hidden recesses of the body.
These two poets describe the early modern body as a virgin land that can dispense knowledge only if its voice is deciphered and its vagueness erased. Once
translated into textual and poetical terms, as suggested by Daniel Featley in his
inaugural plea to the readers ('all sorts to be readers, all readers to be understanders, all understanders to be happie'),[98] the human body can therefore be read as
a text that becomes a source of knowledge. The final goal of this process is, as we
have seen, a form of sovereign power over the world of the self, which is, unlike
many modern experiences of discovery and colonization, surely advantageous.

However, the corporeal 'new world' longed for by Underwood, Fletcher, Benlowes, Featley and Roberts seems to defer any unequivocal definition. The complexity of allegorical associations encrusted around the image of the body that is the central object of Underwood's and, more strikingly, Fletcher's poetry demonstrates that the geography of the early modern body can be sensed only at the point of intersection among its many different languages, such as anatomy, poetry, moral enquiry and political reflection. In other words, what seems to emerge from Underwood's as well as Fletcher's anatomical poems is the idea that in the early modern age the human body does not speak one single specific language, but stands at the point of convergence of many different interrelated and mutually interfering discourses.

If, therefore, the only possible rhetoric of the early modern body is characterized by a continuous process of progressive accumulation of voices and discourses, how can a poet represent the new 'anatomical' body? What could be said about the early modern body, which appeared as a

> Place too seldome view'd, yet still in view;
> Neare as our selves, yet farthest from our care;
> Which we by leaving find, by seeking lost;
> A forrain home, a strange, though native coast;
> Most obvious to all, yet most unknown to most?[99]

These lines seem to suggest that the only way to describe the human body in the early modern age is that of adopting an oxymoronic rhythm in which every statement is immediately followed by its negation ('too seldome view'd, *yet* still in view'; 'Neare as our selves, *yet* farthest from our care'; 'Most obvious to all, *yet* most unknown to most'). Both *A New Anatomie* and *The Purple Island* try to harmonize the variety of the voices that surround the human body. In so doing they offer the vision of a highly polyphonic entity, whose cognitive boundaries are continually redefined by poetic allegorism, medicine and political enquiry. Such an 'unwonted manner' is, as Underwood puts it, a striking trait of modernity and projects the human body into a semantic universe where its languages are 'anatomically' infinite.

# 5 SUBTLE BODIES: THE LIMITS OF CATEGORIES IN GIROLAMO CARDANO'S *DE SUBTILITATE*

## Sarah Parker

In 1550, Italian doctor and professor of medicine Girolamo Cardano (1501–74) published an important work in the course of his career as physician, mathematician and astrologer, the *De subtilitate, libri XXI*. The work takes on the difficult task of exploring what it calls *subtilitas*: 'My purpose in writing this work is to expound the significance of subtilitas. Now subtilitas is a certain intellectual process whereby sensible things are perceived with the senses and intelligible things are comprehended by the intellect, but with difficulty.'[1] The challenge of studying things that are difficult to perceive with the senses and to grasp with the intellect means that only those with exceptional faculties of intellect and sense will be able to understand the elusive and complex phenomena that *De subtilitate* discusses.

Cardano warns his reader from the opening lines of the book that describing the subtle often means abandoning the dominant Aristotelian model of inquiry, where causes must be discovered before describing their potential effects. In Aristotle's *oeuvre*, the search for cause–effect relationships is often the philosopher's most important job, because it answers the key teleological question: why does this thing exist and function as it does in the world? For Cardano, however, these questions are not always answerable. What is more, the exclusively teleological focus of Aristotelian inquiry leaves the philosopher without a method for understanding a vast number of phenomena that do not necessarily have a clear causal relationship. Rather than restricting inquiry to such causal relationships, *subtilitas* allows the author to explore the contradictions, paradoxes and mysteries that he can locate, even though they are difficult to explain.

Cardano's methodological reworking of the teleological inquiry championed by Aristotle disrupts the classificatory schema central to Aristotle's natural philosophy. In the *Parts of Animals*, Aristotle poses methodological questions important to the natural philosopher: 'the following question about how one is to carry out an examination should not be overlooked – I mean the question of whether one should study things in common according to kind first, and then later their distinctive characteristics, or whether one should study them one by one straight away'.[2] In other words, should an investigation begin with categories into which observed phenomena can be placed, or should the investigation begin with the individuality and particularity of each phenomenon? Aristotle concludes that observation of particulars must precede categorization, while still holding the creation of classificatory systems as an ultimate goal. The philosopher bridges the gap between the observation of particulars and their classification by employing a cause–effect methodology. In order to understand, for example, why some animals have a backbone, it is necessary to understand the purpose of the backbone, what Aristotle would call its final cause. He thus specifies that the backbone must accommodate the dual purpose of maintaining the length and straightness of the animal while also allowing the animal to move its body. Therefore, the structure of the backbone, which is both continuous and made of many parts, permits it to perform the dual function of keeping the animal straight while also allowing the body to move and bend.[3] The combination of these two final causes, in other words the teleological purpose of the backbone, explains why it is made up of individual vertebrae that form a cohesive whole while also allowing for a range of motion. Having understood that the final cause of the backbone allows the natural philosopher not only to account for its structure, but also to set up a classificatory system that separates the many particular animals that have a backbone from the many particular animals that do not. This intimate relationship between teleological explanation and classification requires a methodological approach where understanding cause–effect relationships is a fundamental step in the process of classification.[4]

Aristotle's rigorous attention to logic and taxonomy had a longstanding effect on the development and organization of scientific knowledge. As far as the study of the human body is concerned, this influence is evident in the signal medical writings of Galen.[5] His treatise 'That the Best Doctor is also a Philosopher', argues that part of medical training should include a study of logic which, Galen argues, can be deduced from the pre-Aristotelian writings of Hippocrates. The treatise asserts, 'Hippocrates also pointed out that an inability to distinguish diseases by species and genus leads to the failure of the doctor in his therapeutic aims; his attempt was to encourage us to train ourselves in logical theory', but the logical theory that leads to establishing the species and genus of a disease derives from Aristotelian philosophy, not the Hippocratic corpus.[6] It was Aristotle who established the strategies of logical inquiry that Galen attributes to Hippocrates in his claim that a good physician needs philosophical training in order to examine the body and diagnose its illnesses. Galen passionately argues that a good physician must study philosophy, and more specifically logic, in order to properly understand the classificatory guidelines of recognizing and organizing symptoms for proper diagnosis. Furthermore, Galen argues that such study in turn improves character, promoting the development of qualities such as justice and temperance.[7] Finally, and perhaps most importantly for Galen, proper use of logic allows the physician to understand the work of his predecessors quickly and effectively, so that he can move on to the work of expanding and enlarging upon that foundation of knowledge:

> And, if we practice philosophy, there is nothing to prevent us, not only from reaching a similar attainment [to Hippocrates], but even from becoming better than him. For it is open to us to learn everything which he gave us a good account of, and then to find out the rest for ourselves.[8]

According to Galen, Aristotelian logic is fundamental both to the study of established medical doctrine and to the development of new knowledge.

For Galen, and for the early modern physicians who continued his project, the study of anatomy was an important site for expanding upon the writings of his medical predecessors, such as Hippocrates. Galen's commitment to the organizational schema derived from Aristotelian logic is evident in his anatomical studies. In terms of his own training, Galen was influenced by a number of schools of philosophy, and never considered himself a strict Aristotelian. He does, however, reference Aristotelian philosophy throughout his work, and many of his close friends, patients, and colleagues considered themselves adherents to the Peripatetic school. The historical circumstances that Galen describes in the many autobiographical moments we find throughout his writings illustrate that he was continually surrounded by a group of fellow enthusiasts for anatomy who were also affiliated with Peripatetic philosophy, and it is often at the encouragement of these Aristotelian friends that Galen writes his anatomical works.

Galen's *On Anatomical Procedures* provides an important example of the impact that Aristotelian philosophy had on his work. Around AD 177, Galen gave a series of lectures on anatomy that were compiled and published as *On Anatomical Procedures*. In the beginning of the work, Galen adds a preface detailing the circumstances that led him to compile these notes for publication. He tells a story of friendship between himself and Flavius Boëthus, a prominent Roman citizen who served as a consul and was also appointed governor of Palestine. It was Boëthus who introduced Galen to the Roman court and secured him his most famous patient, Emperor Marcus Aurelius. Boëthus was also a well-known Peripatetic, and he was among several Roman citizens who considered themselves followers of Aristotle and urged Galen to perform dissections and vivisections that would enhance their knowledge of natural philosophy in the Aristotelian tradition. The product of these demonstrations fairly early on in Galen's career was a set of preliminary notes on anatomical procedures in two books that was lost in a fire after the death of Boëthus. Consequently Galen decided to collect his previous notes and add to them his new observations; *On Anatomical Procedures* was the result of this labour.

The genealogy of Galen's anatomical writings illustrates the links that his work had with Aristotelian philosophy, even though Galen would never declare himself an Aristotelian since he was also influenced by other rival schools of philosophy, such as Platonism, Stoicism and Epicureanism. The spur to investigating anatomy, however, he largely attributes to his contemporaries who studied Aristotle, not only Boëthus but also Alexander of Damascus, who was probably the first imperial chair of Aristotelian philosophy at Athens appointed by the emperor Marcus Aurelius,[9] as well as Eudemus the Peripatetic. The earliest audience for the dissections leading up to *On Anatomical Procedures* was a group deeply influenced by the methodology and logic that characterized Aristotelian philosophy. This Aristotelian context for Galen's work influences his writing on anatomy and especially the hierarchical schema that he establishes for discussing the order of the body.

Another of Galen's important anatomical works, *On the Usefulness of the Parts of the Body* illustrates the profound influence that Aristotelian teleology had on Galen's anatomical investigations. In this work, the Aristotelian claim that 'every instrument is for the sake of something, and each of the parts of the body is for the sake of something' determines Galen's investigative methodology.[10] The entire book explains the human body by providing answers to the key Aristotelian question that Cardano would later find unanswerable: why does this thing exist and function as it does in the world? Galen describes each part of the body by explaining its final purpose or teleology, and using that explanation to guide the classificatory schema for his exploration of the body. For example, if the bones share a final purpose of providing a structure and foundation for the body, then Galen groups them together for discussion and explanation.

In the period when Cardano was writing the majority of his *oeuvre*, new developments in anatomy and physiology were challenging certain aspects of the Galenic interpretations of anatomy that had dominated the medical world for hundreds of years. Cardano, who considered himself first and foremost a physician despite his proficiency in many areas of study, was familiar with these debates, controversies and publications. In his autobiographical writings, he consistently touts his skills in medicine, including his expertise in anatomy. Throughout most of his life he lived and worked in northern Italy near the Paduan medical university where many of the greatest physicians and anatomists of the time studied and taught. In terms of his own scholarship, Cardano was familiar with the history of anatomical study from the canonical medical writings of ancient Greece, to the medieval treatises of the Arabic and European traditions, while also maintaining familiarity with the more recently published works of his contemporaries. In the course of his long career as a writer, Cardano published an *oeuvre* that is almost overwhelming. His works, which were collected for an *Opera Omnia* edition printed in the seventeenth century, comprise ten folio volumes of several hundred pages each. Almost half of these numerous publications could be classified as medical.

Despite his impressive output of medical writings and his professional interest in anatomy, Cardano never considered himself an expert in the practice of dissection; and his works do not include an anatomical treatise. He did, however, insist on his particular skills in the procedures that guided dissection as they were passed down from antiquity. In his autobiography *De vita propriis*, written in the last years of his life and first published in 1643, he recounts with pride an anecdote in which he amazes the audience of an anatomical dissection with his knowledge of the Greek text that is guiding the demonstration. This story, which takes place at the university in Bologna, describes the typical pre-Vesalian anatomy lesson guided by the authoritative text rather than the cadaver.[11] The professor of medicine, an eminent anatomist named Fracanziano, presides. Rather than performing the dissection himself, he lectures primarily from his memory of Galen. This faithfully memorized text guides the activity of dissection, most likely performed by an anonymous surgeon. In a discussion of the stomach, Fracanziano gives a citation from the Greek, at which point Cardano speaks up to assert that he has left out the negative particle *où* in his quotation. When the presiding professor brings out the text to check Cardano's correction, the text proves that the citation was in fact as Cardano remembered it. Cardano recounts with satisfaction how his perfect knowledge amazed both Fracanziano and all of the students in attendance: 'He was silenced, amazed, and filled with admiration; the students, who had literally dragged me forcibly to the place, marveled even more.'[12] Cardano prizes his knowledge of the study of anatomy so highly that his ability to show such learning off to a crowd becomes an important moment in the image of himself he hopes to leave with others, from those in attendance at the anatomy lesson to the future audience of his autobiographical writings. He even goes so far as to claim that the embarrassment caused by this incident led Fracanziano to avoid meeting him in public, and that the distinguished professor eventually resigned because of the humiliation of having been publicly proven wrong.

Cardano also put his anatomical knowledge to practical use as a physician in post-mortem autopsies. He considered himself especially skilled at this newly popularized procedure, which usually involved an aristocratic patient who had been attended by multiple doctors at the moment of his or her death. Each of these attending physicians would have a hypothesis as to where the seat of disease had been located, and this theory would have guided the prescribed remedies. The ceremony of opening the body after death was a central moment in the competition among these doctors, for the location of the disease could either vindicate the physician in his theories about the illness and his prescribed remedies or, on the other hand, it could prove a source of embarrassment if those theories were not confirmed by the location of putrefaction in the body. At many points throughout his works, Cardano recounts with satisfaction the number of times that he was proved correct in his identification of the disease and the cause of death when the autopsy was performed. An avid gambler, he even boasts that he was able to make money by betting with his rivals that his prediction would be proven correct on opening the body. In his autobiography, he recounts a number of such successes, posing rhetorical questions to his reader as though these stories would be famous enough to precede him:

> very many, openly eager at first to be able to prove that I had been mistaken, had dissected bodies, as that of Senator Orsi, of Doctor Pellegrini, and of Giorgio Ghisleri. In the last case, does not my prediction that the source of the ailment would be in the liver seem astonishing, when the urine was in no way affected?[13]

As in his story of triumph at the anatomical lectures of Fracanziano, Cardano boasts that his predictions were so unfailingly proven by autopsy that his rivals began to keep their cases secret from him and henceforward avoided accepting his challenge. Finally, in at least one significant instance, Cardano himself performed an autopsy on his friend Gianbattista Pellegrini, which he conducted just one day after Pellegrini died. Afterwards Cardano wrote a lengthy description of the course of his friend's illness and recorded what he discovered upon opening the body.[14] In addition to proving his capacities as a physician and his loyalties as a friend, the work highlighted Cardano's ability to oversee a dissection, even though the occasions when he was directly involved in such dissections were rare.

At the time when Cardano was practising medicine and writing, the most famous among anatomical publications was the 1543 publication of the *De corporis humani fabrica* by his younger contemporary, Andreas Vesalius (1514–64). Cardano knew Vesalius personally and was proud of this acquaintance. He reports in his autobiography that Vesalius had been instrumental in procuring a professional offer that would have allowed Cardano to serve as the personal physician to the king of Denmark. Though Cardano declines this offer because he does not want to move to a colder climate and risk persecution as a Catholic, he nevertheless deems the event significant in his life, as it is included in the 'Brief Narrative' that begins his autobiography.[15] In a later chapter entitled 'Concerning my friends and Patrons', Cardano specifically mentions Vesalius as one of only two 'highly esteemed' professional associates, and he describes Vesalius as 'the foremost exponent of his day of the science of anatomy'.[16] Cardano's admiration for Vesalius is evident in his inclusion of the famous anatomist in his list of one hundred notable people for whom he gives a horoscope in the 1547 publication of the *Liber de exemplis centum geniturarum*.[17]

Vesalius is most famous in the history of anatomy for his anatomical treatise *On the Fabric of the Human Body* (published in Latin in 1543, translated in English in 1998) in which he attacks Galenic anatomy. In the dedicatory epistle to King Charles V, he justifies his critique of Galen on the grounds that his work was based on the dissection of apes and not humans.[18] Since Galen's treatises comprised the major classical precedent to studies in anatomy and physiology, Vesalius's challenge to aspects of Galenic anatomy set off a debate in European medical academies. Many important professors of anatomy took offence at Vesalius's dismissal of Galen, refusing to believe that new discoveries could upset the authority of the classical master. The most famous of these debates took place between Vesalius and his former teacher at Paris, Jacobus Sylvius (Jacques Dubois). Sylvius openly attacked Vesalius, insisting on the accuracy of Galen's writings, and Vesalius responded with a public letter in defence of his discoveries.

Presenting Vesalian anatomy as simply anti-Galenic, however, risks ignoring the fact that Vesalius maintained an allegiance to the works of Galen in other aspects of his anatomical research. Most significantly for this discussion of classification, Vesalius followed Galen's methodology, drawn from Aristotelian philosophy, of ordering the study of the body according to the uses of the individual parts. By using Galen's teleological approach, Vesalius was in fact recuperating elements of Galenic anatomy that had been lost in the medieval period.

In the many years between Galen's writings and the fourteenth century, most physicians and medical practitioners neglected the study of anatomy. Though Galen's texts were assiduously translated, copied and studied in the Arab world, few of these scholars conducted any new research.[19] It was not until the dissections carried out by Mondino de' Luzzi around 1318 in the university at Bologna that students of medicine recommenced the use of dissection to study anatomy and physiology.[20] Mondino published a textbook of anatomy drawn from his dissections but, significantly, he did not follow the classificatory system of Galen. Despite the profound influence that Galen's writings had on Mondino, he opted to follow a different order of dissection and therefore description of the body. Where Galen had created an order based on a hierarchy of purpose, Mondino's ordering prioritized practical necessities rather than philosophical dicta. He began with the areas most prone to quick decomposition, namely the stomach and the viscera, and ended with the bones, the part of the body that one would arrive at last when proceeding from the outside in.

Vesalius's decision to follow Galen's philosophical model in the ordering of his discussion of the body signals a respect for Galen's attention to methodology, despite *De fabrica*'s harsh critique of Galen's lack of experience with human dissection. In fact, Vesalius justifies his assiduous observation of Galen's mistakes by pointing out that Galen often read his own earlier writings with a critical eye and changed or modified earlier statements in his later works.[21] Even as he critiques his important predecessor for making claims about the human body while dissecting animals, Vesalius suggests (albeit not very humbly) that he is in fact continuing a project that Galen had begun and in a similar spirit of inquiry and pursuit of knowledge.

Vesalius's debt to Galen is, as I have already suggested, largely evident in his arguments for the purposefulness of each anatomical structure under discussion. This focus on purpose in turn suggests a proper order to be followed in anatomical study. He expresses admiration for Galen's decision to emphasize this organizational structure of the body in his treatise rather than following a more practically convenient procedure, such as the one used by Mondino. Importantly, this attention to Aristotelian teleology does not necessarily demand adherence to Aristotelian conclusions about the body. For example, Aristotle insists that the heart is the primary organ and the seat of intelligence, while Galen disputes this point and argues, with Plato, that the head and brain are more important. And yet, in his discussion of the head in *On the Usefulness of Parts*, Galen maintains his Aristotelian focus on the final purpose of the head, namely, to hold the eyes. In Galen's opinion, the eyes are the major sensory receptor that could not be located anywhere else on the body, since their primary purpose is to see as accurately and as far away as possible. Whereas other animals have their mouths or ears located in various places, the eyes are always as high up as possible, as evidenced by the fact that some creatures without heads have their eyes at the end of antennae.[22] The human head must therefore be formed for the sake of the eyes. The brain, in turn, is also formed for the sake of the eyes, and he concludes the discussion of the head and the sense organs arguing, 'For the encephalon seems to have been placed in the head because of the eyes, and the other sense instruments to have been placed there because of the encephalon.'[23] Though Galen clearly prioritizes the head, and specifically the organs of sight, over Aristotle's insistence on the heart's importance, he nevertheless employs Aristotle's teleological methodology when making his argument for a different understanding of the body.

Vesalius's discussion of the head follows the Galenic precedent, prioritizing the head over the heart while maintaining an attention to Aristotelian cause–effect logic. The fifth chapter of the first book, 'Why The Head is so Shaped; The Number of Different Shapes', unreservedly agrees with Galen's claim that the head and the brain were both formed for the sake of the eyes.[24] Moreover, his citation of Galen's argument is rather brief and passes over the nuances of several pages of logical development that led Galen to his final conclusion. Vesalius's casual reference to Galen as an authoritative predecessor whom he can quickly point to and move on from offers a sharp contrast to his previous reference to the anatomist 'deceived by his apes'. The positive reference to Galen illustrates that Vesalius valued Galen's use of Aristotelian logic to explain the purpose of each part of the human body, despite his harsh critique of Galen's mistakes in deducing information about human bodies from other animals.

Though he is most famous for revolutionizing the study of anatomy and sparking debates over the accuracy of Galen's claims, Vesalius nevertheless maintained the focus on Aristotelian methodology that had guided Galen's dissections. Such teleological explanations of the body continued to dominate anatomical discussion throughout early modern Europe, even among anatomists influenced by Vesalius's challenges to Galenic authority. One such anatomist, French physician Charles Estienne of the famous Parisian publishing house, published an elaborate anatomical treatise, *On the Dissection of the Parts of the Human Body* (Latin edition, 1545; French edition, 1546). Estienne was so inspired by Vesalius's strategy of combining detailed discussion of the body with rich illustrations that he followed a similar strategy in his work, which, it can be argued, draws on the *De fabrica*.[25] Following the Galenic emphasis on the teleological purpose of each part of the body, Estienne includes the study of the body's cause-and-effect relations in his definition of anatomy. The anatomist therefore not only examines and describes the various parts of the body, but he also uses that knowledge to make claims about the purpose or usefulness of each part of the body. Taking up the very same Galenic example that Vesalius cites in the opening of his *De fabrica*, Estienne references the eye and its teleological purpose to allow vision. The various structures, nerves and 'humours' of the eye contribute to this final purpose, allowing humans to see. The purposefulness of the eye provides the opening, exemplary model that guides the discussion of the human body throughout the work.

In his proem to the first book, Estienne refers to the Aristotelian argument that the purposefulness of the body confirms the perfect logic of a divine maker, an argument that Galen thoroughly explores in *On the Usefulness of the Parts of the Body*. Estienne, like many early modern anatomists, takes up this argument by adapting it to a highly Christianized interpretation. The study of anatomy, he argues, has both practical and spiritual uses; it not only improves our ability to treat the body when it is not working properly, but dissection also illustrates the impressive power of the Christian God. Estienne thus claims a special place for 'the contemplation of man', and claims that the study of this 'unique artifice and work allows us to understand the incredible power of our immortal God'.[26] Though Aristotelian philosophy did not argue for a divine creator intentionally assigning each element of the world a purpose, his philosophy nevertheless lends itself to this theological interpretation. Estienne was not alone in adapting Aristotle thus, as Christian thinkers who had read and interpreted Aristotelian philosophy since the medieval period adjusted it to their cosmology by envisioning a purposeful deity directing the final outcome of each naturally occurring phenomenon.

Aristotelian methodology gives anatomical works like those of Vesalius and Estienne an overarching organization and a coherent purpose. Following Galen's example, the two arrange their discussions of the human body according to the shared purposefulness of the various parts. Both anatomists therefore begin with a discussion of the bones, using the argument that the skeleton serves as a foundational support for the body. This approach seems counterintuitive, considering that the process of dissection begins with the exterior and proceeds inward; but, in terms of the methodological commitment to purposefulness, it makes sense to begin a treatise on anatomy with the skeleton. The treatises of Vesalius and Estienne share an overall organizational structure that emphasizes an orderly and considered progression from one part of the body to another, based on the function or use of each part.

Cardano's treatise on subtlety, by contrast, does not follow an obvious organizational scheme. One the one hand, *De subtilitate* clearly aims at an overarching ontological arrangement that progresses from lowest to highest, with man at its centre. On the other hand, so many asides interrupt this progression that digression seems to characterize the work more than the ontological outline. The opening chapters discuss the most fundamental and basic aspects of the world such as first principles and the elements. Subsequent chapters follow a progression through metals, plants and animals, arriving at the chapters on humanity at the centre of the book. This section is followed by explorations of the heavens and angels, and the work exultantly concludes with a chapter entitled, 'De Deo et Universo'. Within this scheme, the discussion of 'man' finds itself in a central place;[27] yet, all the while, Cardano's focus on *subtilitas* as the guiding thread that connects all of these objects of inquiry troubles this seemingly clear organization. Because the work aims to avoid topics that seem typical, standard, or easy to understand, Cardano's prose is consistently swept up into a fascination for the strange and the exceptional. This desire for digression transforms the book from a generically classifiable work into a complex hybridization of the many areas of intellectual inquiry that captured the attention of Cardano's learned public. From natural philosophy to theology, from architecture to ethnography, from astrology to mathematics, from alchemy to dietary regime, *De subtilitate*'s wide-ranging subject matter attests to Cardano's own broad fascination for a number of pursuits.[28]

When the *De subtilitate* arrives at the chapters dedicated to the human body, Cardano's position as an expert in medicine does not lead to a more systematic treatment of this topic. Indeed, the chapters that focus on the human are just as full of digressions and seemingly unrelated topics as the rest of the book. Though Cardano touches on many of the same aspects of the human body that one finds in the more strictly organized medical writings of his contemporaries, his discussions are not guided by a systematic organization. The tendency towards digression and the juxtaposition of seemingly unrelated topics corresponds, however, with Cardano's claim that *subtilitas* does not allow the philosopher to consider natural phenomena according to the Aristotelian focus on teleology. The organizational scheme guiding Vesalius and Estienne disintegrates, since the various topics under discussion are not necessarily driven by a cause–effect relationship that we can understand.

Guided by the search for the subtle rather than an overarching teleological description of the body, Cardano's work on the human tends to focus on various (often unrelated) aspects of the human body that qualify as 'difficult to understand with the mind or perceive with the senses'. The bones of the skull qualify for Cardano as an example of *subtilitas* manifested in the body. Though a basic tactile encounter with the human head makes it seem as though the skull were one continuous bone, in fact it is composed of multiple bones joined by tiny sutures. Nature has fashioned the skull in such a subtle way, Cardano reasons, for a multitude of purposes. This structure protects the head, 'so that if one part is broken, it is not necessary that the entire structure be compromised and broken'.[29] Furthermore, he argues that the tiny openings allow veins and arteries to pass through the skull while permitting the head to release extra heat or waste matter.[30] Because these sutures are so small as to be nearly imperceptible, they serve these functions while allowing the bones themselves to be thick and strong for the protection of the brain.

Cardano's observations about the bones of the skull are almost identical to the points that both Vesalius and Estienne make in their anatomical treatises. *De fabrica*'s first book enumerates the bones and ligaments that support the body, and its sixth chapter, 'On the Eight Bones of the Head and the Sutures Connecting Them', treats the bones of the skull in great detail. Vesalius cites the same two purposes behind this particular structure for the skull. He contrasts the structure of this unique 'helmet' protecting the brain with a clay pot: while many solidly formed vessels are easily destroyed upon impact, 'if it [the skull] were ever struck and broken, the cracks would not proceed throughout the skull as through an earthenware pot, but would stop at the point where the bone itself ended, at the sutures'.[31] Chapters eight and nine of Estienne's first book also discuss the bones of the skull and make a similar claim regarding the usefulness of the sutures: 'so that if a blow were to fall on the head, it would not split like a pot from one side to the other or in many pieces'.[32]

Vesalius and Estienne also concur with Cardano's second point that the sutures provide a way for the body to release noxious or heated humors, rather than allowing them to get trapped at the top of the head. Vesalius again uses a metaphor to explain this useful quality of the skull, comparing it to a house that requires a chimney. As the domicile of the brain, the head somewhat resembles the roof of a hothouse, in that it forms a receptacle for all sorts of smoky and vaporous waste which rises from below, and since for this reason the head itself requires an even more efficient exhaust system, the wise Parent of everything made the helmet surrounding the brain not solid all over but full of holes and interlaced with sutures.[33]

Vesalius's metaphor attributes teleology to the structure of the head and credits a divine creator with that purposefulness. Estienne too remarks on the need for the brain to expunge its excess humours: 'Such a conjunction of several bones together was also necessary in order to allow the humours of the brain to exit.'[34] And, as with his other anatomical observations, Estienne consistently attributes the proper functioning of the human form to the Christian God.

Though the descriptions of Cardano, Vesalius and Estienne use the same line of reasoning to explain why the bones of the skull are multiple and joined by tiny sutures, Cardano's observations do not rely on a teleological understanding of the body for their foundation. In other words, he does not describe the bones of the skull in order to relate their structure and function to an overall description of the bones, ligaments, muscles and organs that make up the human body. Instead, *subtilitas* guides the work's discussions of physical phenomena, directing the investigation towards those aspects of human anatomy and physiology that are difficult to understand with the mind and to perceive with the senses. This contrast between Cardano's work and that of Vesalius and Estienne is especially evident in *De subtilitate*'s unique organizational structure. On the one hand, both Vesalius and Estienne situate their explanations of the cranium within an overall presentation of the skeletal system, providing detailed discussions of the organization and names of the bones of the skull as these are contextualized by a similarly systematic description of the entire skeleton. Cardano's description of the skull, on the other hand, is not contextualized by a systematic discussion of other bone groups. Instead this section is preceded by an account of a lactating man the author claims to have witnessed first-hand and an ethnographic aside comparing the Spanish conquistadors' claims that the newly discovered 'Indians' have particularly thick skulls to Herodotus's report on Ethiopians in his *Histories*. Where Vesalius and Estienne pursue a linear organizational scheme that logically develops a presentation and explanation of the body, Cardano's work is guided by the potentially digressive relationships that *subtilitas* reveals.

Cardano's discussions of the human body in *De subtilitate* evidence his knowledge of the new developments in contemporary anatomical treatises. As a physician, Cardano was drawn to the epistemological optimism of the classificatory project that Vesalius came to represent with the publication of *De fabrica*. Throughout Cardano's medical, autobiographical and philosophical writings, he is careful to emphasize his own knowledge of anatomy and his mastery of theoretical medicine more broadly. Anatomical classification was, however, deeply indebted to the cause–effect model of Aristotelian inquiry that *De subtilitate* found too limiting. Rather than providing a mode through which all possible varieties of human form could be represented, the anatomical treatise as a genre was indebted to an Aristotelian logic that delimited and restricted discussions of the human body. While Cardano finds certain anatomical topics, like the peculiar form of the skull, fascinating, his work does not group such discussions within the organizational schema dictated by the anatomical treatise. In foregoing these generic restrictions, Cardano opens up the possibility of exploring aspects of the human body that would not necessarily fit within the purview of the descriptions found in Vesalius and Estienne. Cardano's name for this methodology is *subtilitas*. The wondrous experience of seeing a lactating man with his own eyes or the contemporary interest in the relationship between European heads and the heads of newly discovered peoples both provide accounts of non-standard bodies. Presenting these anomalies contrasts with the more or less universal descriptions of the body that anatomical treatises sought to develop. Vesalius and Estienne describe the tiny sutures in the bones of the skull as a universal human feature that fits into an overarching schema of other universal truths concerning the standard human body. Cardano's work acknowledges this universal quality of anatomical makeup, and the title of his chapter on the human body, 'On the Nature and Temperament of Man', implies that there are certain universal qualities that characterize the human body. Nevertheless, the work illustrates a continuous resistance to the strict organizational structure of the anatomical treatise and a fascination for digressive discussions of anomalies and variations in human bodies. Admitting descriptions of these bodily aberrations challenges the fundamental claims of Aristotelian cause–effect logic. While a woman's lactation seems easily explained as the effect of a clear cause (pregnancy and the resultant need to nourish a newborn baby), a male body performing the same function appears inexplicable within this framework. To the modern reader, Cardano's claim to have witnessed such a monstrosity may seem fantastical and even naïve, but it is significant for its challenge to such explanations of human physiology. As L. Daston and K. Park have argued, Cardano's wonder at the variety and complexity of the world is not Aristotelian wonder at the regular and functional aspects of nature, but rather wonder at the infinite multiplicity that he finds in all areas of philosophical inquiry.[35]

As a practicing physician, Cardano was well aware of the many potential variations in human form as well as the seemingly infinite varieties of illnesses that could attack and undermine the body. His challenge to Aristotelian models of inquiry corresponds to this basis of practical knowledge. Though *De subtilitate* acknowledges the usefulness, and even the intellectual pleasure, of anatomical classification, it nevertheless develops a mode of inquiry that allows the natural philosopher to move outside of the potentially Procrustean boundaries set up by the anatomical treatise as it was reimagined by Vesalius and his successors. A great admirer of Vesalius and of anatomical study more generally, Cardano's development of *subtilitas* was by no means a rejection of the systems of classification developed in these anatomical works. In defining *subtilitas* he was, rather, taking up these systems and introducing a new strategy for stretching their capacity to describe a broader array of natural phenomena.

## Acknowledgements

Thanks to the Huntington Library's Evelyn S. Nation fellowship in the history of medicine, I was able to complete the necessary research for much of this essay, and I am especially grateful for the assistance of the Huntington's librarians and staff. Additionally, I would like to thank the UNC Medieval and Early Modern Studies programme for research assistance.

# 6 MIRRORING, ANATOMY, TRANSPARENCY: THE COLLECTIVE BODY AND THE CO-OPTED INDIVIDUAL IN SPENSER, HOBBES AND BUNYAN

## Nick Davis

This essay examines three texts, printed respectively in 1590, 1651 and 1682, which are concerned with establishing a relationship between the symbolic image of an anthropomorphic body and the reader's understanding of individual life's fundamental orientations. They are the Castle of Alma episode from Edmund Spenser's *The Faerie Queene*, Thomas Hobbes's *Leviathan* and John Bunyan's *The Holy War*. *Leviathan* and *The Holy War* have as frontispieces highly significant visual representations of an anthropomorphic figure who dominates a landscape by virtue of scale and position; Spenser's body-castle is described in detail as seen from outside, as internally explored and in its envisaged physical setting. The three texts manifestly have different explanatory and persuasive purposes, but all establish a certain managed ambiguity in their symbolic representation of the body: the anthropomorphic image offered to the reader can be received, variously, as (a) an embodiment of collective knowledge which the reader/spectator already possesses, *qua* member of that collectivity, (b) a novel means of organizing collective knowledge, conceived on the model of anatomy, whose make-up and functioning therefore have to be explicated, and – as a corollary of (b) – (c) a novel means of self-understanding as an individual agent. I shall argue that emphasis on the constructedness of the symbolic body image forms a crucial part of the texts' mediations between the presumptively collective and the prescriptively individual. Considered together, they offer a lens on the large-scale cultural transition, characteristic of early modernity, from predominantly collectivist to predominantly individualist conceptions of selfhood.

The Castle of Alma sequence (*The Faerie Queene*, book 2: canto 9, canto 11, canto 12, stanza 1)[1] invites the reader to take stock of long-standing traditions of symbolic corporeal representation.[2] Here the presented anthropomorphic body is, in the first place, a mirror-like device[3] whose purpose is the recapturing for recognition of attributively collective knowledge or experience; such knowledge or experience is 'collective' in the sense that the having of it obviates the drawing of a distinction between what might be registered by an individual and what might be registered by a group. Medieval to early modern texts metaphorically conceived as mirrors broadly accept a gnosiology in which 'apprehension of the world [is] not regarded as a creative function but as an assimilation and retracing of given facts'.[4] Creativeness here emerges here, theoretically, not in the establishment of pertinent information but in the form of its retracing. Setting up an image of the body as a knowledge-mirror projects the principle – more or less an anthropological universal, as Vico posits – that bodily form and process possess *a priori* validity as a means of organizing cultural data. The collectivist mirror-body is also integrative of knowledge: it is a medium for the simultaneous and somewhat co-ordinated presentation of different understandings of the human. Many passages from *The Faerie Queene* stand in continuity with medieval allegorical writing, most obviously the dream visions of Chaucer and Langland.[5] Like its era's symbolic writing in general the episode centred on Alma's castle creatively explores dissonances and correspondences between discrepant systems of understanding, which are being simultaneously invoked. For example, this castle, which is solidly constructed like a piece of architecture, also shakes apprehensively – so expressing its likeness to a sentient body – when surprised by a sudden noise.[6]

For present purposes it will be sufficient to identify the predominant knowledge schemes, co-ordinated and integrated in some degree by bodily reference, which the episode *qua* 'mirror' recalls. Lady Alma's governance of the castle as chatelaine connotes the proper functioning of the human rational soul that, as in Plato and Aristotle, 'doth rule the earthly masse [i.e. the body, its inferior], / And all the service of the bodie frame;'[7] but the internal divisions of the castle, progressively explored by its visitors in the narrated action, also reference those of the soul itself, traditionally divided into vegetable (presiding over nourishment and growth), sensitive (the arena of feelings) and intellectual (interrelating judgement, imagination and memory). The Alma narrative, linked in of course with the larger emergent design of the poem's second book and of the poem as a whole, seeks to define, I would suggest, a point of crossing between otherwise divergent strands of discourse. Very conspicuously, it sets in play conceptions of the moral life in a broadly classical understanding, where temperance is a finding of balance or the middle way between extremes, but also in a broadly Christian understanding, as projected in metaphors of struggle and the search for salvation. It invokes a transcendent Pythagorean–Platonic mathematics, which is taken to underlie the organization of the real, including that of the cosmos at every level, and which comes to the fore in the well-known *conundra* of the 'mathematical stanza;'[8] what is stated here has clear, iconic internal structure as a conjoining of the circle, the triangle and the square, but its bearing on bodily form as such and on its surrounding symbolic scene is indefinitely open to speculative enquiry.[9] The whole episode's metaphoric conception is partly sustained by the notion of the body politic. More will be said of this shortly, but we may note for the time being the episode's manifest concern with the hierarchical distribution of social functions, and with propriety of behaviour in ordinary social interaction and in warfare. The era's consideration of the polis as a body itself mediates tensions between classically derived enquiry into optimal structures of rule (see Archambault) and the Pauline account of the spontaneous integration of a Christian spiritual community.[10] It has already been observed that the castle carries the double connotative weighting of a nervously responsive living organism and a construction that is robust and enduring;[11] in the second respect it is a piece of well-designed architecture, made following medieval practice and as Vitruvian theory recommends in bodily concordant proportions. The image of a properly constructed castle submitted to determined siege by malign forces sits well with the medieval narrative scheme of the psychomachia, or struggle within and for the human soul.[12] Finally the episode has contemporary national-cultural and geographic reference, somewhat unstable in character: in so far as the castle is under attack, it seems to be in Spenser's Ireland (assailants rise against Arthur and his squire, who have not yet gained admittance to the castle, like 'a swarme of Gnats at euentide / Out of the fennes of Allan;'[13] the castle's fine 'porch' (its chin) is on the other hand made of exceptionally valuable stone 'far from Ireland brought',[14] and therefore self-locates in the England of the poem's publication.

Diversity and discrepancy of symbolic reference as commonly found in the more elaborate allegorical texts of the medieval to early modern period, is not a product of waywardness or carelessness, but a homage paid to the security of traditional collective representations, constructions of cultural knowledge shared on an assumed basis of common experience. Traditional collective representations both assume and avow conditions of intertextuality.[15] Textual commonplaces with a quotient of visual form, their authority has more than one attributed origin and they are open to multiple interpretations as figurings of truth. Familiar examples from medieval culture are the *locus amoenus*, which, in a given instance, may or may not have Edenic significance, the image of the pre-eminent warrior bearing arms that may or may not contextually evoke the Christian armour of Ephesians 6, and the image of the sacral monarch who stands at the apex of social power. Symbolic narrative in the Alma sequence explores several receptions of the image of the body as portal to knowledge, in a spirit of inclusiveness and without disturbing the forms of reception themselves. But, having identified this marked tendency in Spenser's symbolic account of the body, it is possible to identify another, making for the availability of quite a different kind of reading. As a matter of general critical recognition, the optics of *The Faerie Queene* produces several focal resolutions. We turn now to features of the body-castle episodes, which are explicitly disaligned from reference to what can already be established as collective knowledge. Reading on this other track requires the pursuit of disambiguation and the attempted construction of univocal meaning.

Declaration that a working model for ethical temperance has been provided comes not after the description of Alma's castle in canto 9, but after the description of Arthur's struggle with Maleger and his followers in canto 11, where the image of the castle loses its narrative significance. Canto 12 begins with the following narratorial declaration:

> Now gins this goodly frame of Temperance
> Fairly to rise, and her adorned hed
> To pricke [mark, aimed at] of highest praise forth to aduaunce,
> Formerly grounded, and fast setteled,
> On firme foundation of true bountyhed [goodness, virtue].[16]

Temperance's 'frame' as characterized here is anthropomorphically conceived – it has a 'head' – and is also firmly founded like an architectural construction, but correct apprehension of it requires us to take account of canto 11, with its dispersed, relatively chaotic visual scene, and not only the architecturally centred scene of canto 9. It will be necessary to rethink our conception of what I have been terming the body-castle episode since, as Spenser's narrator explains at the start, the human body is symbolically represented here not once but twice. As 'kept in sober government' it is the 'most fair and excellent' of God's works; but as deprived of temperance 'though misrule and passions bace: / It growes a Monster, and incontinent [immediately, with a pun on moral 'incontinence'] / Doth lose his dignity and natiue grace.' In reading the passage we will '[b]ehold ... both one and other in this place'.[17] The episode's human body is the castle under Alma's governance with its demurely polite social etiquette: here the going amusements are restrained flirtation[18] and reading (canto 10). But it is also and with equal insistence the throng of rabble-insurgents who have the castle under siege. I shall attempt to explain why the poem's instructive body needs to be shown in two entirely different forms.

Book 2 describes the moral education of its central figure, Guyon, represented as young and approaching maturation, and is among other things a bid to civilize its reader along characteristic sixteenth-century lines. Individual attainment of civility here necessitates some withdrawal of emotional-cum-intellectual attachment to the universal, collective human body. As Norbert Elias explains, the period's raising of the bar for standards of refinement went with the treatment of ever-growing areas of 'natural' or commonplace behaviour as unmannerly and indelicate. Its implementation of self-distancing from one's own and others' bodily functions involved, for example, the innovatory use of such items as table-cutlery, commodes, handkerchiefs and nightwear. As well as evoking traditional symbolisms, the Alma episode offers an anatomy of newly conceived symbolic structures in a specific articulation. Here 'anatomy' carries its up to date, somewhat Vesalian meaning of a precise, painstaking examination and exposition of bodily forms or processes in their functional interconnectedness; in respect of this procedure the body's most significant analogues are the thoroughly planned building and the machine.[19] A good deal of canto 9 is given to systematic, anatomical description of this particular well-designed and properly functional bodily system.[20] Conceived with topological accuracy as an apparatus that connects mouth and anus (its 'two gates')[21] it takes in guests much as it takes in food; its teeth, for example, are a welcoming corps of disciplined guards.[22] We are informed in some detail about the efficient workings of its digestive tract, culminating in excretion,[23] of its emotional life, leading to thoughtful impasse,[24] and of its cognitive equipment, disposed as three persons who occupy adjoining chambers in the turret.[25] A. C. Hamilton comments, not unreasonably, that some of the body-castle's features seem to be modelled on Spenser's personal appearance;[26] this is an individually originated account of optimal bodily form and function.

To view the passage in this other way, also sanctioned for reading, is to witness a foundering of the metaphorics of the body politic. Insofar as it is a collective body, this is shown to exist partly as a formless horde of '[v]ile caitiue wretches, ragged, rude, deformd, / All threatening death',[27] connoting political misrule (popular insurgency in a government view) and disease as a form of bodily dissolution. The polar opposite of such disorder and its proposed remedy is the passage's anatomical modelling of the disciplined, systemically interconnected and pragmatically functional body. This is introduced as a novel intellectual construction that is to play its part in the ethical forming of the reader. One of the poem's declared purposes is, in the formulation of the 'Letter to Raleigh', to 'fashion (represent, mould, create)' optimal human beings in motion whose compelling example will, like that of Cyrus and his army in the Anabasis, contribute towards the 'fashioning' of readers who can live optimal lives.[28] Vesalius's *De humanis corporis fabrica* (1543) has as one of its objectives the dissemination of anatomical knowledge to all, including relatively unlearned practitioners of surgery and courtiers intrigued by the book's design.[29] *The Faerie Queene*'s exemplary anatomy of the living body is not, on the other hand, for all members of the polis: those given over to 'misrule' have thereby demonstrated incapacity to comprehend it, and are discovered raging in its vicinity.[30] Its meaning as a matter of applicability to individual life, not already assumed to be a given of group experience, is best acquired through a labour and pathos of individual understanding.

This returns us to a question which was raised earlier: why is the 'frame' of Temperance said to come into view after the spatially dispersed fighting of canto 11, and not after the description of an architectural-cum-mechanical structure in canto 9? The answer is, I would suggest, that the significance of the book's modelling of an optimal body is best grasped through reflection on a form of individual experience, one which only an individual can undergo and suitably interpret. Here our vehicle for such reflection is Arthur, who attempts to fight Malegar as leader of the horde that has been besieging the castle. As this episode makes clear, while the collectivist symbolic body is supra-individual and unthreatened by mortality, the individually constructed symbolic body carries significance only in the context of individual life; or, to put it more concretely, we come to value it fully only by learning that we are going to die, and that what it models, however useful or prestigious, can falter in its personal application – we all sometimes become tired or fall ill. The episode of Arthur and Malegar is largely untraditional as narrative allegory (one can source its individual components,[31] but not its whole organization), highly paradoxical as narrative action and,[32] against the background of the larger poem, surprisingly unchivalric in styling, since Arthur nearly dies during the combat (not at Malegar's hand but through the intervention of two hag-like women). Named by the narrator Impotence and Impatience, these project individual, isolating forms of experience, ones that it would be emotionally preferable not to have: as well as being self-governing machine-like structures we are also beings possessed of limited and unreliable powers and, *qua* 'impatient', ones who struggle against acceptance of that condition. Health – classical *salus*, with connotations of salvation and safety – has by this point in the symbolic narrative morphed into a phenomenon that is to be scrutinized and monitored at the individual as distinct from the social level. The poem's image of Temperance gains its fully instructive force as a consequence of the reader's cathartic acceptance of vulnerability to personal suffering in the forms of weakness and illness, reminders of death as terminal dissolution.

I have identified three moments in the reading of Spenser's Alma passage: that of accepting the force of traditional symbolic representations centred on the body, shown in an image that is, however, divided and unintegrated because the body politic itself is divided and unintegrated; that of tracing the interconnections of a novel symbolic body, architectural and mechanical in construction; and that of integrating response to this imposing model body with awareness of individual frailty and mortality. I have also suggested that reading of the passage encompasses these moments sequentially, in the order just set out. Comparable moments also have great importance in the readerly encounter with Hobbes's *Leviathan*; but the argument is structured in such a way as to fold these moments on to one another, setting them before the attention simultaneously.

*

Hobbes has no piety whatsoever towards traditional collective representations, seeing the mentality of ordinary people as a blank sheet apt to be imprinted with such commanding texts or images as the ruling authority chooses:[33]

> Common-peoples minds, unless they be tainted by dependence on the Potent, or scribbled over with the opinions of their Doctors, are like clean paper, fit to receive whatsoever by Publique Authority shall be imprinted in them.[34]

In this spirit his monstrous anthropomorphic creature, Leviathan, forcefully displayed in the text's frontispiece (see Figure 6.1), is being put forward as a new, valid collective representation for the ruling authority to relay to its subjects. This symbolic figure has, I would suggest, a somewhat parodic and subversive relation to the collective symbolic representations of cultural tradition: those are accepted primarily through habit and custom – and have of late, so runs the underlying thought, been much contested and, as part of this process, done a lot of damage; this impressive and threatening image, on the other hand, is well fitted to impose assent; moreover, the items displayed in boxes in the lower half of the image show how this symbolic figure's power, secular and sacral, is put into practical effect; here a fired cannon, for example, is treated as being equivalent to the thunderbolt of excommunication (the forked objects immediately below symbolize weapons of argument). The image so viewed immediately establishes two focuses of political interest: how is sovereign power implemented, once it has been established, in that series of relays which conserves its triumphant force; and, the text's more pressing concern, how does it compel the foundational and spontaneous collective acknowledgement that underpins such implementation?

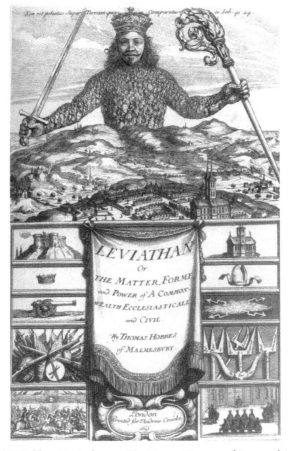

Figure 6.1: T. Hobbes, *Leviathan or, The Matter, Forme and Power of A Common-Wealth Ecclesiasticall and Civill* (London, 1651), frontispiece.

Answering the second question involves paying close attention to the book's rhetorically charged opening statements. In making automata, we are told, human beings give to certain products of engineering 'an artificial life', simulating animals capable of motion in imitation of nature as 'the Art whereby God hath made and governes the World'. But human art can also go beyond this in imitating

> that Rationall and most excellent worke of Nature, Man. For by Art is created that great LEVIATHAN, called a COMMON-WEALTH, or STATE, (in latin CIVI-TAS) which is but an Artificiall Man; though of greater stature and strength than the Naturall, for whose protection and defence it was intended; and in which, the Soveraignty is an Artificiall Soul, as giving life and motion to the whole body.[35]

Aristotle speaks similarly, in the *Poetics*, of *muthos* (plot, story) as the soul that gives life to a tragedy, insofar as we can regard tragic plays as members of an artificial living species that human beings have created. A gigantic fabricated man who supplies protection for a human collectivity evokes ancient stories of Talos, the bronze man who guarded Crete. A figure called 'Leviathan' recalls in name but not in form the Leviathan of Job 40–1 and Isaiah 27.1, variously glossed as a crocodile, a whale, a fish, a snake and a dragon;[36] Leviathan as modern monster, and its scriptural counterpart, can be taken to be alike only in the challenging sense supplied by the Vulgate citation: 'Non est potestas Super Terram quae Comparetus ei' – 'There is no power on earth which is to be compared with him.' Later in *Leviathan* the formulations of the quoted passage are recalled when we are told, in the only other reference to the creature Leviathan, how this engineered construction comes to be – or, as simulated 'man', is born. It has to be imagined that all the members of a collectivity at a certain point say to one another, 'I Authorise and give up my Right of Governing my selfe, to this Man, or to this Assembly of men [i.e. the sovereign power in whatever form], on this condition, that thou give up thy Right to him, and Authorise all his actions in like manner.' Once this is done, explains Hobbes,

> the Multitude so united in one Person, is called a COMMON-WEALTH, in latine CIVITAS. This is the generation of that great LEVIATHAN, or rather (to speake more reverently) of that Mortall God, to which we owe under the Immortall God, our peace and defence.[37]

As the text clearly acknowledges, this is not to be taken as a historical account of a sovereign state's formation. The individuals who compose a given sovereign state, or their forbears, are not to be imagined as having gathered one day to make a verbal contract with one another: that story is provided in order to bring out the political meaning of the contractual principle. Which is to say that the problem concerning a collectivity's spontaneous assenting to the imposition on themselves of a sovereign power is repeated in the problem concerning a collectivity's spontaneous construction of a sovereign power that holds sway over them, as symbolized in both cases by an extremely powerful artificial man or 'Mortall God'. To recapitulate, we have considered *Leviathan*'s putting forward of a new collective representation with political force in the space once occupied by traditional collective representations. And in order to explain what this new representation, 'Leviathan', might be, we have considered the text's account of that constructive act that has produced a mighty artificial man. However, the account of the second has to be received as an explanatory fiction, and it has not yet proved possible to say anything revealing about Leviathan's actual construction, its (or his) engineering, including the fabrication of Leviathan's 'soul', the contractually transferred sovereign power, which is said to give this creature 'life and motion'. Here there is an obvious contrast with Spenser's complex anatomy of the symbolic temperate body. Aristotle's *Poetics*, which is one of Leviathan's intertexts, likewise offers useful information about the optimal form of a tragic *muthos* as well as metaphorically instating it as tragedy's 'soul'.

The resolution of this issue is, however, provided in *Leviathan*'s frontispiece, probably more clearly and certainly more directly than in its written text.[38] Its symbolic anthropomorphic giant represents a human collectivity with a certain grotesque explicitness, since the visible portions of it excepting the head and fingers are composed of a multiplicity of human bodies. These are clothed and, mainly, hatted – that is, wearing their public garb as if at or approaching some form of assembly. Given that Leviathan the creature faces towards us, confronting the reader as if in a mirroring relationship, why are its component bodies, who in some sense represent 'us', facing in the opposite direction? The effect is disconcerting, like that of the Magritte painting ('Réproduction') which shows a man looking at the mirrored image of himself seen from behind, as the spectator already views him. The frontispiece's positioning of the human forms composing Leviathan was evidently not the only possibility envisaged. In a manuscript version prepared by the same artist for the exiled Charles II, and no doubt designed to win his personal approval, the component forms are heads, unhatted, facing outwards from the image and wearing agitated facial expressions suggestive of excitement or fear.[39] This clearly conveys the awed subordination of the collectivity's individual members to the 'artificiall man' whom they compose, a man who bears the trappings of a monarch and does indeed, as in the printed version, look somewhat like Charles. The logic of the bodies' positioning in the printed frontispiece has, however, been convincingly identified by Horst Bredekamp: '[t]he eyes of each one, regardless of position, is directed towards the giant's head and returns through his eyes back to the viewer'.[40] (my emphasis). In other words, a form of mirroring is indeed taking place: what the reader encounters in meeting the eyes of the gigantic 'artificiall man' is his/her own gaze, which is now to be imagined as belonging to the gazing totality made up of the ensemble of readers and ensemble of political subjects, the assembled throng which the image presents. A place has thus been assigned to the individual as a bearer of volition in the same movement that locates him as part of a collectivity living in subjection to the sovereign power, a being whose powers seem to resemble his own in a huge magnification. The artificial construction that makes this paradoxical act of (self-) seeing possible is the argument of the book, the force of which is established in this introductory tableau.

At the centre of *Leviathan* as an act of persuasion there is a moment of uncanny encounter, ingeniously contrived in such a way as to provoke awe and fearful apprehension:[41] in the text's necessary monster, Leviathan, we confront both the implacable character of sovereign power as it bears on the individual subject and the frightful nature of what it has been created to oppose and subdue: our own collective disposition towards anarchy. The sovereign state, considered to be the most impressive of human inventions and a virtual 'man' in its own mode of being, is found to exist in the relay of looks that passes continuously between its component human entities considered as disparate individuals and these same human entities given collective embodiment in the sovereign power, a designated person or assembly. It is not necessary to appeal to a founding contract in order to establish this 'man's' right to exist or principle of existence, much as it is not necessary to make an experimental entry to the state of nature (as in the brilliant evocation of chapter 13) in order to establish that life outside this constructed, non-natural legal-political framework is nasty, brutish and short. Such are *Leviathan's* optical dealings with an issue of political foundation, making for simultaneous individual self-recognition as political agent and political subject. To behold the image of sovereign power in the text's mediation of it is to perceive, immediately, that 'there is no power on earth which is to be compared with him' – Leviathan considered as political artefact identifies as foundational constant a continuing subjective condition of fearful apprehension that also goes on discovering its own remedy.

*

To turn from Hobbes to Bunyan is, at first sight, to return to the sphere of established collective representations. Here the trajectory of symbolic reading more closely resembles the one that has been defined for the Alma episode for *Leviathan*. Nevertheless, the design of *The Holy War* also resembles that of *Leviathan* in that one of its key purposes is to create and sustain a moment of recognition; and in that moment a semiotics of collective representation is brought firmly under authorial control in the interests of fixing a pattern of response. Figure 6.2 shows the book's frontispiece, probably composed like that of Hobbes's text under authorial supervision. It represents what is in important respects an apocalyptic scene, whose focus is the climactic battle of Revelations 10 between the great dragon, identified with the Devil, and the host of God's angels. The portion of the terrestrial globe shown beneath the warring parties makes it clear that the fate of the earth is at issue. But the image of a walled town-cum-body – the obvious bodily features being 'Heart Castle', 'Eargate' and 'Eyegate' – placed at the image's centre cues a narrative of individually-located struggle in the psychomachia's double sense of struggle both within and for the soul: the book will place eschatology within a personal perspective where, as in *The Pilgrim's Progress*, the represented experience of an individual is offered as possessing universal significance. Yet while the text's 'Towne of Mansoul', gendered as female along traditional lines, is by analogy the unitary soul of an individual, its principal narrative concern is the life of the soul as compositely represented by the varied members of a civic corporation; the main actors are agencies of good and evil projected as rival military and occupying forces, and their helpers or enemies among the townsmen whose loyalties they contest. In the frontispiece the most conspicuous figure, larger indeed than the town, the Devil in dragon form or Emanuel as leader of the opposing army, is the recognizable image of Bunyan in the role of author.[42] One of the inferences which may be drawn from this placing of weighty visual emphasis on 'Bunyan' is that it will be the responsibility of the author to explain how a story of conflict and deceit with numerous narrative agents bears analogically on the spiritual life of the individual, since received frameworks of understanding will not necessarily do this with clarity and reliability. In the prefatory poem Bunyan states that reading must be guided by his continuously-provided marginal glosses on the action: 'Nor do thou go to work without my Key, / (In mysteries men soon do lose their way) ... / It lies there in the window.' 'The margent'[43] here is the marginally supplied gloss for 'the window', without whose light the narrative allegory would resist interpretation or be interpreted falsely.

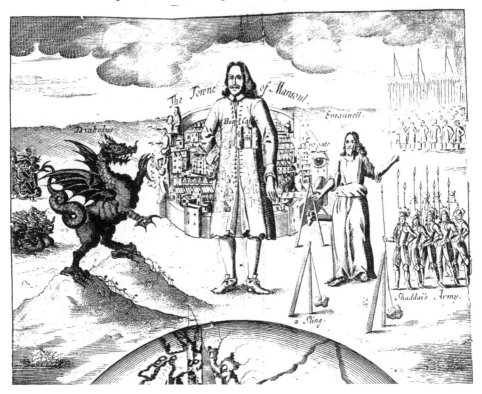

Figure 6.2: John Bunyan, *The Holy War* (London, 1682), frontispiece.

Walter Ong has pointed to the role of the printed book in producing the strong impression that a given text is closed off and separated from other texts, and not locatable within a shared intertextual field; which, in forming the conception and reception of a book with this novel profile, affirms its originality and individuality while conferring the same attributes on its writer.[44] Bunyan aligns himself with the emergent figure of the book author, an act in conformity with a Protestant critique of the traditional, priestly conveyance of doctrine. *The Holy War*'s purpose is to establish, on an individual author's initiative, a novel basis on which certain doctrines can be assimilated at the level of experience by the reader who tracks a specific narrative development. The force of this conception depends partly on the reader's awareness that the attribution to an individual, *qua* author, of distinctive authorizing powers is a cultural practice of recent invention.[45] The narrated action locally includes a critique of the embodiment of doctrine in customary forms: three 'proper men' called Tradition, Human-wisdom and Mans Invention enlist as Emanuel's soldiers, but following capture in a skirmish they join the diabolic army since, as they explain, they do not 'so much live by Religion, as by the fates of Fortune'.[46] The shape of the whole narrative establishes convergent paths between a representation of scripturally charted world history, spanning Creation and the Last Days, and the representation of an individual life that spans the fall into sin via temptation, the experience of redemption, and – the text's distinctive concern – entry into a more fortunate though still imperfect condition of life where grace is operative. Here, crucially, the traditional security of the body imaged as a defensive enclosure has to be relocated on a new conceptual and pragmatic basis. In the context of a broad awareness of the shape of collective human history the reader is offered a representative personal history for the truth of which 'Bunyan' stands as guarantor: the prefatory poem includes authorial declaration that 'I myself was in the Town, / Both when 'twas set up, and when pulling down', and that 'what is here in view / Of mine own knowledge, I dare say is true'.[47] The role of the author, constructed between empirical writer, empirical reader and the text that mediates their activities, is to establish conditions of access to a human ethical-spiritual state that is to be shared as an affective condition. In the terms offered by a traditional mapping of mind onto body it is a condition of heart.

The narrative of *The Holy War* has three phases and leads logically towards a newly inflected account of the contemporary Christian believer's condition. As symbolic narrative it also offers a novel anatomy of the living soul, in that the corporate functioning of a town on a contemporary model, with its differentiated officials and volatile, rumour-led collective awareness, is treated as a vehicle for analysis of the soul's individually assertive and interacting faculties. Among the marks of the allegory's distinctiveness is that it has relatively little use for the potential body symbolism of an architectural structure, or for representation of the soul as this structure's unitary resident, both falling within the convention of 'mirroring': these commonplaces of collective knowledge are acknowledged but also largely[48] ignored in the interests of exploring new forms of insight. The main schemes of action are the following: (1) Diabolus seduces the inhabitants of Mansoul, a town originally established by King Shaddai and, subverting its institutions, gains unremitting control over the town's life. (2) On hearing of this the King's son, Prince Emanuel, directs and finally leads a prolonged military assault on the town, overcoming the followers of Diabolus and freely bestowing mercy on its inhabitants, beginning with the civic leaders who have expected to be put to death; this moment of concord is marked by celebration. (3) There is a further lengthy period of grievous internecine struggle between Diabolonians, who remain lurking within and ready to emerge from 'the outsides, and walls'[49] of the town, and those loyal to Emanuel; though the Prince's followers often fail in vigilance or force, his leading soldiers never lose control of Heart Castle, which is 'the strong hold of the town'.[50] It is made clear, then, that in the third phase, even though it is emphatically one of uncertainty and confusion, the responsibility for resisting Diabolus has in an important respect been transferred to Mansoul, since the heart of the individual has now undergone experiences which enable it to resist deception and capture; this is what the individual is required continuously to recall as a condition of present spiritual well-being. In the frontispiece's striking conception, this insight is figured as a condition of transparent correspondence between the castle-heart of Mansoul, the heart of 'Bunyan', a set of purposes projected in a book, and their counterpart in the text's fashioning of it, the suitably educated heart of the reader: to respond to the text appropriately is to perceive and experience their essential alignment.

Collective representations that are well established in custom and tradition engage what Yeats called 'emotion of multitude': their being actively shared as well as their intersubjective availability is a matter of group significance,[51] they are embedded in familiar practices, they can be variously semiotized in a manner, which connotes social breadth and historical depth. The symbolic image of the body as a defensible enclosure can, as an instance of such a representation, be received as a reminder of knowledge of the human state whose substance is a vast tissue of individual experiences. However, an anatomizing of the symbolic collective body, of the kind which occurs in Spenser, Bunyan and, more abruptly and prescriptively, in Hobbes, implies a re-examination of received cultural knowledge and its bearing on individual action and choice. *The Holy War*, which is of the three most fully conceived as a communication between an individual text and an individual reader, offers a symbolic narrative whose purpose is to mould a style of reception such that it can be received in the proper manner with certain anticipated consequences. It is focally as a story of the heart that this symbolic narrative bids to avoid the hazards of intertextual connection and vagaries of collective use, with a view to conveying a univocal meaning with individual application that should also be reliably transmitted.

# 7 FROM HUMAN TO POLITICAL BODY AND SOUL: MATERIALISM AND MORTALISM IN THE POLITICAL THEORY OF THOMAS HOBBES

## Ionut Untea

The beheading of Charles I signalled the end of the traditional theory according to which the king had two bodies: his own natural, mortal one and also an immortal one – the Commonwealth itself.[1] Drawing from Scripture (Matthew 18:9), James I, Charles I's father, had argued that in times of rebellion the head of the Commonwealth may be forced to cut off some 'rotten members' to preserve the integrity of the rest of the body.[2] He did not foresee that the body would cut off its own head in order to free itself from an unwanted political life. According to Katherine Bootle Atie, Thomas Hobbes (1558–1679) shared the general interest of his contemporaries to resuscitate the metaphor of the immortal body of the state '[i]mbuing political discourse with more vitality than any other writer that century'.[3] This essay argues on the contrary that, after the social and political upheavals of the Civil War, Hobbes had no intention of returning to a conception that was divorced from the new political realities and instead preferred to place in the centre of his political theory the idea of the mortality of the political body. Hobbes developed his political theory in analogy with his materialistic view of the human body. Drawing a close parallel between the natural and the artificial bodies enabled him to build a coherent political theory of the state as an autonomous 'artificial man'. This approach led him to adopt a pessimistic view of politics due to the transfer of some natural passions into the artificial life of Leviathan.

## Materialism and Mechanical Psychology

Hobbes's materialism was not an isolated case among the scientific conceptions of the seventeenth century, where the atomistic philosophy of the ancient philosophers Democritus, Epicurus and Lucretius enjoyed great popularity. Johannes Kepler, a central figure of the new science, initially believed that planets moved because they possessed some 'moving soul' (*animae motrices*), but later reconsidered his position in favour of a materialistic account.[4] In reinterpreting ancient atomism to accord with the science of his time, Pierre Gassendi paved the way for the foundation of modern atomism by Isaac Newton.

Descartes regarded the bodies of living organisms as machines.[5] However, with this conception came also his dualism, according to which, although the human individual is a 'thinking thing', the mind is a substance different from the body, and whose essence is thought.[6] The Cartesian view was quickly adopted by the members of the Royal Society who were not merely scientists but also pious men.[7] Cambridge Platonists such as Ralph Cudworth went on to argue that there was a distinction in ancient atomism between 'theistic atomism', originally propounded by Moses, and 'atheistic atomism', which came from pagan philosophers.[8]

Hobbes refused to add an 'idealistic superstructure' to the dominant mechanical conception of his time.[9] For him human beings, like animals, were made entirely of matter. Surprisingly enough, he based this materialistic conception on certain biblical texts, especially the passage in the Book of Genesis which was often used to sustain the duality matter-spirit in the created world: 'It is said, "God made man of the dust of the earth, and breathed into his nostrils (*spiraculum vitae*) the breath of life, and man was made a living soul"' (Genesis 2:7). His materialistic interpretation follows immediately: 'There the breath of life inspired by God signifies no more but that God gave him life.'[10] Because 'soul and life in the Scripture do usually signify the same thing', Hobbes orients his philosophy on the path of theological mortalism: 'the immortal life ... beginneth not in man till the resurrection and day of judgement; and hath for cause, not his specifical nature and generation, but the promise'.[11] The predominant view on theological mortalism in seventeenth-century England agreed with Early Church Father, Eusebius of Caesarea (*c.* AD 263–339), who had declared it a heretic doctrine introduced among the Christians of Arabia around AD 235–40. Yet, since Queen Elisabeth's Articles of Religion of 1563 had not officially condemned it, there was no reason for Hobbes to ignore it.[12] In actual fact, Anabaptists and Socinians held that the soul remained in deep sleep from the moment of death until the general Resurrection (hence their nickname 'Soul Sleepers'), while Anglicans tended to adopt a more ambiguous position, somewhere between avoiding the issue altogether and embracing Calvin's condemnation of mortalism.[13] Far from having a Calvinistic approach, as Nathaniel H. Henry suggests,[14] Hobbes clearly expresses his mortalist views in chapter 38 of *Leviathan*: 'That the soul of man is in its own nature eternal ... independent on the body ... is a doctrine not apparent in Scripture.'[15]

In view of his popularity,[16] the theological and scientific interpretation propounded by Hobbes was hard to ignore. In 1659 Henry More wrote a treatise entitled *The Immortality of the Soul* against Hobbes's materialism and mortalism. In *The True Intellectual System of the Universe* (1678), Ralph Cudworth criticized Hobbes's conception without mentioning his name. More and Cudworth praised Descartes's dualism, which remained for the seventeenth-century English intellectual life the main alternative to Hobbes's materialism.[17] As early as 1645 Hobbes had entered into a controversy with Bishop John Bramhall on free will and necessitarianism, which were direct consequences of Hobbes's materialism and mortalism. Bramhall argued that without an immaterial soul the human body could not engage in any action nor indeed be a subject.[18] Moreover, he believed that this conception undermined politics itself, since the law would punish someone for an action he could not but do and since any consultation, advice and deliberation would have no effect on human conduct.[19] Thus, according to John Bramhall, in the Hobbesian universe the human body remains exclusively under 'a natural and necessary flux of extrinsecall causes' that have a non-mediated effect on its behaviour.[20]

The view that the human body remains passive under the influence of external causes fails to take into account the specificity of Hobbes's conception of the 'thinking body'.[21] In *De Corpore* (1655) he claims that the distinction between mind (or soul) and body remains one of the 'gross errors of writers of metaphysics', who love abstraction.[22] On the contrary, Hobbes preferred a philosophical vision of a dynamic human psychology. Also in opposition to Descartes he conceived human psychology in continuity with physics.[23] In the *Epistle Dedicatory* of *De Cive* (1642) Hobbes contrasts the rigour and achievements of natural science with the contradictory conclusions in the history of moral philosophy concerning human actions:

> [W]hatever ... distinguishes the modern world from the barbarity of the past, is almost wholly the gift of *Geometry*; for what we owe to *Physics, Physics* owes to *Geometry*. If the moral Philosophers had done their job with equal success, I do not know what greater contribution human industry could have made to human happiness. For if the patterns of human action were known with the same certainty as the relations of magnitude in figures, ambition and greed, whose power rests on the false opinions of the common people about right and wrong, would be disarmed, and the human race would enjoy such secure peace that (apart from conflicts over space as the population grew) it seems unlikely that it would ever have to fight again. But as things are, the war of the sword and the war of the pens is perpetual; there is no greater knowledge [*scientia*] of natural right and natural laws today than in the past[24]

The project of making moral and political philosophy rigorous in the sense of natural sciences was not addressed exclusively to scientists or philosophers, but also to ordinary people. In the epistle dedicatory of *Elements of Law* (1640) he claimed to have laid 'the true and only foundation' of a 'science' of 'justice and policy'.[25] He clearly emphasizes how important to him the reception of his scientific project by common people would be: 'it would be an incomparable benefit to commonwealth, *if every man* held the opinions concerning law and policy here delivered'.[26] Thus, Hobbes' purpose was to educate the entire society according to his scientific principles, to initiate a revolution in psychological, moral and political knowledge, or at least to provide a firm basis for subsequent scientific developments on human nature. The project to make science accessible to every member of the commonwealth partly explains the emphasis on one simple and commonly perceived phenomenon: motion.

In *De Corpore* Hobbes praises Galileo, 'the first to open to us the first gate of universal physics, which is the nature of motion' and claimed that Galileo had been the first to have written anything useful on motion.[27] He was impressed by Galileo's metaphor of the 'book of nature' in *The Assayer* (1623), according to which the universe lies open before the eyes of humans, '[b]ut it cannot be understood unless you have first learned to understand the language and recognize the characters in which it is written'.[28] For Galileo the language was mathematics, the characters geometrical figures and motion the principal application of geometry.[29] This played an essential role in Galileo's investigations of the motions of the earth and the new science of mechanics.[30] Hobbes was influenced by this conception and also by Galileo's account on the production of sensory qualities by motion: heat, for example, was a quality caused by motion not a quality inherent in a given object, contrary to Aristotelian tradition.[31] However, he considered that Galileo had not taken the implications of the science of motion far enough. His conception differed from Galileo's in its materialistic understanding of geometry itself: because Hobbes's materialism excluded any abstraction and understood only bodies as real, geometrical points, lines and figures were not, according to him, ideal objects in the traditional Euclidian sense. By replacing the abstract entities not found in nature with a 'materialistic reading of the science of mathematics', Hobbes arrived at the conclusion that the language of the book of nature was mathematics, but its characters were not something abstract, as in Galileo: they were material bodies in motion, i.e. nature itself.[32] It follows that absolutely everything in nature is the effect of motion and impact, from physical qualities to the emergence of the human mind and to moral and political phenomena.[33]

For instance, in the *Objections* to Descartes's *Meditations* Hobbes shows that denying the existence of an immaterial substance in the constitution of the body does not imply that human beings do not possess a mind, only that the mind is in fact 'nothing but movements in certain parts of an organic body'.[34] Internal motions, which produce the mind, result from external motions:

> The cause of sense, is the external body, or object, which presseth the organ proper to each sense, either immediately, as in the taste and touch; or mediately, as in seeing, hearing, and smelling: which pressure, by the mediation of nerves and other strings and membranes of the body, continued inwards to the brain and heart, causeth there a resistance, or counter-pressure, or endeavour of the heart to deliver itself[35]

Motion produces the mind because the primary organ in human constitution is the heart. Indeed the nervous system, whose basic function is to deliver external stimuli to the heart, can develop more sophisticated abilities only in relation to the impressions that the heart develops in decoding the messages transmitted by the senses and the nerves:

> [W]hen the action of the same object is continued from the eyes, ears, and other organs to the heart, the real effect there is nothing but motion, or endeavour; which consisteth in appetite or aversion to or from the object moving. But the appearance or sense of that motion is that we either call delight or trouble of mind.[36]

In chapter 3 of *Leviathan* Hobbes asserts that the basic function of the human brain, facilitating the 'translation' of motion[37] from an external body to the heart is 'common to man and beast'. Therefore, both are capable of associating an experience or an 'effect imagined' with 'the causes of means that produce it'.[38]

Initially, deliberation appears as a mere 'succession of appetites, aversions, hopes and fears', depending on what a person or an animal feels in reaction to external stimuli interpreted by the heart. At this point, the will is defined as 'the last appetite, or aversion' and is only 'the act, not the faculty, of willing'. Hobbes further argues that the act of willing necessarily occurs also in animal deliberation.[39] What contributes to the emergence of the faculty of willing is that human beings develop passions much more complex than those of animals, which have 'no other passion but sensual, such as are hunger, thirst, lust, and anger'.[40]

Moral sentiments such as pity or benevolence are only developments of simpler passions common to all creatures on earth, seeking pleasure and avoiding pain: 'Grief for the calamity of another is pity; and ariseth from the imagination that the like calamity may befall himself; and therefore is called also compassion.'[41] Here Hobbes shows that his morals, although necessarily based on psychological egoism, can prescribe an altruistic behaviour of human subjects.[42] The limits of such altruism are revealed when one has to choose between preserving one's own life or the life of someone else. Moreover, if one also takes into account the fear of insecurity of every individual in the state of nature,[43] it becomes clear why Hobbes holds that the state of nature sooner or later becomes a state of war. However, even if this kind of *egoistical altruism* does not preclude the apparition of the state of war, it can provide the basis for the covenant by which political life is made possible, since what everyone hopes to obtain by instituting the sovereign is his own security.[44]

When accusing Hobbes of making impossible moral and political life, Bishop Bramhall does not observe that Hobbes's determinism has his own resources to counter a chaotic movement of individuals in nature. Although the brain or any other part of the human body is not moving by itself, but is moved by external causes,[45] Hobbes's 'thinking bodies' are under the influence and generate in their turn an entire range of diverse movements as sense perception, imagination, memory, thought, vital and voluntary movements,[46] moral sentiments and political actions.

## The Political Automaton and Artificial Altruism

In the introduction to *Leviathan* Hobbes gives new meaning to the ancient dictum *Nosce teipsum*, which he translates as *Read thyself*.[47] Ted H. Miller argues that this is 'an oblique reference' to *Nosce teipsum*, the poem by John Davis dedicated to Queen Elisabeth, which was 'the first English work to combine poetry and a systematic philosophical doctrine', although one diametrically opposed to Hobbes's ideas, maintaining that the soul is spiritual, immortal and indifferent to the death of its body. Accordingly, by alluding to *Nosce teipsum*, 'Hobbes may have been subtly suggesting his desire to compete with the famous self-reading of a previous courtly poet-philosopher'.[48] Miller's interpretation, although consistent with the arguments presented in this essay, does not explain Hobbes's unusual translation of the Latin precept. This section explores the implications of the translation 'read thyself' in terms of Hobbes's science of human nature.

Unlike animals, human beings have developed the capacity to 'read' the thoughts and passions that animate themselves. In the state of nature, where nothing guarantees that the security provided by personal means suffices to counter any possible danger, somebody else's predicament naturally gives rise to a feeling of 'compassion', not because of natural man's elevated ideas about human value in general but because he can already read in himself the fear caused by seeing or hearing the consequences of the other's experience. The moral judgement formulated on the basis of this reading of the personal self would suffice for human relations to develop peacefully, even in the state of nature. However, a *human* society remains highly unstable, because of those who refuse to read in themselves, but who 'take great delight to show what they think they have read in [other] men, by uncharitable censures of one another behind their backs'.[49] Stephen H. Daniel argues that the primary reason for Hobbes's reluctance to develop a theory of *human* society is that 'the sociable inclinations of man ... the natural ties of affection, or the pride which might motivate men to do benevolent actions, cannot be treated with the systematic precision demanded by a political science', which deals only with *civil* society.[50] While Hobbes makes this point on several occasions[51], in the Introduction to *Leviathan* he asserts that a science of *human* society would be possible in principle if human beings 'would take the pains' of observing the 'read thyself' principle 'by which they might learn truly to read one another'.[52] Moreover, even if 'the characters of man's heart' are 'legible' in a non-mediated manner 'only to him that searcheth hearts', i. e. God himself (see 1 Samuel 16:7), 'whosoever looketh into himself and considereth what he doth when he does think, opine, reason, hope, fear, etc., and upon what grounds; *he shall thereby read and know* what are the thoughts and passions of all other men upon the like occasions'.[53]

In other words, after the model of Galileo's book of nature, Hobbes views human nature as a book, open before the eyes of every subject endowed with a body, but which can only be deciphered by whoever makes the effort to seek in themselves for the laws of causality governing physiological reactions ultimately translated by the heart into a whole range of psychological and intellectual reactions. This *translation* crucially defines the specificity of the human species because it represents the basis for the evolution from a relatively passive subjection to the laws of necessity (as Bishop Bramhall interpreted Hobbes's position) to a more active understanding of the human dependence of the laws of causality. In *De Cive* Hobbes confirms that psychological egoism motivates individuals in the state of nature, but he emphasizes that their psychological reactions are effects of a necessity comparable to that which governs the motions of inanimate bodies:

> For each man is drawn to desire that which is Good for him, and to Avoid what is bad for him, and most of all the greatest of natural evils, which is death; *this happens by a real necessity of nature as powerful as that by which a stone falls downward.*[54]

Yet, human beings do not remain stuck in passive submission. Using their newly acquired reason, they begin to fashion their own destiny, although within the boundaries imposed by natural necessity: 'And what is not contrary to right reason, all agree is done justly, and *of Right* ... Therefore the first foundation of natural *Right* is that *each man protect his life and limbs as much as he can*.'[55] Given this understanding of individuals' dynamic subjection to the laws of causality, Hobbes asserts in *Leviathan* that the 'asperity and irregularity' making a human being comparable to a stone, which 'takes more room from others than itself fills', can be overcome if one renounces 'those things which to himself are superfluous, and to others necessary'. Only when they exert a strict control over their passions are individuals able to build the social edifice.[56]

The analogy of the building stones might suggest that men would remain passive while all the activity would come from the builders, who select those that are better suited to life in society; yet, this is not an accurate depiction of Hobbes's view. He employs this analogy because it comes from the Scripture: 'The stone which the builders rejected, the same is become the head of the corner' (Matthew 21:42). However, as can be observed, the meaning is reversed by renouncing the second part of the text, which alludes to Christ, and by putting the emphasis on the builders rather than the merits of the rejected stone. By taking Christ out of the equation of earthly politics, Hobbes establishes a clear distinction between human and divine politics. In the latter, men are more passive because Christ is able to bring together and to fit the asperities in the nature of the chosen ones into one body, i.e. one kingdom. Human politics on the other hand results in many kingdoms, not a single one. Besides, in earthly politics men are both 'the matter thereof, and the artificer' without any divine intervention.[57] This explains why, in chapter 15 of *Leviathan*, individuals are depicted more as *living stones*: even before the apparition of the sovereign, in the state of nature, those who are the *matter* of the state agree to restrain their passions (the asperities of their nature) in order to be called 'sociable' by following 'the fundamental law of nature, which commandeth to seek peace'.[58]

Hobbes's dynamic perspective does not stop at the image of a static edifice created by human living stones: at the centre of his doctrine is the state as a *political automaton*. At the very beginning of the introduction to *Leviathan*, the *automata* are defined as 'engines that move themselves by springs and wheels as doth a watch' and their regular movement as nothing but 'artificial life'.[59] Thus, the Commonwealth is a machine whose purpose is to compensate the weakness of 'natural man' who, in *human* society, is incapable of sustained altruism. This happens because in *human* or *civil* society, men's lives are not ruled by the fear of death or simple passions as in the state of nature, but they focus on more abstract goals such as 'knowledge', 'praise' from others during life, 'fame after death', 'eloquence', etc.[60] Yet, because of these '[v]ain, glorious men' fail to attain 'the true knowledge of themselves'.[61] Here again Hobbes uses a biblical metaphor: such men are 'children of pride'.[62] The only way to conduct these 'children' to common consent in social relations is to make them experience the constant necessity to avoid everything that causes aversion and ultimately fear the greatest danger of all: death.[63] Leviathan is the mechanism whereby men have the guarantee that there is at last someone who can 'keep them in awe, and tie them by fear of punishment to the performance of their covenants'.[64] Instead of having a natural altruism based on their own self-reading, subjects are forced to be altruistic by fear of punishment. This is no longer 'compassion' since the subject does not try to understand the other's predicament, but tries only to avoid the pain that would be inflicted by the sovereign if he breaks the law. However, a form of *artificial* altruism remains insofar as the mechanism of the state is self-imposed: in fact the sovereign, the 'artificial soul' of the commonwealth 'giving life and motion to the whole body',[65] is also the representative of each subject.[66] He acts benevolently on behalf of his subjects.

While the sovereign is the representative of the members of the commonwealth, the Leviathan, does not represent anyone. Hobbes names it 'artificial man',[67] not 'artificial person', because for him 'person' means 'face', or 'mask', or 'visard'.[68] Paradoxically, the Leviathan is an artificial mechanism, but it has the dignity of a natural person because its autonomy is characteristic of human beings. Ignoring this distinction between 'artificial man' and 'artificial person' Tom Sorell argues that Hobbes did not intend to compare the commonwealth to a natural body.[69] The analysis presented in this section shows the contrary. The following section argues that the Leviathan, being modelled on 'that rational and most excellent work of Nature, man,'[70] remains potentially subjected to passions similar to those of individuals in the state of nature.

## The Mortal Body of the State and its Artificial Egoism

In the Hobbesian materialistic universe, the difference between humans and animals is not one of kind but of degree.[71] Those attributes that were previously regarded as effects of an immaterial substance present in human nature are now just effects of motions in matter.[72] For instance, 'natural wit' is defined in chapter 8 of *Leviathan* as 'celerity of imagining (that is, swift succession of one thought to another); and steady direction to some approved end'. By contrast, 'a slow imagination maketh that defect or fault of the mind which is commonly called dullness, stupidity, and sometimes by other names that signify slowness of motion, or difficulty to be moved'.[73] Hobbes's psychology makes clear that individuals of slower thinking are nevertheless superior to madmen and children who are on a par with 'brute beasts' (at least in a certain period of their life), because they do not use their senses coherently to produce rapid motions and durable impressions in their brain.[74]

The distinction between natural and acquired wit, also in chapter 8, may first seem superfluous since Hobbes argues that natural wit is acquired by personal experience:

> These [intellectual] virtues are of two sorts; natural and acquired. By natural, I mean not that which a man hath from his birth: for that is nothing else but sense; wherein men differ so little one from another, and from brute beasts, as it is not to be reckoned amongst virtues. But I mean that wit which is gotten by use only, and experience, without method, culture, or instruction.[75]

This conception of natural intelligence indicates that for Hobbes the 'natural' world is already an artificial construct, but, unlike the artificial or social world, one that remains within the limits of exclusively personally developed wisdom or skill. It follows that, according to Hobbes, human dignity cannot be granted to a child although it can be granted to those individuals he names 'savages' from the Americas, even though they realize their 'concord' not by the artificial mechanism of politics, but only by 'natural lust'.[76]

Although wit is acquired by experience, the physical and psychological development of the human individual remains entirely personal and is not inherited. Children born within the *civil* society nevertheless stand a better chance to acquire human dignity, since knowledge - and even faith, another product of the passion of curiosity[77] – is cultivated in them by 'study and reason', by 'hearing' and by 'education, discipline, correction'.[78]

Like the child's cognitive development, the 'thinking body' of the state evolves continuously from birth, although not through education and correction since the state does not belong to a political body of a superior order. It can nevertheless become part of an international political family. From the moment of its birth, the Leviathan relies on the resources of its 'artificer',[79] namely the experience and 'wit' acquired in the state of nature by the individuals who decided to create it. There is, therefore, no guarantee that every state has an equal chance to survive and become a 'mortal god'.[80]

At the beginning of chapter 29 of *Leviathan* Hobbes presents a doctrine that can be considered to prefigure Darwin's natural selection, although with a major distinction: Hobbes puts the emphasis on the *internal* factors that determine evolution. Every political mechanism created by human beings in different parts of the world and at different moments of the state of nature seems perfectly fit to perform its task of protecting its creators from external dangers, at least for a certain time. The problem is that no such mechanism is created perfect. Originally it is designed 'to live as long as mankind, or as the laws of nature, or as justice itself' but 'nothing can be immortal which mortals make'. If the artificer is not 'a very able architect', the result is merely a 'crazy building' which provides safety for one or two generations but 'must assuredly fall upon the heads of their posterity'. No more than 'madmen' does the 'crazy building' rise up to the standards of an autonomous – though artificial – 'man'. The problems that such a state has to face are not typically external: they tend to 'resemble the diseases of a natural body, which proceed from a defectuous procreation'.[81]

Even diseases stemming from external factors are regarded as having internal causes. Thus, Hobbes describes malaria (*ague*) tentatively as a condition whereby the veins 'are not (as they ought to be) supplied from the arteries' because of 'venomous matter', blocking blood circulation. As a result, 'there succeedeth at first a cold contraction and trembling of the limbs; and afterwards a hot and strong endeavour of the heart to force a passage for the blood'.[82] Hobbes's view that the soul is the life of the body differed from Harvey's view, which proposed that it was the blood itself.[83] This is why in *Leviathan* he identifies two different correspondents for the soul and for the blood of the political thinking body. If the sovereign is regarded as the soul of the commonwealth, the circulation of money in a state is analogous to the circulation of blood in a living organism. Accordingly, as the circulation of the blood needs the heart, monetary circulation needs a 'public treasury'. When the symptoms of the 'ague' are applied to the political body, almost nothing changes, except that the cause of the disease is internal, the 'tenacity of the people', who hamper 'the passage of money to the public treasury'. As a result, the Leviathan 'struggles with the people by stratagems of law to obtain little sums, which, not sufficing, he is fain at last violently to open the way for present supply or perish'.[84] Hobbes gives other examples of diseases affecting Leviathan that are due to internal factors. One is 'pleurisy', caused by the formation of monopolies which concentrate the social blood 'in too much abundance in one or a few private men', a phenomenon usually accompanied by 'fever and painful stitches'.[85] Another example is worm infestation: when a town or a region becomes increasingly autonomous, thus resembling the 'worms in the entrails of a natural man'. [86]

Among the diseases listed, 'epilepsy' seems to have an external cause, but, from the way Hobbes describes it, the cause is secondary, because what matters most is the submission of the subject to the 'power of the soul in the brain'. Political epilepsy appears when a 'spiritual power' tries to exercise control over the political body by 'giving greater rewards than life, and of inflicting greater punishments than death'.[87] There is but one case where the cause may be regarded as somewhat external and that is when the Pope tries to exercise control over sovereigns.[88] Here indeed there is an identifiable external 'unnatural spirit or wind in the head that obstructeth the roots of the nerves'.[89] However, Hobbes's argument applies to any religious authority that would attempt to subjugate the real brain and soul of the state.

There are also cases when the causes of the disease lie not in various parts of the political body, but in its very soul. For instance 'the insatiable appetite, or bulimia, of enlarging dominion', which causes states to wage wars where they receive 'incurable wounds' from their external enemies.[90]

The artificial life of the Leviathan is therefore largely analogous to that of a 'natural man', albeit with the essential difference that the causes of its diseases are mainly internal. So the state is permanently on the lookout for any possible internal threat that has an impact on the political relations between the sovereign and his subjects. The analogy between the artificial body of the Leviathan and the natural human body led Hobbes to express his preference for authoritarian regimes in the chapter where he gave examples of the state's diseases.[91] In chapter 30, however, he precludes any extreme interpretation of his views by indicating that the laws concerning the 'ease and benefit' of the subjects have to 'look only inward'. Thus the sovereign's effort to fight internal disease must not necessarily be seen merely as a display authority but also as 'compassion'. Therefore Hobbes argues that any law must be inspired 'from the general informations and complaints of the people of each province, who are best acquainted with their own wants'.[92]

Yet Hobbes's emphasis on the idea that the laws of a state should be concerned primarily with the welfare of its subjects does not negate the state's artificial egoism – quite the reverse, since the state is only interested in welfare as a means to prevent internal diseases. Material well-being can also lead to an increase of population that is potentially dangerous for the life of the Commonwealth in view of its limited resources. Chapter 24 of *Leviathan* offers a number of solutions for such cases: importation, trade, sending subjects to work in another state, colonization and even 'just war'.[93] Hobbes's argument about colonies is also an analogy with human development: 'The procreation or children of a Commonwealth are those we call plantations, or colonies.'[94] This echoes the view earlier in the same chapter regarding a child's 'wit':

> [W]hen a colony is settled, they are either a Commonwealth of themselves, discharged of their subjection to their sovereign that sent them ... in which case the Commonwealth from which they went was called their metropolis, or mother, and requires no more of them than fathers require of the children whom they emancipate ... which is honour and friendship; or else they remain united to their metropolis.[95]

In other words, like human children, colonies are their parents' property, devoid of the dignity of autonomy until their emancipation. More specifically, if granting that autonomy is not in the interest of the state, which is both mother and father, colonies are no more than 'worms in the entrails of a natural man'. However, where autonomy is granted, privileged relations have to be maintained with the parent. This means that a state with an increasing number of children solves its demographical problems and contributes to the creation of a family of states where knowledge and 'commodities' can be exchanged.

The scientific exploration of the physiological and psychological processes that occur in the body of a 'natural man' helped Hobbes to formulate a political 'science' of the mortal body of the Leviathan. In doing so he hoped to give a firm grounding to moral and political philosophy, after centuries of 'wars of the sword' and 'wars of the pens'. The limits of such a conception are that in some instances he did not establish a perfect parallelism between the body of the state and the human body. For instance, if relations between states in the international state of nature are based mainly on self-interest and reduced 'family' ties (children to parent), then Hobbesian international communities cannot form greater and diverse families (such as husband and wife, adopted children, communities based on cultural ideals, etc.). Hobbes created a theoretical argument by which a state has to recognize the human dignity of another state's subjects and even to those individuals who are in the state of nature, provided they can prove that they have attained human dignity due to the concord provided by 'natural lust': 'The savages of America are not without some good moral sentences; also they have a little arithmetic.'[96] However, the political relations with those 'savages' cannot go beyond the state's artificial egoism, according to which a *civil* society can justifiably acquire the surplus of the land of a *human* society through war: 'The multitude of poor and yet strong people still increasing, they are to be transplanted into countries not sufficiently inhabited; where nevertheless they are not to exterminate those they find there; but constrain them to inhabit closer together'.[97]

In short the insufficiency of the Hobbesian international political life stems from the fact that the artificial body of the state is both mother and father for its children. Although it can be subjected to a range of human passions and sentiments, unlike human beings it cannot feel love for someone different from itself. The absence of such a sentiment leads Hobbes's political theory to a pessimistic view of the political destiny of the human species: '[a]nd when all the world is overcharged with inhabitants, then the last remedy of all is war, which provideth for every man, by victory or death'.[98] One cannot see how this 'final' war 'would close a cycle so that a new one could begin'.[99] Insufficient global resources will preclude the start of a new cycle of human history under the protection of the artificial body of the Leviathan. According to this pessimistic view, the remaining members of humanity ultimately cannot escape from a life 'solitary, poor, nasty, brutish, and short'.[100]

# 8 VISUALIZING THE FIBRE-WOVEN BODY: NEHEMIAH GREW'S PLANT ANATOMY AND THE EMERGENCE OF THE FIBRE BODY

Hisao Ishizuka

Although almost forgotten now, fibre attracted enormous interest among medico-scientists throughout the long eighteenth century. It is no exaggeration to say that if the nineteenth century was the age of the cell, then the eighteenth century was the age of fibre. Setting fibre as the ultimate building unit of the animal body, many eighteenth-century medico-scientists developed various theories based on the concept of fibre and the fibre body. That the two pillars of eighteenth-century medical sciences, Herman Boerhaave (1688–1738) and Albrecht von Haller (1708–77), were the eminent proponents of fibre theory speaks to its importance during that period. Although this theory was fully established with the systematization by Boerhaave's medical doctrine in the early eighteenth century, there were significant contributions to the formation of the theory and the idea of the fibre body by anatomists, physiologists, natural philosophers and microscopists of the later seventeenth century. Among others, Nehemiah Grew (1641–1721), a plant anatomist, made a crucial step towards the emergence of the idea of the fibre body by most explicitly articulating the two constituent features of fibre theory – the idea of the fibre as the minimum constituent of the body and the idea that the whole body is variously interwoven of nothing but these fibres.

Focusing on his anatomical works, this essay illuminates the significance of the new understanding of the body as fibre-woven textiles fully visualized in Grew's plant anatomy, which helped to crystallize into a coherent whole the fragmented ideas of the discrete anatomists and microscopists who studied the organs of the body. By visualizing the complete fibrosity of the body and by exploiting the metaphor of textiles in describing the hidden fabric of the inner body, Grew paved the way for the emergence of fibre theory and the fibre body, to which most anatomists and physiologists of the Enlightenment subscribed. This essay also attempts to show that Grew's image of the fibre body as something that is interwoven and interconnected by and through fibres provides an antidote to the weakening of the societal bonds of late-seventeenth-century

England and gives impetus to plausible knowledge for eighteenth-century understanding of society as a network-like system that sympathizes within itself. In doing so, this essay suggests an alternative way of thinking about the origin of the culture of sensibility, which is usually traced back to Thomas Willis's brain neuro-anatomy.

## The Prelude to the Fibre-Woven Body

The question, what is the minimum building unit of the body, seems to be peripheral to anatomists from classical times to the early modern era. Most accepted the crude division of the body that Aristotle first proclaimed – the 'similar part' that could be divided several times but still retain the same nature, in contrast to the 'dissimilar parts' that are composed of various similar parts.[1] Aristotle's division was the most popular in the anatomical texts and survived well into the seventeenth century.[2] There did not seem to be a driving force that made anatomists explain the composite of the body starting with the minimum unit of the body.

There was, however, another Aristotelian doctrine both important and useful for understanding the minimum unit of the body – that is, *minima naturalia*, the smallest particles fixed by nature. In Aristotle's account, the minima, a concept inseparable from the theory of substantial form, were supposed to be only the temporary state of matter and the vehicle of form; once mixed, they lose their separate entities to merge into the homogeneous compound. In the Middle Ages, however, the minima came to acquire a more direct physical meaning; and though still distinguishable from atomistic particles, the minima were closer to atomistic particles in meaning. Julius Scaliger (1484–1558), for example, thought of minima as the first building blocks of a whole.[3] When the corpuscularian philosophy gained momentum in the seventeenth century, the scholastic *minima naturalia* were increasingly replaced by, or conflated with, the minima of atomistic particles endowed with three-dimensional physical qualities. As R. Boyle pronounced, *minima naturalia* 'must have [their] determinate *bigness* or *size*, and [their] own *shape*'.[4] Corpuscularian philosophers hoped to discern the particular sizes and shapes of the minute particles, so far only hypothetical entities, with the help of microscopes.

Although the philosophers' expectations were not realized, the application of the microscope to the living body led some anatomists to search for a still smaller unit of the body, which was, as it were, equivalent to the physicist's atom, and to recast the scholastic minima (already conflated with the biological unit) into the constituent unit uniform in the living body. Hypothetical entities that signify minima, such as Leeuwenhoek's globule, Malpighi's gland (the glandular follicle), and Grew's fibre, all emerged in this context.[5] In a rather short span of time towards the end of the seventeenth century, however, the fibre, rather than the other two candidates, gained its place as the possible theoretical limit (minima) of the living body. There are several plausible reasons for this; among others, two points are significant in relation to the formation of the fibre body, that is, the vascularity and the texture of the body.

## *The Body as Vessels*

In the latter half of the seventeenth century, anatomists began to discover hitherto unseen vessels in the inner space of the body, combining the new technique of anatomical injections with microscopic inspections. Harvey's discovery of the circulation of blood and the Cartesian renovation of the body as a hydraulic machine constituted the background for the development of the injection technique.[6] In particular, this technique was propounded by Frederik Ruysch (1638–1731), the professor of anatomy at Amsterdam whose superb technique of injections came to be known as the 'Ruyschian art'.[7] Ruysch's method enabled him to discover and clearly show the unexpected vessels in almost all living tissues, from bones to ligaments to tendons to membranes. He became the most influential proponent of the vascularity of the body, the idea of which had already circulated among the Dutch medical circle.[8]

The vascularity of the body was also demonstrated by another instrument, the microscope. Malpighi had discovered the capillary blood vessels in the lungs as early as 1661, and Leeuwenhoek much more closely examined their marvellous distribution and appearance throughout the whole body over many years.[9] Following the discovery, many anatomists began to examine the ever-finer texture of various organs such as the liver (by Glisson), the heart (by Lower), the glands (by Wharton and Malpighi), the kidney, the lungs, the tongue (by Malpighi), the brain (by Willis) and the genital organs (by de Graaf), the results of which were incorporated in the magnificent atlas of *Anatomia humani corporis* (1685) by Bidloo.[10] The successive discoveries of the hidden vascularity of the body served to establish the new perception that the body was wholly composed of vessels. It is important to note here that the new understanding of the vascularity of the body demands the figure of the fibre rather than the atom as the minima of the solid body.

## *The Body as Textiles*

Around the same period when the anatomists discovered the vascularity of the body, the microscopist amply observed the finely woven texture of micro-worlds. The success and popularity of Hooke's *Micrographia* (1665) undoubtedly lie in its outstanding details of the subtle texture of matters (both in verbal and pictorial – but the visual representations are more striking). As the newly emerged world revealed by the microscope was entirely new and unexpected, the microscopist had to borrow from the common language or employ metaphors to make sense of the otherwise unintelligible microworld.[11] A set of metaphors from the textile and weaving industries was an apt choice, for the substance (especially the living body) was, in closer analysis, seen to be woven like embroidery or a garment. As a result, descriptions of the microscopic world are fraught with 'textile' words peculiar to woven fabric, such as 'text(ure)', 'context(ure)', 'intertext(ure)', 'cloth', 'wool', 'lace', 'warp and woof', 'knitting', 'spinning', 'weaving', 'interweaving', 'thread', 'filament', and of course 'fibre'. Hooke, for instance, having examined several kinds of mushroom, compared their texture to 'a kind of cloth', and found 'their texture to be somewhat of this kind, that is, to consist of an infinite company of small filaments, every way contex'd and woven together, so as to make a kind of cloth'.[12] The sponge (a kind of zoophyte) was seen to consist of an infinite number of the small fibres, 'curiously jointed or contex'd together in the form of Net'.[13] Seeing the surface of rosemary, Hooke concluded, 'Nature in this [is], as it were, expressing her Needle-work, or imbroidery.'[14]

It is no wonder, then, that anatomist contemporaries of Hooke also appropriated the world of textiles for the complicated but marvelously contrived micro-structure of the living body. Edmund King, an English anatomist, finding the parenchymous parts consisting wholly of vessels 'curiously wrought and interwoven', compared them to 'a piece of fine Cloth (which consist of so many several minute Hairs, call'd *Wool*)'.[15] F. Glisson, another anatomist of the era, also found the textile metaphor useful for his description of the texture of the skin.[16]

The visual representations sometimes even more effectively exhibit the anatomists' perception of the textile body. Edmund King's figure of the 'Embroidery of Veins and Arteries of the Testicle' (see Figure 8.1) gives clearer evidence of how he perceived the texture of the testicles in terms of textile embroidery. Displaced onto the two-dimensional space, the texture surprisingly resembles a piece of textile. Another example can be seen in Willis's scheme of the nervous system of the neck, which is like a transparent piece of textile. Other examples from anatomical illustrations amply show the textile image of the body. These include *Bibliotheca anatomica*, a valuable collection mainly selected from later seventeenth-century anatomical writings in Europe, ranging from Bartholin, Glisson, Lower, Malpighi, Willis, Diemerbroeck and Bidloo to Ruysch. An appendix attached to the first volume of James Drake's *Anthropologia nova* is, in its scale, a more comprehensive collection of the anatomical illustrations, drawing on the same sources as in *Bibliotheca anatomica*. Thomas Willis's gorgeous plates for *Pharmaceutice rationalis* (1679) are more compelling in the size, detail and vividness of the images of the specimen. At times, the anatomical specimens are displayed in the form of a piece of cloth (see Figure 8.2), which indicates that the micro-texture of the membranes is closely related to the textile fabrics. The textile-like patterns embedded in these anatomical tables are clearly shown in some of these figures as if they were an anatomical pattern book of the human body. What these anatomical illustrations lay bare is that the animal/human body is dexterously stitched by Nature's needles into finely woven textiles. Going deeper into the hidden recess of the invisible space of the living body, strangely the anatomists found themselves beholding the external coverings (the woven clothes) in which the living body is ordinarily enclosed.

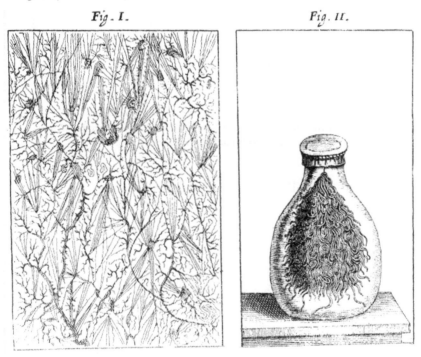

Figure 8.1: 'The Embroidery of the Veins and the Arteries of the Testicle', from 'Some Observations Concerning the Organs of Generation, Made by Dr. Edmund King', *Philosophical Transactions*, 4 (1669), pp. 1043–8, on p. 1048; reproduced with permission of the Royal Society of London.

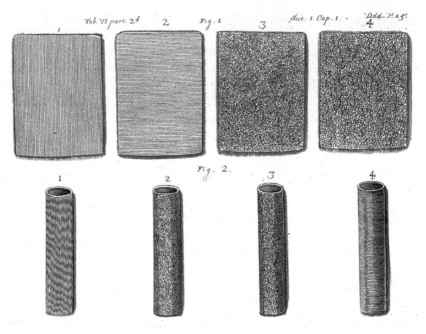

**Figure 8.2: 'The Four Distinct Coats of the Artery', from Thomas Willis,**
*Pharmaceutice rationalis* **(London, 1684), table 6, pt 2; reproduced by**
**permission of British Library.**

## Grew's Plant Anatomy and the Fibre Body

*Grew and Fibre*

When Nehemiah Grew compiled his 1670s works into the *Anatomy of Plants* (1682), the metaphor of embroidery, textiles and weaving, on which he heavily relied in depicting the anatomical structure and texture of plants, was already familiar to anatomists. And yet, it was Grew who gave a decisive step towards the notion of fibre theory and the fibre body by presenting a lucid and comprehensible understanding that the whole living body was variously knit and interwoven by an infinite number of fibres, which were thought to be the minima.

In the *Anatomy of Plants*, Grew clearly distinguished the two types of tissue (or structural unit) – the parenchymous and the ligneous ('the *Pithy Part* and the *Lignous Part*').[17] All the parts of the plant are composed of these basic tissues; but more fundamentally, the two types of tissues are distinguished by, and therefore built up by, two basic elements: the more or less spherical units called bladders and the elongated vessels. And yet, more importantly, both basic elements consist of 'Fibres'. He concludes the discourse with an illustration of the texture of the pith and by extension of the whole plant:

> [A]s the *Vessels* of a *Plant, sc.* the *Aer-Vessels* and the *Lymphaducts* are made up of *Fibres*; according to what I have in this discourse above said; so the *Pith* of a *Plant*, or the *Bladders* whereof the *Pith* consists are likewise made up of *Fibres*. Which is true also of the *Parenchyma* of the *Barque*. And also of the *Insertions* in the *Wood*. Yea, and of the Fruit, and all other *Parencymous Parts* of a *Plant* ... Whence it follows, that the whole *substance*, or all the Parts of a *Plant*, so far as *Organical*, they also consist of *Fibres*.[18]

Thus, Grew established fibre as the minimum unit of the plant structure.

In his last work, *Cosmologia Sacra* (1701), a religious and philosophical treatise, Grew rendered in a more lucid expression that the whole plant was composed of 'two Species of Fibres', and argued that 'all the Parts, from the Root to the Seed, are distinguished one from another, only by the different Position, Proportion, and other Relations and Properties, of those two sorts of Fibres.'[19] Although these fibres were ultimately invisible, therefore, hypothetical, he alleged that even those parts that were neither formed into 'visible *Tubes*, nor into *Bladders*' were 'yet made up of Fibres'.[20]

Searching for the invisible texture of the plant's fabric, Grew employed the metaphor of the textile and weaving more amply than any other anatomist. For example, he described the roots 'as a piece of Cloath', and the parenchyma of the skin 'as a Glove is to the Hand.'[21] They are only the tip of the iceberg. The notable example among others is the texture of the pith, whose 'Contexture' is totally '*Fibrous*'. Here Grew made an explicit analogy between Nature's work and '*Needle work*':

> [T]he *Vessels* running by the length of the *Root*, as the *Warp*; by the *Parenchymous Fibres* running cross or horizontally, as the *Woof*: they are thus *knit* and as it were *stitched* up together. Yet their *westage* seemth not to be simple, as in *Cloath*; but that many of the *Parenchymous Fibres* are *wrapped* round about each *Vessel*; and, in the same manner, are continued from one *Vessel* to another; thereby knitting them altogether, more closely, into one *Tubulary Thred*; and those *Threds*, again, into one *Brace*: much after the manner of the *Needle work* called *Back-Stitch* or that used in Quilting of Balls.[22] (See Figure 8.3)

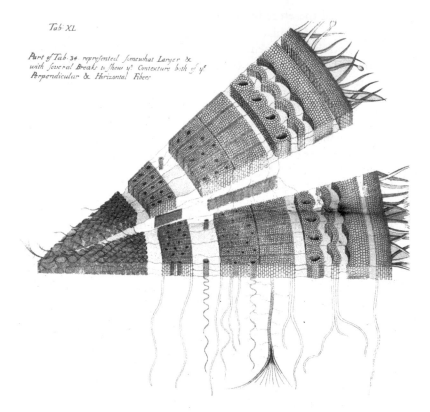

Figure 8.3: 'The Contexture of Perpendicular and Horizontal Fibres', from Nehemiah Grew, *The Anatomy of Plants* (London, 1682), table 40; reproduced with permission of the Peter H. Raven Library, Missouri Botanical Garden.

Grew's text, as it were, is stitched and closely embroidered by the cluster of textile metaphors. And, indeed, Grew was highly conscious of employing the textile trope. When he compared the whole body of a plant to a piece of '*fine Bone-lace*' in explaining the 'true *Texture* of a *Plant*', he explicitly referred to women working on a cushion, because both the texture of a plant and '*Cloth-Work*' are contrived in the same way.[23]

Just as Hooke's *Micrographia* was praised for the minutely detailed visualization, so Grew's work owed its success to the gorgeous pictorial representations of a plant's structure. The illustrations amply demonstrate the fibrosity of the inner and outer structures of plants as wonderfully woven fabrics (see Figures 8.4 and 8.5). Both in the verbal description and in the pictorial representation, he succeeded in visualizing the inner structure of plants as a textile fabric.

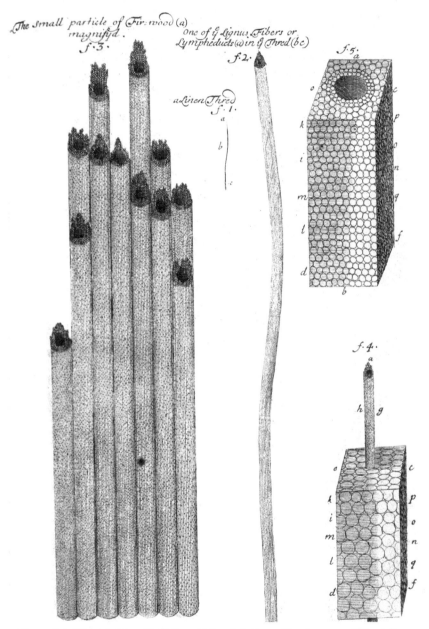

Figure 8.4: 'Threads Magnified', from Nehemiah Grew, *The Anatomy of Plants* (London, 1682), table 39; reproduced with permission of the Peter H. Raven Library, Missouri Botanical Garden.

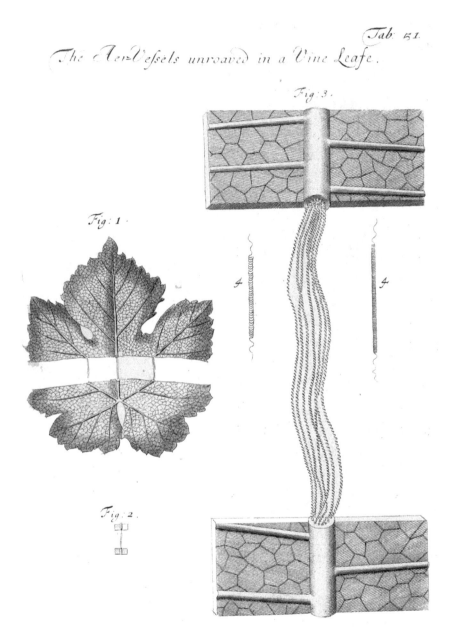

Figure 8.5: 'The Air-Vessels Unroaved in a Vine Leaf', from Nehemiah Grew, *The Anatomy of Plants* (London, 1682), table 51; reproduced with permission of the Peter H. Raven Library, Missouri Botanical Garden.

## Plants and Animals: The Comparative Method

The idea of the fibre-woven body seems to be restricted to the vegetative world, and not to be applied to the animal one, whose complex structures make difficult an easy adaptation. So, how can Grew extend the fibre body to the animal kingdom? The key lies in the analogy and comparison of the plant with the animal. Indeed, Grew had studied animal anatomy before he engaged in plant anatomy, and one of his aims in his study of plant anatomy was to demonstrate that plants had similar organic structures to those of animals, and by extension that plants were contrived in the same manner as animals ('*a* Plant *is, as it were, an* Animal *in Quires; as an* Animal *is a* Plant, *or rather several* Plants *bound up into one* Volume'.[24] The rationale for the analogical thinking was the principle of uniformity of nature: that is, nature has a uniform plan to contrive natural creatures. This view seems to have been shared widely among anatomists and microscopists at that time. The marvellous micro-structure of the tiny insects seen through the microscope (they had a whole set of the same organs as those of other animals) may have promoted this view.

The analogical relation between plants and animals was always present in his mind.[25] For example, Grew's distinction of the two types of tissues in plant anatomy was based on a traditional classification of the body in animal/human anatomy (for example, the division of the body into the spermatic parts and the fleshy parts, or into the vascular parts and the parenchymous parts). Moreover, the correlation of the vessels between plants and animals appeared to be obvious, for 'as the *Sanguineous Vessels* in an *Animal* are composed of a number of *Fibres*, set round, in a *Tubulary Figure*, together: so are these *Lymphaducts* or a *Plant*'.[26] The apparent lack of some organs in plants correlative to those of animals did not mean that plants were inferior to animals; even though in some cases plants were not endowed with organs identical to those of animals, they were instead supplied with organs analogical to those of animals. Grew explained away the apparent lack of viscera in plants with recourse to the comparative method: 'what the *Viscera* are in *Animals*, the *Vessels* themselves are in *Plants*. That is to say, as the *Viscera* of an *Animal*, are but *Vessels* conglomerated: so the *Vessels* of a *Plant*, are *Viscera* drawn out at length.'[27] Finding a great agreement between the animal and the plant, Grew implied that the body of animals was also composed of fibres, and argued that the fibres composing the body of an animal were 'of two general Kinds' as in the plant.[28]

Around the time when Grew's last writing was published, the idea of the fibre body had just entered into the realm of human anatomy, to which Grew's analysis of plant anatomy had a great contribution. Therefore, we should revise the Whiggish interpretation of Grew that the analogies and metaphors he employed 'misled' him to concentrate on cell walls (the woven fabrics), rather than their content, as J. Bolam argues – the view that mistakenly puts him in the place of the unfortunate precursor to the discovery of cell.[29] On the contrary, the textile and weaving metaphor and the analogy between plants and animals – Grew's analytical tools for plant anatomy – would rather make Grew's account more plausible and cogent for the late seventeenth-century anatomists, who, in another realm, discovered the complete vascularity of the animal/human body, whose organs were spun with finely woven textiles. To put it differently, Grew's view of the complete fibrosity of the plant's body would serve to consolidate into a coherent whole the otherwise fragmented and isolated vision of anatomists of the discrete organs of the animal/human body.[30]

## Atheism and Re-Weaving the Social Body

There is no doubt, as many historians have argued, that especially in later seventeenth-century England there was a vivid apprehension and deep fear of phenomena that people called 'atheism'; however, these phenomena were extremely shadowy, despite the exaggerated rhetoric used by accusers. The Puritan Revolution left a deep psychological scar on the minds of those who shared a widespread revulsion against political radicalism and religious 'enthusiasm'.[31] Hobbes's materialism and Epicurius's atomism were perhaps the main strands of the heterodoxy of the time (the later seventeenth century added to them Spinoza's pantheism).[32] New science, with its association with atomistic philosophy (a chance-driven world of the fortuitous concourse of atoms), was always in danger of acquiring the label of heresy, although Restoration atomism was considered by its defenders to have been baptized along the line set by Gassendi and Charleton (God had endowed matter with an internal principle of motion at Creation).[33] Many mechanists took up Gassendi and Charlton's stratagem of the rehabilitation of atheistic atomism. Corpuscularian mechanism could easily raise the spectre of a materialist view of the world totally devoid of intelligent beings.[34] Many supposed that God's direct intervention was not necessary; therefore, it often was regarded as atheism.[35]

Natural philosophers defended against charges of atheism in the form of natural theology (or physico-theology) – the argument from design, an attempt to prove the existence of God by pointing to the complexity and beauty of the natural world. The newly invented microscope provided powerful evidence that proved the incredible beauty and regularity of the natural world and the purposefulness of God's design in nature. Microscopic research into living nature and anatomical observations of the body of living creatures were essential to demonstrate divine providence and an end in nature, to purge any implication of atheism from their philosophy. Natural philosophers thought that as a divine architect God must have a design, which was made visible in His products of living nature thanks to the modern engine, the microscope.

In this context, what the above-mentioned microscopists-cum-anatomists discovered was not only the fibre or the texture of the body but also God's unmistakable intelligence and existence in nature, which were embedded in the wonderfully woven fabrics of the body. The fibre body enabled precisely that which atomistic matter theory attempted but could not accomplish: namely, to purge as completely as possible the atheistic innuendo of their philosophies. This is one reason why the atomistic particle was not adopted as the minimum or the theoretical limit of the living body, even though many anatomists believed that the fibre was formed of atoms (earth particles) held together with a glue-like substance. The fibre of living beings, rather than the atomistic particle of matter, was an appropriate choice for many apologetics.

The shift from atom to fibre, placed in a broad social perspective, is also symptomatic of a change from the chaotic social and political order of the Civil War period to the relatively stable social regimen of the Restoration. The familiar parallel between the physical body and the social body could be easily evoked in these periods – the potentially fortuitous atom and the chaotic social order in which the 'individual' atom (the Greek word 'atomos' means 'undividable') purposelessly moves and 'dances' around.[36] As Stephen Clucas argues, the radical instability of matter (atom) with its potential for disintegration and consolidation, which would unconsciously raise the deep-seated anxiety of social and moral disorder, was the focal theme in seventeenth-century discourses on atomism.[37] It is a short step from a Demo-critic to a demo-cratic view of atomism, as John Evelyn's lines show:

No Monarch rules the Universe.
But chance and Atomes make this All
In order Democraticall
Without design, or Fate, or, Force.[38]

Seen in this context, Grew's vision of the fibre body is considered to emerge as a social antidote to the apparent weakening of societal bonds, which atomistic philosophies could not remedy (on the contrary, the atomistic mechanism seemed to escalate the debilities of the social body). It could be argued that the formation of the fibre body at that period was interrelated with a broad social and cultural concern for restoring and re-constituting the social order, and with the pressing need of re-binding and re-weaving the relation of the individual to the society as a whole. This would probably explain the fact that the fibre body in its most explicit form was first articulated by Grew, whose country witnessed unprecedented turmoil throughout the seventeenth century.

## Conclusion: The Fibre Body as Another Origin of Sensibility

At the end of the seventeenth century, a small anatomical text written by James Keill was published, which in the following century became one of the most popular and standard textbooks on human anatomy. Keill's text assumed a new look in deliberately avoiding the pedagogic definition of the division of the body, with which the traditional anatomical text usually opened. For Keill, it was sufficient to provide the reader the simple fact that '*All the Part are made up of Fibres*':

> I purposely pass over the various Definitions of a Part, as being of no great Use; and of the same Reason I will not trouble the Reader with the several Divisions which Anatomists make of the Parts of the Humane Body. It is sufficient to know that all the Parts are made up of Threads, or Fibres, of which there be different Kinds.[39]

This is, perhaps, the first entry of fibre theory in an anatomical textbook written in English. Following Grew's vision of the fibre body, Keill viewed the human body as composed of nothing but fibres. Although Keill's version of fibre theory is far from the most sophisticated one, he at least sets the fibre as the starting point of his anatomical text. For more than a century to follow, fibre theory and the fibre body stayed at the heart of 'human' anatomy and physiology to which 'plant' anatomy, to a significant degree, contributed. As the eighteenth century continued, the idea of the fibre body gradually stretched beyond the bound of the medical circle to the cultural sphere. To conclude this essay, I want to briefly address the thorny issue regarding the origin of the culture of sensibility in terms of the fibre body.

It is now commonly assumed that the defining feature of the Age of Enlightenment is the culture of nervous sensibility. There, a Man of Feeling and a Woman of Sensibility enjoyed their sweet lives with pitying tears for their fellow beings in distress and often wiped their tears by doing good to them; there, sentimental readers dampened with tears every page of sentimental novels and experienced their delicate feelings and involuntary quivering. It is a truism of the age that delicate sensibility and finer feeling required correspondingly finer nerves. From a medical front, especially from the middle of the eighteenth century onwards, as the nervous system and the brain gained strength in the medical world via Scottish medics such as Monro, Whytt and Cullen, nervous sensibility was regarded as a vital property for living creatures. To live is to feel, and to be sensible is to be alive; in order to feel, one has to possess nerves. Thus, culturally and medically, nervous sensibility became the key to unlocking the hidden dimensions of living beings, who were defined as nervous creatures.

The origin of the nervous paradigm that posited nerves in the midst of human beings is usually traced back to Thomas Willis's investigation into brain anatomy during the mid-seventeenth century: Willis limited the soul to the brain and argued that nerves alone were to be held responsible for sensory perceptions and human knowledge. This thesis, first proposed by G. S. Rousseau,[40] has had a tremendous impact on subsequent studies on sensibility. The thesis has, however, some difficulty dealing with the compatible picture of the development of the fibre body. Although Rousseau includes fibres in the paradigm of the nerves (as a kind of subcategory) as well as animal spirits,[41] strangely a detailed explanation of the fibres is totally missed in his explanatory picture. Moreover, the privileged status of the brain and the nerves in the anatomical research of the latter half of the seventeenth century seems to be overemphasized. As mentioned above, the dominant feature of the anatomical research of the era was to search for an ever-finer texture of the body, which many anatomists began to think consisted of an infinite number of fibres. Willis's anatomical research of the brain was only one of such investigations into the fibre-woven body. Almost all eighteenth-century physicians subscribed to the idea of the fibre-woven body as the theoretical matrix of medicine: they construed the body to be interwoven with the innumerable threads as Grew saw it. George Cheyne, one of the most fashionable nerve doctors of the eighteenth century, postulated the fibre doctrine as follows:

> All the solids of the Body ... resolve themselves, or may be separated into such Fibres at last. They are probably platted and twisted together ... to make the larger sensible Fibres; and these again are either united in Bundles to form the *Muscles, Tendons, Ligaments*, &c. or woven into a fine *Web*, like cloth, to make the *Membrane*, the coats of the Vessels, &c.[42]

However important a place the brain and the nerves occupied in the later eighteenth century, the fibres rather than the nerves, the fibre body rather than the nervous body set the starting point to provide plausible knowledge for the culture of sensibility.

The alternative view of the culture of sensibility that posits the fibre body as another origin more properly fits eighteenth-century knowledge of society and the body epitomized as sensibility and sympathy. For one thing, although to *feel* is to involuntarily vibrate or quiver according to the degree of sensibility of the nerves, for the sensitized body to properly vibrate, the body should be composed of something like threads or strings (note that the nerves were commonly thought not to be solid or tense like strings, but to be so soft and pulpy not to perform vibratory action[43]); the image of the fibre-woven body precedes the nervous one as an explanatory model of sensibility. The recurrent image of the body compared to a musical string instrument throughout the eighteenth century was founded upon the same epistemological matrix of the fibre body. The set of terms related to the fibre-thread property such as 'tone', 'tension', 'elasticity', 'vibration', 'oscillation', and many others that frequently propped up in eighteenth-century medical and cultural discourses also indicate the enduring legacy of the fibre body. For another, the idea of the fibre body physically corresponds to the principle of sympathy, a distinguishing feature of eighteenth-century culture. Theorists of the fibre body imagined the body as a vast network-like structure composed of a cellular texture. The web-like continuity woven out of the cellular substances supports the consent of parts, medical sympathy, which if extended to social body furthers and embodies the principle of moral sympathy. The principle of moral sympathy – for which interconnectedness, continuity and sociability are indispensable – could be visualized as thread-like fibres: as Tiphaigne de la Roche, a French medical theorist of sympathy, held, individuals are linked to others by the infinite number of threads through which sympathy acts.[44] As Grew's vision of the fibre body worked for the pressing need to re-bind the dangerously fragile society, the eighteenth-century version of the fibre body fed into knowledge of sympathy and sensibility, two pillars of Enlightenment culture.

# 9 FORMS OF MATERIALIST EMBODIMENT

## Charles T. Wolfe

The materialist approach to the body is often understood in 'mechanistic' terms, as the view in which the properties unique to organic, living embodied agents are reduced to the properties of matter as a whole, allowing for mechanistic explanation. Indeed, from Hobbes and Descartes in the seventeenth century to the popularity of automata such as Vaucanson's in the eighteenth century, this vision of things would seem to be correct. In this essay I aim to correct this inaccurate vision of materialism. On the contrary, the materialist project on closer consideration reveals itself to be an *embodied* discourse, significantly if not exclusively, (a) focusing on the contribution that 'biology' or rather 'natural history' and physiology make to metaphysical debates, (b) much more intimately connected to what we now call 'vitalism' (as indicated by the presence of Théophile de Bordeu, a prominent Montpellier physician and theorist of vitalism, as a fictional character and spokesman of materialism in Diderot's novel *D'Alembert's Dream*), and ultimately (c) an anti-mechanistic doctrine which focuses on the unique properties of organic beings. To establish this revised vision of materialism I examine philosophical texts including La Mettrie's *Man a Machine* and Diderot's *D'Alembert's Dream*; medical entries in the *Encyclopédie* by physicians such as Ménuret; and clandestine combinations of these such as Fontenelle.

> That the mind possesses such a corporeal nature need not be feared as a blow to our self-esteem.[1]

## I.

We tend to think of the emergence of modern materialism as somehow an outgrowth, albeit a more fiery and impassioned one, of the forms of mechanism that flourished in the Scientific Revolution. Now, mechanism itself comes in a variety of forms or programmatic statements, as we can see in the following broad definitions from some representative figures. For Robert Boyle, the basic properties or 'qualities' of things can be exhaustively explained in terms *of*, if not reduced *to* 'the motion, size, figure and contrivance of their own parts', with new qualities being produced by 'changing the texture or motion' of these basic parts.[2]

As applied to the body, and thus at a more macroscopic level, Descartes states that he will assume that the body is nothing other than 'a statue or machine made of earth', to which he adds famous analogies with the machinery of fountains comprising moving hydraulic statues and other sorts of clockwork.[3] Most broadly of all, Herman Boerhaave, the great Leiden professor of medicine, stated in a 1703 lecture revealingly entitled 'On the Usefulness of Mechanical Methods in Medicine' that 'the nature of the human body is the same as that of the whole of the Universe;'[4] he certainly does not mean that the body has a life like that of the world-soul, or even that it is part of the one total substance of the universe as in Spinozist substance monism (a view held by committed materialists such as John Toland, for whom 'every material Thing is all Things',[5] or Diderot, for whom 'everything changes, everything passes ... only the Whole remains').[6] Rather, Boerhaave is restating the essential claims of mechanism in ontologized fashion: it is not just that matter itself can exhaustively be defined in terms of shape, size and motion, or that the body can (and should) be studied as if it were a mechanistic arrangement of matter – or a machine, whichever comes first to mind – but that the body is itself the same *in essence* as the rest of the universe: mechanical.

If materialism really was an outgrowth of mechanism, a typical example would be La Mettrie's 'man-machine', which is often described, presumably by authors unfamiliar with his writings or otherwise blinded by the prevalence of older interpretive schemas, as simply the Cartesian *bête-machine* extended to humans.[7] This narrative of progression or decline (depending on whether one is a positivistically inclined historian of the behavioural sciences intent on tracing a line from Descartes to cybernetics via La Mettrie[8] or a moralistically inclined philosopher intent on showing how the triumph of mechanism and/or materialism spelled the death of 'meaning and value'[9]) can also be told in more theoretical terms, in which the increasing complexification of Cartesian mechanism is a necessary component of every major step forward in physiology, through Lamarck and Claude Bernard.[10] However, the point to retain here is that if we consider these narratives from the standpoint of *embodiment* – of our existence as embodied beings – it would appear that we have ended up with an atomistic, reductive, depersonalized way of relating to our bodies, or rather to the fact of our embodiment. This is often decried by theorists who think something was lost at a certain historical conjuncture, a historico-destinal moment of 'dehumanization' or alienation,[11] or historians who wish to retrieve something of the 'lived body'.[12]

Whether we like it or not, or whether it matches our 'phenomenology', in the sense of our experience of what it is to be in a body – the pain, the enjoyment, the ineffable subjectivity and so on – we have ended up, in this tale of the Fall, with what Ian Hacking recently called 'Cartesian bodies': no longer machines governed by immaterial souls, but nevertheless fully mechanical assemblages of replaceable parts, whether prostheses or artificially grown biological parts.[13] Of course, there have been other responses to the growing complexity of mechanism and its materialistic outgrowths besides desperate appeals to the respect of the sovereignty of the flesh: some thinkers have celebrated the potential for hybridization between body and machine,[14] while others in a more historical vein have emphasized the particularly *heuristic* role of automata such as Vaucanson's duck.[15] However, I would like to suggest a different response to this narrative, one which partly seeks to correct it on historical grounds: that there was such a thing as a *specifically materialist sense of embodiment*. In other words, materialism was not merely an obsessive reiteration or heightened performance of the 'mechanistic' vision of the body, whatever that might be: reducing it to isolated parts or defining it in accordance with general mechanical laws, but in any case factoring out the rich, fluid, *personal* sense of what it is to be in a body.

This is not just because materialists frequently repeated like a mantra that everything that is real is (a) body. Granted, we should not ignore these proclamations – consider Hobbes's 'That which is not body is no part of the universe', 'there is no motion save of corporeal substance',[16] or Bacon's 'In nature nothing exists besides individual bodies, performing pure individual acts according to a law.'[17] Diderot gives a more explicitly reductionist cast to the claim that 'all is body', when, in a major unpublished work which occupied him during the last decades of his life, the *Elements of Physiology*, he explains that 'the action of the soul on the body is the action of one part of the body on another, and the action of the body on the soul is again that of one part of the body on another' and, in his marginal commentary on Hemsterhuis's 1772 *Lettre sur l'homme*, 'wherever I read *soul* I replace it with *man* or *animal*.'[18] Similarly, La Mettrie in his first philosophical work, the *Natural History of the Soul* (1745, later revised as *Treatise on the Soul*), declares 'he who wishes to know the properties of the soul must first search for those which manifest themselves clearly in the body'.[19] It makes sense, then, that a word that was used as a synonym for 'materialism' in the late seventeenth century, albeit not so frequently, was 'corporealism'. Ralph Cudworth describes 'Corporealists' as those who 'acknowledge no other *Substance* besides *Body* or *Matter*'.[20] Furetière's influential *Dictionnaire* defines materialists, in an entry added to its 1727 edition (it first appeared in 1690) as 'a kind of philosophers who claim that only matter or the body exist, no other substance in the world; matter or body is eternal, and from it everything else is formed'.[21]

Trumpeting that 'all is body' or that 'wherever I read "soul" I replace it with "body"' is not, then, tantamount to a discourse of embodiment. But what is embodiment? Obviously, if we are to decide whether or not materialists had a concept of embodiment, we need a working definition of the term. I will suggest such a definition, borrowing hints from two distinct and influential intellectual traditions of recent decades. Very briefly, in the study of cognition, 'embodied mind' perspectives reject traditional computational approaches and present our cerebral life as necessarily occurring within a body, understood both as a dynamic system and as something fundamentally *my own* in the sense of Maurice Merleau-Ponty's *corps propre*.[22] The emphasis here usually falls on how an embodied agent inhabits the world, not as one body amongst others (atoms and asteroids and Fanta cans) but as a *subject* in her own environment. In cultural studies, embodiment connotes a complex, twofold relation between historicity and gender, in which 'subjectivity [is] profoundly experienced as interrelated with the physical, and societal changes or structures influenced the ways in which the body was perceived',[23] through scientific discourses but also in many other ways, often with a stress on the *local*, contextual character of embodiment.[24] Both of these perspectives share a sense (an intuition? a theoretical commitment?) that the body exists outside of the fully spatialized, quantified pronouncements of modern science; the extent to which this is a subtle or even satisfactory portrayal of modern science is open to question. After all, quantification in the history of 'embodied' sciences such as medicine is a case where oppositions between the 'fluid, lived, emotive body' and the measurements of 'laboratory technicians' fall flat: consider the case of Sanctorius (1561–1636), who was one of William Harvey's professors of medicine at Padua. Sanctorius designed a special chair to measure what he called the 'insensible respiration' of the body by frequently weighing himself, all that he ate, drank and excreted. Where do cold mechanical measurement and 'warm' humoral complexity respectively 'sit' here?[25]

Regardless, the 'lived body' we encounter in contemporary embodiment discourse is the body in pain, or in a state of enjoyment; in a reflexive, indeed intimate relation to itself – quite different, according to embodiment theorists, from the more generic body in space. They maintain that the lived body (which really is *the* body for embodiment discourse) exists at least in part 'outside of physical space'.[26] Thus the living body – indeed, any organism – 'is an individual in a sense which is not that of modern physics'.[27] This is often presented in cultural studies as an insight countering 'Cartesianism', with the rise of a Cartesian mechanistic world-picture often described: 'As a machine, the body became objectified; a focus of intense curiosity, but entirely divorced from the world of the speaking and thinking subject.'[28] It is hard to separate this from contemporary embodied-mind assertions such as, 'Life is not physical in the standard materialist sense of purely external structure and function. Life realizes a kind of interiority, the interiority of selfhood and sense-making. We accordingly need an expanded notion of the physical to account for the organism or living being.'[29] As I will be suggesting, this 'expanded notion of the physical' has always been present; it is rather the picture of 'standard materialism' that needs to be revised.

At first blush, a deeply subjective body, or at least one in which subjectivity is somehow 'irreducible', does indeed seem a far cry from both iatromechanical and materialistic approaches to the body. But what are these?

Iatromechanism was an influential school of medical thought in the late seventeenth and early eighteenth centuries, under the twin influences of Descartes's *Traité de l'homme* (1648, published 1662) and Borelli's *De motu animalium* (1680). It is here that we encounter the celebrated descriptions of the body as a set of small interlocking machines: funnels, pulleys, windmills and the like. For Boerhaave, amongst the 'solid parts of the human body', 'some resemble Pillars, Props ... some Axes, Wedges, Leavers and Pullies, others Cords, Presses or Bellows; and others again Sieves, Straines, Pipes'.[30] Giorgio Baglivi, the celebrated Roman anatomist and surgeon who was also a Fellow of the Royal Society in London from 1697 onwards, seems to recommend an *approach* to bodies rather than an ontological claim about their nature, suggesting they be studied according to 'Geometrico-Mechanical Principles', but he adds that if the body's structure (*fabrica*) is approached thus, the observer

> will really meet with Shears in the Jaw-bones and Teeth ... Hydraulick Tubes in the Veins and Arteries, a Piston in the Heart, a Sieve or Straining-Holes in the Viscera, a Pair of Bellows in the Lungs ... the natural Effects of an animated Body can't be accounted for ... any other way, than by those Mathematico-Experimental Principles, by which Nature speaks her own Mind.[31]

The London anatomist and founding member of the Royal Society William Croone says it succinctly, but without the useful metaphors: 'We shall consider the living body to be nothing else but a kind of machine or automaton.'[32]

Indeed, when we speak of mechanisms, the machine analogy, or in this case the specifically medical theory of iatromechanism, we feel that we have some broad intuitive grasp on the issue: a machine is a system of inanimate parts, presumably without a central controller, and certainly without an internal 'vital principle'. Hence, when a living body, whether animal or human, is described as being *like a machine* (or more assertively, as in Croone, 'nothing else but a kind of machine or automaton'), we may trust that we know what is happening: the various properties of organic life – the real, basic properties of what it is to be alive and in a body: self-maintenance, goal-directed behaviour, and on some accounts intentionality or consciousness (these two tend to be associated) – are being redefined as, or reduced to, basic mechanical properties. Notice that even this definition of a higher-level entity in terms of a set of 'lower-level' properties is less straightforward than we might think: are living, embodied properties being defined in favour of *the properties of machines* as they are understood at a given time and place (like Descartes's fountains), or in favour of the basic *properties of nature understood mechanically*? It is after all different to say that the heart is *like* a pump, the lungs *like* a pair of bellows, and to state as Boerhaave did that 'the nature of the human body is the same as that of the whole of the Universe'.[33]

Instead of examining the diversity of mechanistic and reductionist explanations (to which I return below), however, I wish to suggest a different point: that our intuition, our confidence in opposing 'machines' to 'bodies' is misplaced in an important way. After all, 'machine' was often used to simply mean 'body',[34] and mechanical models of life such as Vaucanson's duck were attempts to understand that very thing – life.[35] Conversely, when we turn to the writings of the group of Montpellier physicians known as 'vitalists' – some of whom, such as Théophile de Bordeu, were in close association with materialist philosophers such as Diderot, to the extent that Bordeu becomes a major fictional character in Diderot's experimental philosophical novel, *D'Alembert's Dream* (written in 1769, not published during Diderot's lifetime)[36] – we find, not invocations of a vital principle over and above the workings of the body, but the will to explain 'the mechanism which subserves the functions of the animal economy', a mechanistic level 'chiefly founded on anatomical observations;'[37] even if the same author some pages later adds that movement and sensation are basic, non-reducible features of the body.[38] Of course, this goal to explain the specific workings of our organic body with appropriate concepts, rather than simply retranslating those workings into the vocabulary of simple machines, is two-edged: on the one hand it is indeed exclusively structural, like a kind of expanded or enhanced mechanism;[39] but on the other hand it focuses specifically on the *organic* structure of the body. As another Montpellier vitalist, Ménuret, notes in his fascinating essay in Diderot and D'Alembert's *Encyclopédie*, 'Œconomie Animale', the mechanists, *les Méchaniciens* (referring to iatromechanists as a whole) 'did not even pay attention to the *organic structure* of the human body, which is the source of its main properties'.[40]

## II.

The next point I wish to make about materialist embodiment – my central point – is twofold. First, unlike the approach to the body that sees it as just so many funnels, pulleys and bellows, or that seeks to ascertain basic mechanical laws of the body and the rest of nature, the embodied-materialist approach is 'visceral', figuratively and literally. It is a materialism of vital fluids, touch, affects and passions – which, if we think of the role played by animal spirits in Cartesian neurophysiology, seems to have also been true of various forms of 'mechanism'.[41] But second, this approach, if it is to be legitimately qualified as 'materialist', necessarily has a *reductionist* component, in the sense of the ambition to explain a higher-level phenomenon X in terms of lower-level processes Y: 'where I read *soul* I replace it with *man* or *animal*'. Notice, however, that if 'soul' is reduced to 'animal', the reducing theory or level of explanation is still something *alive*. I will now describe these two contrasting dimensions – the visceral or spirited and the reductive – in more detail, before concluding with some remarks on how they hang together.

The 'visceral' character of early modern materialism takes several forms. One is its privileging of medicine, natural history and the other sciences of 'body' at the expense of physics and mathematics, which are usually presented as abstractions. In what is almost a trope, La Mettrie declares in *L'Homme-Machine* that 'Medicine alone could [effect a] change in the mind and in people's mores, with the Body.'[42] Whether it is problems of good and evil, our knowledge of the external world, or venerable philosophical topics such as life and death, La Mettrie beckons, not to the old motif of the doctor as philosopher or medicine and philosophy as 'sisters' (as in the Alexandrian saying *philosophia et medicina duae sorores sunt*[43]), but to the idea that 'the doctor knows best', even to the extent that 'the Doctor is the only Philosopher who deserves the praise of his country'[44] and by the same token, that it would be best 'for there to be only excellent Doctors to serve as Judges, for only they could distinguish the innocent from guilty criminals'.[45] Not just knowledge of the body or the soul but metaphysics itself gets suffused with this medical flavour: as the vitalist Fouquet writes in an important work on 'the clinic', 'not only is metaphysics not foreign to medicine, it belongs to a large extent to medicine. Medicine alone can extend and perfect metaphysics.'[46]

Another basic sense in which the materialist understanding of body is not restrictively physicalistic or mechanistic, in the sense of Baglivi or Boerhaave as quoted above, has to do with its usage or invocation of entities such as animal spirits, and its emphasis on affects and passions. However, this presents us with a problem of genre, for (philosophical) materialism seems to effortlessly move from (medical) materialism to traditional philosophical debate and back again, with body, soul, humours, spirits, passions and the like being 'located' in the interstices of all of these.

Consider anatomy itself. Inasmuch as it is a mechanistic, demystifying kind of project that reduces the body to parts and layers, we might think of it as appealing to the materialist, perhaps in a kind of post-Cartesian vein. Thus Guillaume Lamy's *Discours anatomiques* (1675) uses anatomy to rebut finalism and teleology in interpreting the structure of the human body. Such a project has its own radical allure,[47] but anatomy is also a problem for the materialist who does not want the body to be defined in exclusively structural, positional, static terms. From Bacon and Locke to La Mettrie and Diderot, despite the various differences between them, we can see a clearly expressed hostility or at least scepticism towards the idea that the anatomical perspective expresses a fundamental 'truth' about the body. In an early manuscript entitled 'Anatomia', which is diversely attributed to Locke or to the physician Thomas Sydenham, with whom Locke worked in the mid-to-late 1660s, we are told that

> All that Anatomie can do is only to shew us the gross and sensible parts of the body, or the vapid dead juices all which, after the most diligent search, will be noe more able to direct a physician how to cure a disease than how to make a man ... The anatomist

will hardly be enabled to tell us what changes any particular medicine either makes or receives in the body.[48]

Similarly, Bacon already criticizes anatomy for a lack of attention to what we might call 'function' or 'physiological process': 'In the inquiry which is made by Anatomy, I find much deficience: for they inquire of the *parts*, and their substances, *figures* and *collocations*; but they inquire not of the *diversities* of the *parts*, the *secrecies of the passages*, and the *seats* or *nestlings of the humours*'[49] – even if he also, and more influentially, wrote that 'Founding a real model of the world ... cannot be done without dissecting and anatomising the world.'[50]

The 'particularities' of certain medicines, the 'diversities' of the parts, the 'secrecies' of the passages; it is not so much the mystery of individuality that is being defended here, but the sense that the dynamic, flowing character of the living body cannot be grasped by 'anatomising' it. This is very much the sort of quarrel that Diderot has with more physicalistically inclined materialists like Helvétius (we could add Hobbes), who think that there is only one kind of cause, physical cause.[51] Diderot is sometimes described, rather anachronistically, as a supporter of self-organization (itself a chemically oriented theory of life), not because he fails to recognize the importance of selection processes in the evolution of life, but because he is concerned with the production of life rather than with its basic structure. He certainly did not worry about the sanctity of life; in his writings on painting he recommends painting from corpses and elsewhere approves of the idea that prisoners condemned to death could be used for scientific experimentation.

I mentioned animal spirits (*pneuma psychikon*, *spiritus animalis*) above. These appeared frequently in various medical treatises of the period, notably in the works of Descartes and the Oxford neuroanatomist Thomas Willis, who described them as 'the most subtle particles of matter', which flow through the spinal marrow into all nervous fibres; they are 'dispersed throughout the body, and as they are distilled in the brain and cerebellum they constitute the Sensitive Soul'.[52] That materialist embodiment is simultaneously vital and reductive – 'visceral', as it were – appears quite clearly in the case of animal spirits, which also usher in a new kind of determinism, summed up by thinkers like La Mettrie and later Sade as the claim that *I am determined by the blood that flows in my veins* (even if strictly speaking animal spirits were not the same as the blood itself, but were rather carried by it).

Early texts of the clandestine tradition display a recurrent usage of animal spirits within a radical, materialist setting and project. For instance, in Fontenelle's little-known subversive piece of 'neurological determinism', the *Treatise on the Freedom of the Soul*, which appeared anonymously in 1700 and was only attributed to him sixty years later; it achieved notoriety once it was republished in the 1743 clandestine collection *Nouvelles libertés de penser*, although it has recently been discovered that copies were burned in Paris in 1700 on order of the Parliament.

(Fontenelle was better known as the long-serving secretary of the Académie Royale des Sciences and author of sparkling works such as the 1686 *Conversations on the Plurality of Worlds*.) The core thesis of this treatise is that the 'soul' (for which we can read 'mind'[53]) thinks 'according to the dispositions of the brain', which are described in terms of animal spirits (the text appropriates sources including Malebranche and Willis). Conversely, any object that becomes an object of thought, including purely mental objects (*objets spirituels*), leaves traces in the brain – not a trace of the object itself but of its representation *qua* object of thought.

It is a specifically *embodied* form of determinism: Fontenelle insists from the outset that cerebral processes are not to be reduced to the events of the physical world as a whole: we are *neurologically* determined (again with ambiguities: is it more the material dispositions of my brain or the quantity and intensity of animal spirits in my nervous vessels?) rather than physically determined by the states of the universe as a whole. Indeed, to articulate a vision of mind and brain in which the two belong to a single embodied whole is radical enough, without specific determinist clauses being added; this was noted in the later eighteenth century by Joseph Priestley, another fellow-traveller of materialism:

> I rather think that the whole man is of some *uniform composition*, and that the property of *perception*, as well as the other powers that are termed *mental*, is the result (whether necessary or not) of such an organical structure as that of the brain[54]

What Priestley calmly discusses as 'uniform composition' was generally a rather scandalous idea. That my mental life is directly the result of the behaviour of animal spirits, implies that my actions are not free in any traditional sense, and further, that even the loftiest thoughts I think are themselves conditioned by an affective, passionate and indeed bodily reality – as we also are told at the beginning of the substantial entry on the passions in Diderot and D'Alembert's *Encyclopédie*:

> Tendencies, inclinations, desires and aversions of some intensity [*vivacité*], along with a blurred sensation of pleasure or pain, occasioned or accompanied by some sort of irregular movement of the blood and of the animal spirits, that is what we call passions. They can eradicate all use of freedom, state in which the soul is in some way rendered passive – hence the name passions.[55]

Hence it should not be a surprise that materialism was also viewed as a philosophy of embodiment in the worst sense! In 1758 the *Nouvelles ecclésiastiques*, an important Jansenist publication, said of Helvétius' work *De l'Esprit* that it should really have been entitled '*Of Diversely Organised Matter*, and even better ... *Of the Flesh, Particularly the Dirtiest, Most Impure Flesh*.'[56] This is not just a hostile projection of 'dirty' hedonism onto an austere metaphysics of matter, a scientism, a theory about mind and cognition. On the contrary, faced with the judgements of various sorts of idealists who felt quite strongly, like Auguste Comte in the nineteenth century, that 'materialism explains the higher in terms of the lower',[57] thinkers like La Mettrie or Diderot were quite happy to opt for 'base materialism'.

La Mettrie wrote several works either in Epicurean ethics broadly conceived or more specifically on pleasure,[58] and as discussed above, even his concept of the 'man-machine' is very much more of a 'desiring machine' than just a set of cogs, funnels and pulleys. Desire is presented in strong terms: 'if you are not content to excel in the art of pleasure, and crime and debauchery aren't strong enough for you, then filth and infamy remain yours for the glorious taking: wallow in it, as pigs do, and you will be happy like a pig'.[59] What La Mettrie leaves open here is whether it is a matter of our happiness being 'like' that of pigs in the sense that an opera lover is just as happy at the opera as a pig is, in filth, or if true happiness – materialist happiness, precisely – is *only* the latter kind.

Equally reductive but less dangerously immoral is Diderot's comment in his correspondence that 'there is a bit of testicle at the bottom of our most sublime sentiments, and our purest [feelings of] tenderness'.[60] And throughout his work, but especially in the two essays devoted to the metaphysics of the senses (the *Letter on the Blind* and the *Letter on the Deaf and Mute*) and his various aesthetic writings, Diderot insists on the primacy of touch, which he also describes as 'the most philosophical of senses', in direct opposition to classical doctrines in which sight of course deserved that honour; he deplores the fact that 'the hands are despised for their materialism'.[61]

Whether or not all of this is commendable, or characteristic of all forms of materialism, it does nevertheless indicate a strong presence of embodiment, implying that many forms of materialism prior to the later nineteenth century were not synonymous with 'physicalism'. Again, my claim is not that every form of materialism was necessarily non-mechanistic or fully centred on embodied beings; but that any genuine understanding of a doctrine that in its early modern forms, and well until the early twentieth century, was often described as voluptuous (in the literal sense of pleasurable), indicates that it is a far cry from what Friedrich Engels influentially described as 'mechanistic materialism'. Indeed, it may be that there was no such thing.[62] In the late nineteenth century, Engels contributed what became for a long time, and in different intellectual quarters, an official story about materialism:

> The materialism of the past century was predominantly mechanistic, because at that time ... only the science of mechanics ... had reached any sort of completion. ... For the materialists of the eighteenth century, man was a machine. This exclusive application of the standards of mechanics to processes of a chemical and organic nature – in which the laws of mechanics are also valid, but are pushed into the background by other, higher laws – constitutes the specific (and at that time, inevitable) limitation of classical French materialism.[63]

Scholarship has continued, particularly in the middle of the twentieth century, to insist that materialism was fundamentally *mechanistic materialism*, the reduction of all change to motion, and of all motion to mechanistic motion.[64] We have seen several reasons why this is false, ranging from the problem of defining mechanism itself with respect to the body, to the various ways in which materialism does not accept strictly mechanistic accounts of the body, whether it is because of its more fluid, passionate understanding of bodily function, or also its hedonism.

In contrast to this received view, we need to take seriously statements such as Diderot's 'of all the physical sciences to which one has attempted to apply geometry, it appears that there are none in which it penetrates less than in Medicine'.[65] A variety of kindred spirits such as Buffon, Maupertuis, La Mettrie and Bonnet (who rejected materialism as a metaphysics) concur in *denying* that the body is something that could be *mathematized*. This can be described as a kind of 'vital materialism'.[66] Yet at the same time this outlook is reductionist, as shown by the example of animal spirits and the theme of my being 'determined by the blood that flows in my veins'.

## III.

Recall Diderot's method in reading the manuscript of the Dutch scientist Hemsterhuis: 'wherever I read *soul* I replace it with *man* or *animal*'.[67] This is a venerable trait of materialisms going back at least as far as Lucretius. The anonymous, clandestine tract of the 1720s entitled *The Material Soul*, mentioned earlier, gives a very personal translation of a passage from *De rerum natura*, which becomes in this version, 'the soul is to the body as scent is to incense'.[68] To use Lockean language, the soul here becomes a secondary quality of the body. La Mettrie is a little more aggressive and also tilts the strategy towards eliminativism (or is it a reduction without elimination?): 'The soul is just a pointless term of which we have no idea and which a good mind should only use to refer to that part of us which thinks.'[69]

Contemporary terminology distinguishes between reductionism and eliminativism,[70] in the sense that there is a difference between the two following sorts of claims, both of which have a respectable materialist pedigree. One claim – eliminativism – holds that the soul and all of its properties that have been described and argued over from, say, Aristotle and Galen to Stahl and Swedenborg *does not exist* and indeed *none of these properties are real;* thus, what *is* real would be the brain, or the heart, or the stomach, and so on. Another claim – reductionism – holds that the soul (to stay with the same example) is indeed not something that exists in any traditional sense; but notice that when La Mettrie, in the above quotation, says we really should only use the word to refer to 'that part of us which thinks', he is not saying mental faculties do not exist but that we need to rethink what their 'seat' is, where they come from, and the extent to which they are independent from the rest of bodily processes, or not.[71] However, he is not suggesting a weaker thesis, which would be that soul/mind might be autonomous in some sense but could be 'defined in terms of' bodily processes.

As I will discuss below, the forms of materialist embodiment discussed here share a commitment to reductionism, but not to eliminativism (although the extent to which this distinction is clearly applicable to the texts at hand is unclear). Reductionism is a common trait of materialist philosophies from Lucretius to d'Holbach and onto Ludwig Büchner – a refusal of spiritual entities such as an immortal soul (without this necessarily having to entail atheism, as in the case of Priestley or earlier, mortalist physicians such as William Coward.[72] The German 'vulgar materialists' of the nineteenth century such as Büchner and Vogt constantly repeat that our present knowledge of the nervous system authorizes us to explain that the word 'soul' really just refers to such functions, including in Vogt's famously crude formulation that 'thought is to the brain what bile is to the liver or urine to the kidneys'.[73]

This fervid reductionism, however, is, once again, not always a matter of reducing a 'free', thinking substance to a fully determined, material entity. Early modern determinism was not necessarily of the sort that would become, by the late eighteenth century, 'Laplacean' determinism. It was, at the risk of over-using this word, what I have called an *embodied* determinism, that is, not a Laplacean vision in which the universe is composed of basic particles which could then be mapped out exhaustively in a mathematical form, but instead, a biologically and psychologically complex account of what it is to be an embodied agent, acting in the midst of a variety of causal chains, some fully internal, some external – like Hobbes's 'endeavours' or La Mettrie's vision of our state of desire as uneasiness as like 'a bird on the branch, always ready to take flight'.[74]

The biological make-up of an individual is an irreducible feature of that individual. As such, it can serve as a set of identifying features that pick out what is unique about her, but it is also a *limit* to her corrigibility. Helvétius had described to Diderot how severely he was punished for his earlier work *De l'Esprit*, with the consequence that he would 'rather die than write another line again'. Diderot responds in his 'Refutation of Helvétius' with a long tale about two cats he saw from his window, who fell from a roof: one died from the fall, the other got up, bruised and bloodied, and said to himself, 'I would rather die than ever climb on the roof again. What am I looking for there? A mouse that is not worth the tasty morsel I could get from my mistress, or steal from the cook.' However, as soon as the cat feels better, he climbs back up on the roof again. Just as the cat cannot but obey his own constitution and drives, similarly, Helvétius has no choice but to go on writing.[75]

All forms of materialism are deterministic, but in different ways: nothing compels the materialist to accept that the body, its fluids (including the animal spirits), its *organization* and the accompanying structure of the passions, is deterministic *just like* a simple machine. Unsurprisingly, a lot depends on how *causes* are understood, and how much weight they are meant to bear in both an ontology and an account of action. Thus it is quite possible, like Helvétius, d'Holbach or Hobbes before them, to hold that there is a fixed, stable and predictable relation between our sensory input, our mental life and consequently our 'temper' and our actions: 'As a being that is organized so as to think and to feel, you must feel pleasure or pain; you must love or hate in accordance with the way your organs are affected by the causes surrounding you or within you.'[76]

## IV.

We have seen that a major objection to materialism, or to any claim that it has a concept of embodiment, is the seeming absence of any 'centre' or 'self' within the system of living parts. To be sure, a number of materialists, who we might call 'vital materialists', are deeply concerned with providing an account of the organism – of the body as something other or more than a set of interlocking, solid parts, although this 'something other or more' is *not* understood as either 'soul' or 'vital force'. As titles of works such as *The Material Soul* convey, their goal is less to explain life in terms of the basic properties of matter (what we would today call physicalism) then to give a material basis for life and animation. If we no longer have an autonomous, immaterial soul controlling the motions of a mechanically defined body, we need a more unified – more 'immanent' – picture of vital activity. Ménuret observed this quite sharply, in his ambitious, programmatic article on the 'animal economy':

> This idea that the soul is the efficient cause of phenomena because it is the origin (*principe*) of vital motions is not an undeniable truth. It is true that if our body was a brute, inorganic machine, it would necessarily have to be directed by some other agent, maintaining and powering its motions. And I do not think the errors of the mechanists stem from anything else than the fact that they do not hold animals to be living, organized composites.[77]

And we saw Ménuret earlier arguing for a more complex, nuanced, almost overlapping relation between 'machine' and 'body' in structural terms than most of our historiographies would generally recognize. Here he is describing the nature of living beings as a type of 'composite' which cannot just be explained in terms of either its constituent parts or its motions (as in Hobbes's definition in the introduction to the *Leviathan* that 'Life is but a motion of limbs'[78]). However, this 'living and organized composite' – in other words, what we would call the organism or, in Ménuret's vocabulary, the 'animal economy' – might still be a 'meat machine', in the sense that it lacks a 'self', a 'historicity', both of which imply a certain kind of unity.

What does it mean for us to be able to look into a person or animal's eyes and sense, as Daniel Dennett has put it, that 'someone is home?'[79] Can the materialist sense of embodiment comprise something more than a history of impulses, drives and instincts, as is often claimed (typically by people who think that if materialism is not just a crude variant of mechanism, its way of accounting for 'life and mind' must necessarily reduce these to the above sorts of factors)? Consider the following portrayal of materialism – which comes from a sophisticated treatment of Diderot:

> Materialism as a working philosophy, used as a tool in the scientific investigation of the material universe, is appropriate and highly effective. Intended for the objective analysis and description of the world of externals, it yields disastrous results when applied to the inner, subjective world of human nature, human thought, and human emotions.[80]

As we have seen, there is something gravely wrong with this picture. Soul, mind, intentionality need not be denied in favour of body, although the materialist has a variety of strategies at her disposal. One strategy – eliminativism broadly construed – is to deny that there is such a thing as the soul. On this view, irritability and other basic physiological properties account for the visible phenomena that we attribute, falsely, to a purely mental agent, a 'sailor in the ship' of the body.[81] Another strategy – reductionism of the more mechanistic and less embodied sort – is to say like Hobbes and Hartley, that 'soul' and its processes are real inasmuch as they can be assimilated to or explained in terms of basic mechanical laws (d'Holbach: 'our minds are subject to the same physical laws as material bodies'[82]).

It is not that the embodied materialist denies that our mental processes are subject to basic laws of physics (although there was very little talk of such laws at the time, d'Holbach's confidence notwithstanding). Rather, the corresponding form of reductionism she defends, the *embodied* version, when presented with a phenomenon such as the sense of self, or appetite, or desire, does not look for strictly mechanistic ways of explaining it but rather seeks to embed it in a general account, employing medical, biological and physiological perspectives on what it is to be that sort of living agent. This is what the materialist physician Abraham Gaultier means when he writes that there is no soul separate from the body, because the soul is simply the body and its workings.[83] It is also the kind of reductionism at work in Diderot's assertion, not that there is no soul, but rather that 'I challenge [you] to explain anything without the body.'[84]

If materialism is not merely mechanistic (or even mechanistic at all, or is such in an expanded, fluid sense far removed from Engels's definition), but instead seeks to articulate an *embodied* account of mental life, the will and action, that does not mean it will provide an account of intentionality or 'first-person' states of experience that will satisfy everyone. Yet such states may in fact be nothing other than certain kinds of narratives or projections. Diderot himself describes the brain as both a book – a source on which information is imprinted, like a mass of sensing, living wax – but also a reader, and ultimately a book 'which reads itself'.[85] Conversely, if our nervous system produces such states, it gives them a kind of reality.

What does it mean to be an 'embodied reductionist'? That is, if there is a materialist form of embodiment, yet all materialists are reductionists of one sort or another, it follows that there is a particular sense of reduction in which the mental is reduced to, or explained in terms of something bodily rather than the basic physical facts about the universe. What does this difference imply and entail? If we think back to the judgement quoted above on how materialism may be useful as a kind of handmaiden of scientific activity, but produces 'disastrous results' when applied to the mind, the person or selfhood, we should be able to see a difference.

Granted, some materialists (such as Hobbes, d'Holbach and Hartley) think that mental life is itself simply a species of motion. Others, speaking about action, motivation and desire rather than about mechanical versus organismic properties of entities, describe us as if we were no better than pigs wallowing in filth. But where are these 'disastrous results' when materialism turns to the inner life? Just because the materialist cannot go along with the idea that 'the mind does not use the body, but fulfills itself through it while at the same time transferring the body outside of physical space'[86] does not have to mean that materialist bodies are just piles of flesh, mere 'aggregates' in the language of the period. After all, living bodies do possess a variety of senses of their inner life, including what Patricia Churchland has elegantly called 'awareness of visceral circumstance'.[87] Leibniz himself entertains this possibility in the *New Essays Concerning Human Understanding* (1704), suggesting that 'something does happen in the soul in response to … the internal motions of the viscerae',[88] perhaps in response to Descartes's remarks in the *Sixth Meditation* on the fact that I have a 'personal' experience of bodily processes including 'twitching in the stomach';[89] but Leibniz quickly adds that the soul is actually unaware of such movements.

That we can have awareness of 'visceral circumstance' does not mean that the materialist sense of embodiment is restricted to the spirits, the humours and the guts. It simply implies that we have what D. M. Armstrong terms 'a route of epistemological access' to our own body which others lack, and thereby also to our mind.[90] D'Holbach seems actually quite sensitive to this: 'I can only be aware or assured of my own existence by the motions I experience in myself;'[91] 'to be what we call intelligent, one must have ideas, thoughts, volitions; one must have organs; to have organs, one must have a body'.[92] But such routes or pathways of access to 'one's self' are not themselves foundational for the materialist and must be *explained*: 'there remains a genuine obligation on the materialist's part to give some account of the subjectivity or … point-of-view-ness of the mental'.[93]

Is there such a thing as subjectivity for the materialist? If there is, it will be essentially synonymous with embodiment. Dreams, hallucinations, out-of-body experiences and challenges to embodiment such as phantom limb syndrome are always traced back – for the materialist – to the interrelations of brain and body, desire and affect. I have argued that the materialist form of embodiment is not just the reduction of body to an entity in space among other entities. Yet at the same time, the materialist body is not the virtual, phantasmagoric body, nor the extraordinarily intimate and private body dear to phenomenologists. It has a unity and a continuity *qua* organism, but it is a unity and continuity which do not rest on a foundational subjectivity, a 'me-ness' which the inquirer or the scientist cannot grasp. In addition, as we saw with respect to mechanism and reductionism, the materialist does not fear the 'componential' gaze upon the body. In response to the assertion of the concrete irreducibility of a living, experiential body, the materialist can always reply that a body is 'only *provisionally* simple; it has remained undecomposed until now, but tomorrow may yield to a new means of analysis'.[94]

## Acknowledgements

Thanks to John Sutton and Brian Keeley for their advice.

# 10 VISUALIZING MONSTERS: ANATOMY AS A REGULATORY SYSTEM

## Touba Ghadessi

This essay considers the constructive intellectual system revealed by the method-ical examination of monsters' visible anomalies during the early modern period. The images and texts that resulted from the study of monsters provided a model of anatomical knowledge that became a valid alternative to the normal ideals promoted by anatomists like Andreas Vesalius, who upheld the idea that truth lied in practice-based processes and their textual and visible translations. The ways in which monstrous bodies were explored echoed these practices and thus reinforced the epistemological maquette proposed by early modern dissections of normalized human bodies.

The question of 'monsters' engaged several fields of knowledge in the sixteenth century: medical traditions from ancient and medieval to early modern sources; theological disputes from antiquity to the Middle Ages; mythological writings from ancient authors and their fantastic adaptations in the Middle Ages; and finally, popular culture informed by selected samples of medical, theological and mythological themes. As medical inquiries grew stronger during the sixteenth and seventeenth centuries – fuelled by first-hand anatomical observations – the second, third and fourth components that defined the monstrous grew weaker in published works.[1] The causes of monstrousness were not understood solely as the results of the opposition between devilish and divine forces, or only as the product of sympathetic magic during pregnancy. Increasingly, methodical expla-nations were used to shed light on the origins of physical deviance. Ultimately, in the nineteenth century, the acknowledged science of teratology emerged, and was explained and defined by Isidore Geoffroy Saint-Hilaire (1805–61).[2]

Fascination with monsters was a part of sixteenth- and seventeenth-century European court culture.[3] Culturally and visually, physically deformed individu-als were prized because their anatomical rarity elicited a wondrous reaction in the minds of early modern audiences. Their marvellous characteristics turned them into collectible objects and when collecting the actual monster was not feasible, images and essays about said monster served as an acceptable replacement. Because they were seen as theological omens and curiosities of nature, attention was paid to documenting the specific anatomical features that made these people into objects worthy of courtly attention. Consequently, their representations held subtexts that highlighted these qualities, so as to justify the interest given by the educated elite to nature's anomalies. The systematization of anatomical particulars provided early modern philosophers, scholars, doctors, scientists and courtiers with a grounded method for the validation of monstrous bodies as new bodies of knowledge.

The early modern development of anatomical knowledge was at its peak in the middle of the sixteenth century with the publication of Andreas Vesalius's *De humani corporis fabrica* (1543) and its emphasis on a normative body.[4] Following the drive for a regulated body, many studies and images of monsters adopted these normalizing standards to examine and describe physical anomalies. In doing so, they presented readers and viewers with visual testimonies of observations akin to anatomical inquiries.[5] The texts related to and the representations of these abnormal beings dramatically highlighted the flaws that made them monstrous, but did so in a meticulous fashion, thus exhibiting their deformed bodies as alluring objects of study. Falling between the search for general rules in science and the need to deal with actual anomalies, works on monsters were the sites of a conflation between the two. The language adopted in these treatises and images allowed the 'irregular' to become familiar and effectively tamed the anatomically unusual.

As new scientific methods developed, the importance of the senses grew and visual representations occupied an increasingly important role. Thus, the primacy of the sense of vision in the quest for truth infused dissection practices. Before Vesalius, Berengario da Carpi (1460–1530) established the importance of the *anathomia sensibilis*, a type of anatomy in which the senses play a central role. Vision in particular served as ultimate proof of knowledge.[6] Through his commentaries, Berengario implemented an epistemological shift in the demonstration, acquisition and transmission of knowledge by insisting that true knowledge was mostly gained by seeing rather than by reading or hearing.[7] As a result, public dissections became associated with a discourse related to true knowledge, as they occurred in a locale meant to enhance visual access. The audience – composed of anatomists, notable men or artists – of a dissection occurring in an anatomical theatre witnessed the truth of the knowledge that was being obtained from accessing the inside of the body. To a degree, the focus on the *inside* of the individual body protected the *surface* of the broader social body from being overly scrutinized, to say nothing of being disaggregated, weighed, measured and found wanting. That is, because the body functioned as a site where the proof of the visible and scientific fact at once constituted and propagated one another, so too could it effectively naturalize the production and enforcement of norms that emerged not from the corpse but from the audience.

The acquisition of knowledge about the normative human body acquired through dissections could be and was circulated through the production of images, this at a time when the ascendancy of perspective had newly secured the truthfulness, verisimilitude and objectivity of visual representation. What we see emerging, then, is a nexus in which science and art combine to effectively transmute physiognomy into physiology, a move that in turn facilitated the application of anatomical knowledge and the staging of public dissections to the study of *visibly* non-normative (i.e. monstrous) bodies. Perhaps ironically, superimposing the scientific authority upon which human dissection depended onto the study of monsters meant that the collection of monsters and/or representations of them expanded beyond mere curiosity or fascination with their marvellous characteristics (though this remained, as I discuss further below). Rather, these pursuits became tantamount to discovering the truth about monsters and monstrousness.[8] Again, this derived from the primacy of the visual. Textual descriptions of monsters emphasized graphic traits for the reader, and, along with visual representations, were meant to be both titillating and instructive. Indeed, as scientific interest in monsters' anatomy lent representations of monsters an element of documentary authenticity, one might say that these representations stood in as visual dissections, not only of monsters but of monstrousness itself, making their wondrousness and deformities accessible to multiple viewers who felt comforted, via their sense of sight, that they were presented with accurate and true knowledge.

Monsters only gradually became systematic objects of inquiry. One of the most important characteristics of the early modern discourse on monsters is the multiplicity of sources that touch upon the subject. The diversity of visual representations and textual descriptions that invoke monsters ensures that the study of these is proportionally complex and multifaceted. Typically, various authors and publishers reproduced mythical images and just slightly rewrote accounts found in ancient texts. In addition, however, a great number of new images and texts dealing with recently-discovered monsters were produced, thus pushing the interest in the monstrous further. These accounts serve as a testimony to the changing understanding of the relation between Man and the Divine, as defined by Nature, and provide information regarding the place of the marvellous, of the curious and of the scientific within the early modern conception of the world.[9]

Even though the interest in the marvellous, the rare, the curious and the inexplicable did not wane, rational scientific accounts added a new component to this pursuit. A vacillation between popular imagination and systematic, medicalized explanations actively structured the public's and the experts' attention to and understanding of monsters from the early modern period and beyond. For instance, the story of the monster of Ravenna in the early 1600s touched the imagination of many people, from Florence to Munich.[10] Fascination with physical deformities was echoed across periods. In the nineteenth century monstrous bodies, which were often delineated with medical terms such as 'pathological', served as references to the given norms of life, yet maintained their fantastic appeal.[11] These different understandings of monsters were in fact not in competition, but rather complemented each other. As L. Daston and K. Park have argued, it would be false to assume a clear teleological evolutionary schema that exclusively categorizes monsters according to the time period. For instance it would be misleading to claim that the medieval monster was seen solely as a sign of theological superstition; or that the early modern monster was understood only as a source of delight and pleasure; and that, suddenly, in the late sixteenth and seventeenth centuries, the monster became an object of medical and scientific inquiry. Rather, these epistemologies tend to overlap – often in socially or culturally expedient ways. This is particularly evident in early modern (re)configurations in which the monster began to comprise an alternate body of knowledge that served, in part, to strengthen anatomical standards, such as those put forth by Vesalius. The normalizing discourse that framed anatomical inquiries – especially in the wake of Vesalius's *De fabrica* – turned the slightest deviation into an object of inquiry. Such deviations provided the exceptions needed to reinforce the structure of a new canon: departures from the norm that served strategically to delineate the boundaries of the very norms beyond which they were doomed to remain.

In 1543, Vesalius published the first edition of *De humani corporis fabrica* (*De fabrica*), a work that combined artistic originality with radical anatomical inquiries. A compendium entitled the *Epitome* was published in tandem with the *De fabrica* and was meant to give an introduction and a topographical approach to the novice in medicine.[12] Although the significance of this publication was great for subsequent inquiries about the human body, anatomical treatises had existed prior to its publication. While the paradigmatic significance of the treatise remains undeniable, ascribing any kind of absolute authority to Vesalius's text is restrictive. The first writings on human anatomy were part of the *Corpus hippocratum* that circulated in Greece around 400 BC.[13] About a hundred years later and for approximately two centuries during the Hellenistic period, actual human dissections occurred, allowing the 'black box' of knowledge to be opened and reveal its secrets.[14] Yet, in spite of this early foray into an empirical experience of the human body, it is the imprint of Galen of Pergamum (130–200) that influenced the transmission of anatomical knowledge from antiquity to the sixteenth century. Prior to becoming the physician of Emperor Marcus Aurelius (121–80), Galen worked in a gladiator school and treated severe wounds, which he used as 'windows into the human body'.[15] While justifying his thoughts on nature and, consequently, his inquiries and writings on the human body through Aristotelian teleological philosophy and empirical methods of investigation, Galen might never have actually practised human dissections.[16] As a result, his descriptions of human anatomy often lacked practical accuracy and the mistakes presented in his *On the Usefulness of the Parts of the Human Body* (*c.* 175) were repeated over time, perpetuating anatomical errors.[17] Human dissections were officially reintroduced into Western teaching practice at the end of the thirteenth century in Bologna;[18] but the logical confrontation of the visual knowledge of the body with the erroneous Galenic textual tradition did not occur overtly until Vesalius addressed it in his *De fabrica*.

Vesalius emphasized direct observation, made this practice part of the curriculum of academic teaching and finally challenged the hegemony of the Galenic tradition.[19] A student of Guinterius Andernacus (1505–74) and Jacobus Sylvius (1478–1555) in Paris in 1533, Vesalius performed dissections that broke with tradition: he eliminated the varied channels that stood between the student of anatomy and the immediate knowledge the dissected body proffered. This methodology allowed him to appreciate the numerous errors made by Galen and to challenge the textual basis of medieval medicine.[20] *De fabrica* not only changed the ways science and anatomy were taught and learned, but it also provided a strong paradigm for anatomical illustrations that would last approximately two hundred years.[21]

In *De fabrica*, Vesalius established a new way to anatomize and made clear from the outset that this treatise and his inquiries were distinct from his predecessors.[22] Notably, in spite of his insistence on an empirical examination and understanding of individual bodies, Vesalius still believed in the principle of a normative body.[23] The Vesalian thrust towards a normative ideal – followed for centuries by various anatomists and physicians – was one that purposefully did not take the physically deviant into account.[24] This was not the case, however, for everyone working within the Vesalian paradigm.

Concomitant with intellectual and scientific developments pertaining to an ideal human body, attention to anatomical irregularities grew from a marginal interest to a defined science. In fact, awareness of physical deviance was fed by the normative ideals promoted by Vesalius and adopted by his followers. The Vesalian body became the new standard 'body of knowledge', and departures from its strict norms fuelled interest in anatomical deviance by creating a parallel scientific pursuit that used the heuristic tools Vesalius had publicly asserted.

Gradually, during the early modern period, a medical lens was added to popular and theological beliefs and monsters began to be studied in a rigorous and systematic scientific manner. Early modern emphasis on empirical examination was employed to explain both normative and unusual natural phenomena; anatomical deviance and its visual symptoms did not escape this pragmatic scrutiny.[25] The intellectual strategies that controlled the understanding of ordinary bodies found resonance in the investigation of extraordinary physical attributes. A few attempts at listing extraordinary humans, animals, organic matters and fantastic beings and stories were made throughout the sixteenth century; the first of such attempts may have been in 1503 with the publication of Jakob Mennel's *De signis portentis, atque prodigiis*. In 1566, Pierre Boaistuau (*c.* 1520–66) published his *Histoires prodigieuses*, in which he combined stories from Greek and Latin classical authors, imaginary biblical occurrences and fantastic animals, with actual congenital diseases.[26] Even though Boaistuau's organizational scheme came close to an actual classification, there was no direct attempt at defining categories. He provided verbal and visual descriptions and an elaboration on the idea of the bizarre and the imaginary, but did not demonstrate a scientific causality for the existence of unusual beings. In addition, the title, preface, dedication and the entirety of the text were in French, rather than Latin. This choice is interesting as Boaistuau meant to target an elite audience; however, the fact that the book is dedicated to a scientific novice, the noble lord Jean Rieux, Seigneur d'Assérac, may justify the vernacular use over the scientific Latin. The preface, though, left no doubt as to the courtly pretensions of the text and the illustrations, through which Boaistuau intended to flatter his patron:

> Your Highness, among all things that may be seen under the skies, nothing touches the human spirit more, nothing pleases the senses more, nothing horrifies more, nothing generates more admiration or terror to creatures than the monsters, prodigies and abominations in which we see the errors of Nature or only assumed, reversed, mutilated and shortened, but (in addition) we discover most often a secret judgment and scourge of God's wrath, through the object of things that are presented, which make us feel the violence of his justice, which is so bitter that we have to look inside ourselves and hit our consciousness with a hammer, peel away at our own vices, be appalled by our wrong-doings, particularly when we read in sacred and secular stories that sometimes the elements were heralds, trumpets, ministers and executors of God's justice.[27]

Shortly after the publication of *Les histoires prodigieuses*, Ambroise Paré (1510–90) wrote and edited several editions of *Des monstres et prodiges*, first published in 1573. Though also written in the vernacular French, the first page of the twenty-fifth book established the more rigorous claims being made by Paré. Paré was fully aware of the risks of using the vernacular French to write a book on scientific or medical matters. In fact, in the preface, he insists that his decision to write in French is a conscious one, meant to ennoble the practice of medicine by enriching it with the knowledge of things such as monsters.[28] In addition, unlike Boaistuau, whom he cites as a provider of some of his case studies, Paré provides a definition of monsters and distinguished the various terms he used:

> Monsters are things that appear outside of the course of Nature (and are most often signs of some misfortune to come) such as a child who is born with one arm only, another with two heads, and other limbs that are out of the ordinary. Prodigies are things that happen against Nature, such as a woman giving birth to a snake, or to a dog, or to anything that goes against Nature ... The mutilated are the blinds, one-eyed

people, hunchbacks, lame people, or people having six fingers or toes, or less than five
fingers or toes, or fingers and toes joined together, or arms that are too short, or noses
that are set too deep like those with crooked noses, or lips that are big and reversed ...
or anything that goes against Nature.[29]

Paré's work fell within a trend that spoke to the growing interest in natural marvels. Indeed, the increase of published works dealing with medical cases in the
sixteenth century signalled the rising interest of laymen and men of sciences for
published accounts of various wonders, including monsters.[30] His many illustrations deal with various monsters, whose medical validity varied from conjoined
twins, to limbless individuals, and finally to imaginary hybrid creations.

Through the preface and through the rest of the *livre*, the reader was presented with case studies accompanied by illustrations, therefore with a guarantee
that the work at hand dealt with true knowledge. Paré's training as a barber-
surgeon, his experience while practising surgery during various battles and his
position as the official surgeon to several kings of France certainly determined
his medical view of the body and its possible variances. Furthermore, after Henri
II's fatal tournament accident on 30 June 1559, Paré met Vesalius, who came
to Paris with the hope that he could heal the dying king.[31] Undoubtedly, the
practiced-based methods of the famous anatomist influenced the royal surgeon.
While *Des monstres et prodiges* is not considered a strict medical assessment of
the pathologies that led to anatomical deformities, it was a step towards medi-
calizing the discourse on monsters and using them as an alternate body of
anatomical knowledge.

Notwithstanding his medical assertions, Paré upheld his belief that monsters also represented what happened to those who faced God's wrath.[32] In fact,
Paré played with the etymological origins of the term 'monster' to support his
theological assumptions. The origin of the word 'monster' is found in the Latin
*mostrare*, to show.[33] Paré himself discussed the monster as 'a being that one
shows'.[34] One of the most famous instances described by Paré was that of conjoined twin sisters born in Verona in 1475. These sisters 'were carried through
several cities in Italy' by their poor parents who thus earned a significant amount
of money thanks to the 'people who were very eager to see this new spectacle of
nature'.[35] The essence of the monster as a creature 'meant to be shown' was here
presented as beneficial since it relieved the family from financial stress. It also
reinforced the concept of the monstrous body needing viewership to exist and
the importance placed on the sense of sight to assert the truth of the spectacle of
knowledge being witnessed. In addition to its ties to the verb *mostrare*, the noun
*mostro* has also been related to the word *monere*, to warn.[36] Hence Paré, Boaistuau and Conrad Lycosthenes (1518–61) among others included the notion of
warning in their definition of monsters. In the same vein, most authors in the
sixteenth century saw monsters as a sign of *remonstrance* from God. Tracing the

etymological route attached to the word monster shows that systematic methods of inquiry used to understand that monsters as phenomena outside the normal course of nature co-existed in time and thought with theological understanding of monsters as signs of divine wrath or omens.[37]

One of the first early modern authors to have provided a more strictly conceived scientific treatise on monsters was Fortunio Liceti (1577–1657) in 1616. Liceti, a physician from Padua, expressed his disbelief in monsters as portentous theological signs and insisted on their importance as living beings that expressed certain truths of nature through their unusual physical appearance.[38] By doing so, Liceti also privileged the sense of sight as a means to acquire true knowledge, since it was the outer appearance of these individuals and creatures that justified the scientific investigation of their bodies. Liceti saw monsters as beings whose deformities elicited the most wonder and the most admiration; he was thus not surprised that men were so intrigued by them and sought to understand their origins.[39] Liceti abandoned the idea of the monster as an ominous divine sign and, rather, justified its existence not as mistake made by nature, but as a necessary difference in the face of adverse conditions. His work demonstrates that monsters in the seventeenth century began to be seen as variations of nature, as indispensable contrasts to the normative body described by Vesalius, and as valid epistemological alternatives. The approach adopted by Liceti exemplifies the construction of notions such as abnormal, deviant or pathological by men. The categories defined by men and assigned to nature are taken much later by Michel Foucault (1926–84), who explained early modern scientific difference. In his project, Foucault explored the inception of monsters not as simple errors of nature, but rather as a Liceti-type of constructed ideals. According to this conceptual model, monsters became required deviations. These deviations would in turn allow nature to preserve its continuum by allowing difference to exist not in *opposition*, but *parallel* to its own course:

> The monster ensures in time, and for our theoretical knowledge, a continuity that, for our everyday experience, floods, volcanoes, and subsiding continents confuse space ... On the basis of the power of the continuum held by nature, the monster ensures the emergence of difference. This difference is still without law and without any well-defined structure; the monster is the root-stock specification, but it is only a sub-species itself in the stubbornly slow stream of history ... Thus, against the background of the continuum, the monster provides an account, as though in caricature, of the genesis of differences[40]

Liceti's adherence to an Aristotelian view of nature, as well as the defined categories he gave his reader turned this work into the result of a physician's gaze upon the explainable anomalies of nature.[41]

Increasingly, the tension between monsters as medical objects of inquiry and monsters as theological warnings became more palpable. While its resolution

– if resolution there needed to be – did not imply the foregoing of one idea for the other, the position taken by anatomists and scientists for the stronger authority of methodical examination often settled the conflict, once again echoing the rationalization of knowledge, truth, and direct observation championed by Vesalius. Realdo Colombo (1510–59) explored the anatomical anomalies of otherwise normative human beings in the fifteenth book of his *De re anatomica* published posthumously in 1559.[42] Colombo took on Vesalius's position as the chair of anatomy at the University of Padua; his medically-guided approach to the study of monsters is thus no surprise since he was teaching anatomy and was immersed in medical treatises during his explorations of anomalous bodies.[43] Unlike Paré, Lycosthenes or Boaistuau, Colombo never mentioned monsters as portentous signs; he did not attack those who had treated them as such, but he purposefully omitted any reference to the prophetic dimension of monsters. One could infer that Colombo's treatise, by virtue of its deliberate exclusion, was one of the few and first teratological treatises that dealt with monsters as pathological anomalies *only*.[44] The dissections that Colombo performed, particularly that of a hermaphrodite, turned his fifteenth book into more than a series of illustrated case studies – it made him and, by proxy, his readers witnesses to the anatomy of monstrous bodies as valid bodies of knowledge.[45]

In spite of the numerous avenues opened by treatises on monsters on the medical, the theological or the philosophical front, an exact and universal name for the science of studying monsters did not appear until the nineteenth century. Following in the footsteps of his father who was a renowned zoologist, Isidore Geoffroy Saint-Hilaire (1805–61) wrote a treatise dealing with monsters in 1832, titled *Traité de tératologie*.[46] From the onset of his book, Saint-Hilaire positions teratology as a distinct and separate science from physiology and related sciences. He confirms the validity of studying monsters, not only as a branch of pathology or philosophical anatomy, but also as an independently justifiable inquiry.[47] Saint-Hilaire denounces previous authors, who purport to study monsters while constantly attaching them to different branches of zoology or embryology. Saint-Hilaire's work builds upon centuries of inquiries; nevertheless, he validates the study of monsters as a uniquely scientific endeavour by not only attributing an exclusive technical term to the study of monsters, but also by renouncing any kind of supernatural claim pertaining to the formation or presence of physically deviant individuals. Though Saint-Hilaire was aware of the major leap he was proposing, he was nonetheless certain about the legitimacy of his claim.[48] He finalized the numerous attempts made before him by offering an exhaustive study of teratology based on his ultimate goal: to understand the modification of the normal order.[49]

Ultimately, Saint-Hilaire's scientific study was the result of numerous intellectual confluences, many of which were born of the original wonder felt in the presence of monsters or in front of their representations.[50] This wondrous feeling was explored and exploited during the early modern period, as exemplified in collections of curiosities amassed by princely, regal and scientific collectors alike and in the portrayals of monsters found in those collections. The anatomical experience and the revealing of the true knowledge of the body during dissection was prolonged and refined by the collection.[51] Further, anatomical collections and the collection of curiosities often carried the stamp of truth beyond the theatre because of their association with the visual experience of dissection. For instance, as one of the most eminent figures in Bologna, the naturalist Ulisse Aldrovandi (1522–1605) gathered a personal collection of over twenty thousand paintings, objects, plants and prints that were housed in a public studio as well as in a private museum in his home.[52] In 1595, Aldrovandi described his collection as follows:

> Today in my microcosm, you can see more than 18,000 different things, among which 7,000 plants in fifteen volumes, dried and pasted, 3,000 of which I had painted as if alive. The rest – animals terrestrial, aerial and aquatic, and other subterranean things such as earths, petrified sap, stones, marbles, rocks, and metals – amount to as many pieces again. I have paintings made of a further 5,000 natural objects – such as plants, various sorts of animals, and stones – some of which have been made into woodcuts. These can be seen in fourteen cupboards, which I call the Pinacotheca.[53]

Establishing specific *tabulae* to organize his entire collection, Aldrovandi emphasized the different links between nature and knowledge in his writings as much as in the physical organization of his collection.[54] In addition, in accordance with an Aristotelian system of thought, Aldrovandi stressed the importance of direct observation in order to better grasp the relationship between natural philosophy, medical knowledge and sensory experience.[55] Aldrovandi's interest in anatomical and pathological rarities comes as no surprise, since monstrous individuals allowed curious scientists to apply at once their medical, natural, and sensory knowledge.

Just as dissections served as epistemological maquettes for the knowledge of a normalized body, portraits of monsters provided the best sensorial model to transmit knowledge of anatomically deviant bodies, by making them visible. Again, we see the convergence of modes of display – here, artistic portraiture and scientific illustrations – within the visual register allows these portraits to celebrate and validate monsters' anatomical difference to assert the exhibited monstrous body as proof of its physical existence, which resides in and is produced through a discourse based on sensory experience *qua* truth.

Portraits of monsters, however, were still distinct from their engraved and printed equivalent in treatises on monsters or single leaf *avvisi*.[56] Whereas a treatise such as Paré's dealt with images of monsters as additional evidence for their textual assertions, portraits stood as independent visual creations. They were neither mere traditional portraits, nor systematic scientific illustrations, nor solely *mirabilia*. For instance, the idealization – and at times allegorization – that was present in portraits of monsters distinguished them from scientific records like Liceti's, which focused on cataloguing physical traits. While comparable in subject matter to many visual documents that were produced in the context of collecting scientific evidence, portraits of the physically deviant integrated an aspect that was absent from these visual records: namely, they highlighted a tension between idealization and likeness specific to the genre of portraiture.[57] In addition, they were independent from textual explanations, as they inherently incorporated a visual subtext meant to serve as scientific truth. Furthermore, the intentional pictorial language employed in these portraits (the compositions, references and formal elements) was that used in canonical court portraiture, in spite of the *Wunderkammer*-quality of their subjects. Portraits of monsters were not mere extensions of curiosity collections. Rather, they existed as a combination of two worlds: they blended visual court conventions with those of the cabinet of curiosity.

Understandably, the popularity of monsters within scientific circles and court culture was the main driving force behind the production and the possession of portraits of monsters. Since these portraits were painted to resemble the authentic sitters, the motivation behind their production could be linked to the fascination with actual deviant bodies. Because monsters had become an object of scientific inquiry, their deviance became circumscribed by and within a normative discourse, which in turn allowed the elite to collect and be fascinated by deviant bodies without that fascination itself seeming deviant. Rather, their interest was attributed to an interest in science itself and to the prestige associated with rarity as codified and established through science, which ensured that collecting monsters was not debased or frivolous, but a suitable pursuit. However, portraits added another dimension to the mere wonder experienced when viewing a monstrous body or a monstrous thing/being in a collection. They called upon the conventional senses of the viewer who recognized the setting – an official courtly portrait – but could not directly associate him or herself with the subject. Akin to staring into distorted mirrors, portraits of monsters afforded both wonder and uncertainty to the viewer, who was taught to trust his or her sight. While the exploration of the monstrous body could provide scientific knowledge, the official framing of the portrait – literally and figuratively – made this body of knowledge a vexed one. These portraits played with the anatomical *nosce te ipsum* by questioning it; they positioned the viewer in a visually doubtful scenario where inserting him or herself inside this independent visual conversation became increasingly uncomfortable.[58]

By incorporating monstrous subjects into the controlled vocabulary of ana-tomical knowledge, anatomists, artists and early modern scientists not only provided an alternative way of understanding human bodies, but they also expanded what constituted cultural conformity. Ultimately, the resulting texts and images dealing with bodies of monsters speak to the lack of linear cultural hegemony and highlight inevitable intellectual exchanges inevitable during a time of self-fashioning and scientific developments.

The fascination with monstrous bodies was articulated through a vocabulary of difference that allowed norms to define themselves against their own bound-aries. The reciprocity between monsters and normal humans grew within a discourse of social regulation and scientific discoveries. The subsequent treatises on monsters intervened in this discourse as active visual markers of such interac-tions and the subjects of these works confronted the viewers with the reality of their monstrous anomalies and with the actuality of their human presence.

# 11 ANATOMY, NEWTONIAN PHYSIOLOGY AND LEARNED CULTURE: THE *MYOTOMIA REFORMATA* AND ITS CONTEXT WITHIN GEORGIAN SCHOLARSHIP

Craig Ashley Hanson

Weak tho' I am of limb, and short of sight,
Far from a lynx, and not a giant quite;
I'll do what Mead and Cheselden advise,
To keep these limbs, and to preserve the eyes.
Not to go back, is somewhat to advance,
And men must walk at least before they dance.
  – Alexander Pope, *The First Epistle of the First Book of Horace Imitated*
  (1737)

In these familiar lines from the *Imitations of Horace*, Alexander Pope references two of Georgian London's most famous medical men, Richard Mead and William Cheselden. Both were familiar to anyone knowledgeable of science, medicine or fashionable society in the 1730s, when the poem was written. Pope consulted each of them, and the lines suggest the intimate, advisory character of the period's medical practice. In an age when medical intervention counted for little in terms of combating illness, good advice was often the best one could hope for.[1]

If not quite relegated to obscurity, Mead and Cheselden perhaps require some introduction today. As physician to King George II, Richard Mead (1673–1754) was an influential figure within the Royal Society, a respected patron of scholarship and an important collector of art and antiquities. William Cheselden (1688–1752) was one of the most celebrated surgeons of his day, well known for his skill in dealing with cataracts and his swiftness in cutting for the stone. Both men attended Pope in the final weeks just before his death in 1744. The poem, as well as the realities of Pope's deteriorating health, upholds these medical practitioners for their counsel; and the personal refrains of the poet's life bear out even more: friendship.[2]

However, in addition to the esteem Mead and Cheselden garnered in terms of medical practice, each could also boast substantive anatomical achievements, each man's subsequent success at least in part depending upon this initial basis of professional credibility. For Cheselden, the surgeon, the connection is understandable. For Mead, a respected physician celebrated for his refinement and mastery of ancient theory, it may appear less obvious. While Cheselden will resurface towards the end of this essay, it is on Mead's relationship to anatomy that I want to concentrate here. Accordingly, I explore his support of the second edition of William Cowper's *Myotomia reformata* published in 1724, contextualizing the book in relation to Cowper's other publications and Mead's own medical training and early career ambitions. A joint effort coordinated by Mead with help from James Jurin, Joseph Tanner and Henry Pemberton – all men with Newtonian commitments – this atlas of the muscles exemplifies Newtonian approaches to medical studies, while underscoring the attendant challenges, especially as related to tensions between anatomy and physiology. The story of the publication indicates the international component of eighteenth-century medical practice – in this case, particularly Anglo-Dutch relations. And finally, with a history of the book in place, I suggest that the lasting significance of Newtonian conceptions of the body are to be found not in the history of medicine but rather in more diffused terms through eighteenth-century conceptions of learned and artistic culture, characteristic of Mead's circle.

William Cowper (1666–1709) published the first edition of *Myotomia reformata, or, A New Administration of all the Muscles of Humane Bodies* in 1694.[3] He was in his late twenties and it was his first major work, appearing just three years after he was admitted to the Company of Barber-Surgeons. Although it points to Cowper's early professional aspirations, in comparison to the 1724 edition, it is modest. An octavo volume with just ten plates, it opens with a preface outlining the history of myology and a twelve-page introduction describing the morphology of muscles and their relationship to tendons, arteries, veins and nerves. The following thirty-six chapters treat the muscles from the abdomen to the toes. Chapters 2 and 3, on the muscles of the testes and the penis, are supplemented with an appendix 'Containing a Description of the Penis and the Manner of its Erection' – notable since Cowper is widely known today only for his identification of the two urethral glands at the base of the penis, still described as Cowper's glands.[4] The text also includes the first publication of the preputial and coronal glands of the penis as reported by Cowper's mentor Dr Edward Tyson.[5] The atlas, in fact, is dedicated to Tyson (as well as Roger Knowles and Edward Brown), and the two went on to collaborate on subsequent projects, including Tyson's treatise on the anatomy of the orangutan, published in 1699.[6] It was Tyson who nominated Cowper for election to the Royal Society later that same year.

Over the next few years, Cowper contributed several articles to the Royal Society's *Philosophical Transactions* including an account in 1702 of a remarkable set of anatomical tables donated by John Evelyn to the Royal Society thirty-five years earlier. While these mounted human specimens are entirely static, Cowper's article uses them to discuss the circulatory system and the movement of blood from the arteries to the veins – employing references to Antoinie van Leeuwenhoek's microscopic work on fish and dogs and the usefulness of wax-injected specimens, a process especially associated with the Dutch anatomist Jan Swammerdam. Utilizing an iatro-mechanical framework, Cowper presents the veins and arteries as a system of pipes arranged in size and location to balance the effects of gravity and the blood's weight.[7] It was, incidentally, around this time that a young William Cheselden began his anatomical studies – under Cowper.

However, by the early eighteenth century Cowper was well known for a second major anatomical atlas that has exposed him ever since to charges of plagiarism. His book, *The Anatomy of Humane Bodies*, printed in Oxford in 1698, includes 105 engravings after the Dutch artist Gerard de Lairesse, prints cut by Abraham Blooteling that had earlier been used to illustrate Dr Govard Bidloo's *Anatomia humani corporis* of 1685, along with a Dutch edition from 1690. Cowper supplied his own original text and nine additional plates engraved by Michael van der Gucht. Two of these images were drawn by Henry Cook; the others likely were by Cowper himself. Although Cowper makes passing mention of Lairesse and Bidloo, it could scarcely count as fair acknowledgement. That the title page substitutes Cowper's name for Bidloo's with a clumsy, pasted cut-out could not have helped matters. As Dániel Margócsy notes, Hendrick Boom, one of the four Dutch publishers backing Bidloo's *Anatomia*, contracted with the London booksellers Samuel Smith and Benjamin Walford for an English edition, supplying them with 300 copies of Lairesse's illustrations. Bidloo and Boom, however, were expecting a straightforward English translation, not a new publication.[8] Both men were furious, the physician outraged that his work had been taken over by another, the publisher fearful that an expanded edition would lower the price of the original. Bidloo responded publicly with a denunciation addressed to the Royal Society, but to no avail, as the institution quietly avoided the fray. Today the whole episode is most interesting for the light shed on the social frameworks of knowledge production in the early modern period, rather than as an exercise in assessing moral breeches of intellectual property, notwithstanding twentieth-century scholars' fixation on the latter.[9]

If our own notions of plagiarism (closely tied to modern copyright) did not yet exist, the basic concept of intellectual property generally did. If straightforward piracy often occurred, it was also heavily criticized. One distinguishing factor in the Bidloo–Cowper case stems from the image-text relationship. For Bidloo, the plates were an essential component of his atlas and thus could not legitimately appear elsewhere. For Cowper – whose first edition of *Myotomia reformata* had included just ten plates – they were compelling images that could be put to much better use with a better text.

From our vantage point, it may seem strange that Lairesse, the artist actually responsible for the extraordinary images, is rendered incidental (Bidloo's claims are hardly that Lairesse had been wronged). In fairness to Bidloo, the basic visual strategies of the plates likely originated with the anatomist rather than the artist. These illustrations, known for their stark 'reality-effect' and their lack of idealization were, ironically, produced by one of the Netherland's most classically-grounded painters, an artist often compared to Poussin. As argued by Rina Knoeff, this emphasis on 'the deadness of the dissected body' was perfectly consistent with Bidloo's larger project, which she convincingly associates with an early modern Mennonite emphasis on the spiritual value of suffering and martyrdom.[10] That Lairesse later distanced himself from the project reinforces the claim that the conception of the illustrations came from Bidloo. And yet the degree to which the work of the artist is simultaneously prized and devalued as simple transcription of the thoughts of another is remarkable.

By the time Cowper's anatomical atlas appeared in 1698, Bidloo had achieved enormous professional success while at the same time managing to alienate nearly all of his medical colleagues. Having come to the attention of William, the Stadholder, in the 1680s, Bidloo accompanied the prince upon his invasion of England in 1688. Through William's patronage, he was placed in charge of all civil and military hospitals in the Netherlands starting in 1690. While spending substantial amounts of time in England where he waited on the king almost daily, Bidloo was nevertheless appointed professor of anatomy at the University of Leiden, replacing the celebrated Newtonian physician Archibald Pitcairn who had returned to Scotland.[11] This prestigious position came also through the patronage of William, who since the 1670s had managed to exercise a growing influence over university appointments. Exasperated, the other members of Leiden's medical faculty urged William either to send Bidloo back to the Netherlands or to appoint a replacement. The king did neither. Finally in 1701 Herman Boerhaave, who had been, in the 1690s, first a student and then tutor to those behind him, was hired as a lecturer.[12]

Even prior to the conflicts over the Leiden appointment, Bidloo had been embroiled in a heated dispute with his former teacher Frederick Ruysch. Bidloo took issue with Ruysch's claims for the utility of wax-injected specimens as a faithful representation of human anatomy. As outlined by Margócsy, Bidloo instead privileged paper atlases, in part, on the grounds that anatomical preparations appear deceptively alive, a point that fits nicely with Knoef's observations regarding Bidloo's emphatically morbid aesthetic.[13] However, in addition to the serious epistemological concerns raised by the debate, the controversy reinforced

Bidloo's public persona as an acerbic annoyance. For all of his professional accomplishments, the outspoken and caustic Bidloo had few professional friends.

That a second, posthumous edition of Cowper's *Anatomy of Humane Bodies* (still in English) was published in Leiden in 1737 reinforces the primacy of Cowper's atlas over that of Bidloo's – precisely the concern of Hendrick Boom, Bidloo's publisher. Edited by C. B. Albinus, a brother of the more famous anatomist, Bernhard Siegfried Albinus, this edition was also available in London, with a Latin translation soon appearing – an indicator that the book had come to be viewed as a standard text in the field. Interestingly, Boerhaave spoke well of it.[14]

Given Bidloo's favoured status with King William, one might speculate about the role of politics in the Bidloo–Cowper conflict. At the very least, the Dutch physician must have been struck by the disparity between what William's support could and could not achieve. Notwithstanding the official appointments, his patronage was of little help (and perhaps a hindrance) in shoring up professional support in both England and the Netherlands. And yet, perhaps Bidloo's close ties to the king did give members of the Royal Society pause in defending Cowper too enthusiastically.[15] The general silence on the issue might be interpreted not as an embarrassed rebuke to Cowper but guarded caution that Bidloo should be quietly ignored (*The Anatomy of Humane Bodies* must have helped secure Cowper's election as a Fellow of the Society, just one year after its publication). Also relevant are the political ends Bidloo provided for William. Although the Scottish Dr Pitcairn occupied the position of anatomy professor at Leiden for just one year, he was immensely influential, and as demonstrated by Anita Guerrini, his loyal following from Tory sympathizers challenges facile identifications of Newtonianism with Whig ideology in any exclusive manner.[16] Bidloo, on the other hand, had shown himself a vocal supporter of the House of Orange (in part through publication of political pamphlets), and perhaps William was perfectly happy to have an absent, loyal anatomy professor holding the Leiden position in his absence. But even without explicit evidence, such speculations underscore the degree to which the reception of Cowper's text and the controversy it occasioned played out within a social and political framework. Assessing the conflict as if it were a present-day case of intellectual property law tends to miss this crucial point.[17]

Developing the social and political framework further requires us to consider Mead's place in the narrative. Introducing him into the story much earlier than scholars have typically is crucial since Mead's personal involvement with Dutch physic began long before he took over editing the second edition of *Myotomia reformata* in 1709.[18] Just before the 'Glorious Revolution', in 1686 his father, Matthew Mead, a celebrated dissenting minister, fled to Holland, suspected of aiding the Rye House Plot to assassinate Charles II. Within a few years, Richard, at age seventeen, also moved to Holland, studying first at Utrecht under Johann

George Graevius and then in 1693 matriculating at Leiden's medical school, just a few months before Pitcairne moved back to Scotland, a year before the post was filled by an absent Bidloo. Thus, in his two years at Leiden, Mead experienced directly the difference between these two anatomy professors. Despite the brief overlap between Mead and Pitcairne, the two eventually became friends, and in 1715 Mead helped secure the release of his former teacher's son, imprisoned for participating in the Jacobite uprising of the that year. There is no evidence that Mead ever reached out to Bidloo. Instead, the other key relationship formed at this time was his friendship with Boerhaave; for a brief period the two were housemates in Leiden, and they maintained a correspondence after each became successful physicians.

In 1698 when the Bidloo–Cowper conflict erupted, Mead was establishing himself as a young doctor and we know little about his professional life, but in 1703 he published his first book, *A Mechanical Account of Poisons in Several Essays*, explaining in the preface that he wanted to see

> how far I could carry mechanical considerations in accounting for those surprising changes which poisons make in an animal body, concluding (as I think fairly) that if so abstruse phaenomena as these did come under the known laws of motion, it might very well be taken for granted, that the more obvious appearances in the same fabric are owing to such causes as are within the reach of geometrical reasoning.[19]

The application of mechanistic approaches to the body was in keeping with Cowper's work from the previous decade, an extension generally of Cartesian strategies, even as Mead struggled to formulate a Newtonian-based model of iatromechanism. It was the same direction a handful of colleagues who had studied under Pitcairn – especially William Cockburn and George Cheyne – had been pushing medical theory more broadly; for Mead's generation, Newtonian mechanics promised a way forward for medicine.[20] If the scientific payoffs of *The Principia* and the forthcoming *Opticks* were rich (indeed for many revolutionary), transforming natural philosophy at the level of method and results, why should there not also be medical applications? Particularly given that seventeenth-century anatomical accomplishments had done little to improve medical theory or practice, Newtonian approaches to medicine offered the potential for meaningful progress and, at least among Newton's supporters, garnered for its proponents credibility and the mantle of reasonable innovation. For Mead, the Newtonian orientation certainly worked: he was elected Fellow of the Royal Society in 1703, and from there his star only rose over the next five decades.

Thus while we do not know what Mead thought of Lairesse's images or of Cowper's use of them in the 1698 *Anatomy of Humane Bodies* (in addition to the latter, he owned a copy of Bidloo's 1685 Latin text), it is clear where Mead's personal and professional sympathies lay.[21] As a result of Cowper's mechanistic orientation, he could be fitted into a narrative that culminated in a Newtonian school of physic of which Mead was a vital part. By contrast, Mead likely viewed Bidloo as a throwback of simple political favouritism that, in fact, interfered with the business of medical training and practice and at least threatened to interject the most blatant sort of state politics into the medical profession.[22] Quite apart from ethical issues resulting from Cowper's use of Lairesse's images, this socially-structured intellectual framework must be kept in mind. There simply was no cause for concern in Mead's attaching his name to the second edition of Cowper's *Myotomia reformata*; misgivings over Cowper's reputation in both England and the Netherlands did not exist in the early eighteenth century.

1703 was an important year for Mead's early career, not only because of his election into the Royal Society, nor because of his publishing debut; that spring he also was appointed physician to the newly rebuilt St Thomas's Hospital in Southwark, an institution that would prove crucial for the careers of many eighteenth-century physicians and surgeons including Cheselden and Tanner. Mead would spend the better part of the next twelve years there. In August of 1711 he was appointed anatomy reader to the Company of Barbers and Surgeons, and in December of the same year, he lectured for three days on the muscles.[23] If – as stated in the advertisement of the 1724 edition of the *Myotomia reformata* – Cowper turned over the revised manuscript to Mead just before his death in 1709, the atlas and its images must have been on Mead's mind as he approached these pedagogical demonstrations. Mead filled the position for the Barber and Surgeons for the next four years.

Mead's success as a physician resulted from multiple factors, his own social skills and intelligence playing a crucial part, as well as the patronage he received from several powerful sectors of the English establishment. It is difficult, however, to overstate the utility of his alignment with Newton, both philosophically and personally. Mead's 1704 book, *A Treatise Concerning the Influence of the Sun and the Moon upon Human Bodies*, may at first strike modern readers as hardly an approach one would expect from a young doctor brandishing his learned grasp of medical theory, but in a world where Newton's mastery of the celestial realm counted for much, Mead's second published volume made perfect sense. Interestingly, Pitcairn, in his inaugural lecture at Leiden, had likewise looked to astronomy as a basis for modern medicine, thrilled at its mathematically derived certainty.[24] Moreover, as Anna Marie Roos has stressed, the book shows Mead recasting ancient medical ideas in the new garb of Newtonianism, firmly anchoring himself with one foot planted on the solid terrain of established tradition, the other on the fashionable ground of the period's most up-to-date thinking. While Mead's 'actual medical treatments and causal explanations of disease were entirely traditional', he nonetheless appeared to be pointing medicine in the new direction of the New Science of the Royal Society.[25] Mead wanted to have his cake as an Ancient, to eat it as a Modern – and remarkably he was, in his lifetime, judged to manage both successfully. He was widely regarded as an authority on traditional medical theory built on the foundations of Hippocrates and Galen. And as for the living, he benefited in no small way from Newton's personal patronage. In 1717, for instance, he was appointed by the mathematician to one of the Royal Society's vice-president positions. That Newton consulted Mead as a physician in matters of his own health was perhaps an even stronger endorsement.

Generalizing about the larger group of 'Newton-struck' physicians, Theodore Brown makes the same point as Roos:

> Iatromechanism [inspired by Newton] itself was a desperate attempt to make physicians *appear* modern and up-to-date while keeping traditional methods of diagnosis and therapy intact. Physicians of the late seventeenth century ... had slapped new corpuscular labels on their traditional remedies. Hydraulic 'Newtonianism' gave physicians of the next generation a sense of methodological improvement, moral uplift, and optimism for the future as well as a rhetoric which might please Newton and his disciples and otherwise prove useful in winning a Newton-admiring and nationalistic British clientele.[26]

Ironically – given that part of the appeal of Newtonian approaches to medicine hinged on mathematical certainty – the practical payoff of medical Newtonianism for eighteenth-century physicians stemmed from its flexibility. The conceptual toolbox of matter, motion, forces and pressure could be deployed in myriad ways. In the words of Andrew Cunningham, 'it is striking how many different explanations, and how many different conclusions, could be built on Newtonian physical principles, depending on what aspects of Newton's works one privileged'.[27]

And the strategy held ramifications for doctors outside of Britain, too. In making the case for Boerhaave as a turning point, after which most anatomists came to see 'anatomical pathology of one kind or another as part of their disciplinary roles', Cunningham notes, for instance, Boerhaave's own ability to synthesize older traditions with more current models: 'Boerhaave managed to take on board and to teach an anatomy and physiology that embraced both the older pathology of fluids, together with the Malphighian and the Newton-influenced pathology of solids of more recent days.'[28]

Such flexibility, however, at least potentially threatened to undermine the traditional authority of physicians, and Mead, in particular, appears to have grasped the dilemma of embracing the methods of the New Science, premised on empirical observation, and yet maintaining one's distance from contemporary practitioners who treated symptoms rather than the causes of illness, practitioners lacking university training in medical theory, practitioners often described as *empirics* (and this at a time when even the word *empirical* was more likely to connote quackery than what we now think of as scientific observation). In *A Mechanical Account of Poisons*, Mead describes his own experiments with snakes, offering an iatromechanistic account of poisons consistent with the latest Newtonian ideals, but as a bulwark to preserve the traditional authority of the physician, he establishes two crucial requirements: classical languages and mathematics. The latter would serve as a path to a 'new animal oeconomy', proof 'that the most useful of arts, if duly cultivated, is more than either meer [*sic*] conjecture or base empiricism'. Neglect of the former was for Mead simply unthinkable, and it serves as the baseline for evaluating mathematical proficiency: 'he who wants [lacks] this necessary qualification will be as ridiculous as one without Greek or Latin'.[29]

Before turning to see how this mathematical emphasis frames the second edition of *Myotomia reformata*, we should consider one other point: the distinction between anatomy and physiology. As Cunningham usefully notes in *The Anatomist Anatomis'd*, his recent book on the disciplinary history of anatomy in the long eighteenth century, there was an important difference, even if medical history has tended to confuse the two.[30] Prior to 1800, anatomy (literally dissection) was an experimental discipline, 'an art and a science', forged to address structures of the body open to sensory experience, a discipline centred on '*what?, how?* and *whether?* questions'. By contrast, early modern physiology was a speculative enterprise, a theoretical discipline that 'asked *why?* questions'.[31] In the eighteenth century, the two were understood as related since sound anatomical observations were seen as the necessary foundations for any legitimate physiological explanations; yet, whereas after 1800 anatomy would come to be viewed as subordinate to physiology, with experimentation playing a relatively minor role in the production of anatomical knowledge, in the early modern period, 'it was the anatomist who was at the forefront of research in medicine and in the whole world of life and living creatures'.[32] It is an important distinction, for according to this model, there could be no Newtonian anatomy, only Newtonian physiology.

The distinction is especially interesting in accounting for Henry Pemberton's introduction to the second edition of *Myotomia reformata*. For the most part, the content and organization of the main body of Cowper's text itself is unchanged. There are, however, three key alterations between the two editions: as already noted, the size (the text grows from octavo to folio); the quality and number of images (whereas the 1694 edition has just ten plates, the 1724 edition has sixty-six); and the introduction (Cowper's original brief introductory remarks are replaced by a seventy-seven-page introduction from Pemberton).

In some ways we should by now know what to expect of Pemberton, as his CV perfectly qualified him for the task of introducing this text that was being refashioned under Mead's direction as a luxurious Newtonian landmark of anatomy. Pemberton studied at Leiden under Boerhaave, taking his MD in 1719. He spent time at St Thomas Hospital, though he never practised medicine in any serious manner after completing his education. He was a Fellow of the Royal Society, sponsored by Mead in 1720, and in fact, came to the attention of

Newton through Mead. The latter passed along a paper by Pemberton confuting Leibniz's account of the force of moving bodies, and Newton, according to Pemberton's biographer, 'was so well pleased with it, that, as great a man as he was, he condescended to visit the doctor at his lodgings, bringing along with him a confutation of his own, grounded on other principles'.[33] Pemberton's article, presented as a 'Letter to Dr Mead', was published in the *Philosophical Transactions* in 17²²⁄₃. He soon became a trusted colleague of Newton's, editing the third edition of the *Principia* in 1726 (just two years after the second edition of the *Myotomia reformata*), and that apparently at Mead's urging.

Pemberton's lengthy introduction is divided into two parts, both of which are filled with increasingly complicated geometric diagrams. In part 1 (pp. v–xxxiii), Pemberton attempts to explain the force of muscular activity via mathematics, in several instances challenging the claims of his seventeenth-century predecessor, the mathematician Giovanni Borelli, whose *De motu animalium*, published posthumously in 1680–1, established the major early modern terms of debate for muscular motion. With twelve diagrams, Pemberton schematizes the force of the muscles in relation to the range of movement of the joints. The crucial precedent here is Nicolaus Steno who, as argued recently by Domencio Meli, adapted the work of Galileo to the body, employing illustrations as experiments in his study of the muscles from the 1660s.[34]

The principle grist for the Newtonian millstone, however, appears in part 2 (pp. xxxiv–lxxvii) as Pemberton 'enquires into the Cause of the Contraction of a muscular Fibre' in light of 'one or two of the most received opinions concerning that matter'.[35] And here he specifically addresses the leading scholars to have weighed in on the issue: not only Borelli and Steno but also Giovanni Battista Morgagni, William Croon, James Keill and Johann Bernoulli. Again proceeding from geometry, Pemberton challenges the widely accepted inflation or ebullition theory of the muscular contraction, a theory that posited open, inflatable chambers within the muscles and, through 'vesicular' notions of fermentation and effervescence, explained movement in terms consistent with Aristotle's mechanical axiom that *anything which moves is moved by something else*.[36] Central to Pemberton's motivation in writing part 2 was Johann Bernoulli's 1694 medical dissertation, completed at Basel and translated into English in 1698 as *Mathematical Disquisitions Concerning Muscular Motion*. As stressed by Troels Kardel, it was the first instance of differential calculus employed in biology; not only did it depend upon Leibniz, the dissertation was apparently reviewed by the celebrated mathematician, and the two men soon embarked upon an extensive correspondence.[37]

Here, we come to one of the crucial subplots of the 1724 edition of *Myotomia reformata*. In the intellectual climate of Georgian England, when Newtonian approaches to medicine held such promise, it made sense that the Newton–Leibniz conflict would play out in the realm of anatomy (probably not insignificant was the fact that Bernoulli's text was itself republished in 1721).[38] Pemberton follows Bernoulli's application of calculus to the study of muscles but in order to challenge the ebullition theory. In several cases he praises the work of Newton ('that great Philosopher, whose chief Glory consists in having banished all Uncertainties from his Inquiries into Nature') and twice refers to 'Sir Isaac Newton's Method of Differences'.[39] However, if Pemberton is eager to refute the mechanical inflation model of muscular movement, he is also reticent to advance a theory of his own. As the essay comes to a conclusion he interprets his own caution as an indication of sound thinking, precisely the sort of wisdom that, for him, characterizes Newton's explorations into the 'Depths of Nature', in contrast to Cartesian speculations, an 'imaginary Empire in Philosophy'. In the penultimate paragraph Pemberton explains that he 'chose in this latter part of the present Discourse only to set out, in the plainest manner I was able, how insufficient all Conjectures have hitherto been at the Cause of muscular motion, without hazarding to augment the Number of Errors by recommending any new Conceit of my own'.[40]

The contrast with Bernoulli is reinforced with the appearance of the essay as an introduction to Cowper's anatomy of the muscles. For in Bernoulli's foreword, the Swiss mathematician writes that

> it is not my intention to present here a special description and anatomy of muscles. This has assuredly been done more than enough by the most prestigious anatomists who have Excelled in this century and do excel still now. And, if I wished, the scope of this short dissertation would not allow me to do it. It is our purpose to outline a general concept of the structure of the muscles as much as necessary properly to explain their mode of action and the resulting animal motions.[41]

The texts then of Pemberton and Bernoulli can be seen as doubly diametrically opposed: the former uses the method of the latter (reclaiming the calculus for Newton) to argue against the claims for an ebullition theory, and whereas Bernoulli sees the 'description' of the muscles as redundant, the second edition of the *Myotomia reformata* insists upon the value of precisely such a project.

To be clear, I should emphasize that there is nothing explicitly Newtonian about Cowper's anatomy. Instead, under the direction of Mead, the text is refashioned through the introductory apparatus as a Newtonian treatise. Returning to Cunningham's distinction between physiology and anatomy, we might observe the degree to which Pemberton's introduction and Cowper's anatomical images and descriptions bear out the two categories. And yet, because Pemberton refuses to advance a theory of his own (notwithstanding a passing allusion to Newton's ether), what counts as 'Newtonian' physiology here is not precisely concerned with explanations of *why*, as Cunningham characterizes most physiological aims but in explaining how other accounts of *why* must be rejected. Curiously, we are left with a defensive physiology that stresses the importance of anatomy, even as that very physiology works hard to establish ties to the more productive applications of Newtonianism.

Yet, if it is clear that Pemberton as Newton's own editor was perfectly positioned to stake out a Newtonian position on muscular motion – if only to show what a Newtonian method could be used to refute rather than affirm – we are still left with accounting for Mead's interest in the second edition. His own Newtonian commitments – social, intellectual and professional – were congruent with Pemberton's, but there was, I believe, an additional motivation for Mead that usefully opens up anatomy as a way of knowing more generally. As much as Mead aimed to update the *Myotomia reformata* vis-à-vis Newtonianism, he also went out of his way to make the book visually impressive. He wanted to see his edition of the book literally take its place on the bookshelves of the learned beside the canonical volumes of anatomy. The illustrations are numerous and impressive, and the decorated initials especially call to mind Vesalius.[42] If we are safe in assuming Mead was aware of Boerhaave's work on the great folio edition of Vesalius, which appeared in 1725, we might have a way of explaining why after such a long time, the second edition of the *Myotomia reformata* appeared when it did.[43]

This Janus-like sensibility is perfectly consistent with Mead's larger conceptions of knowledge production. For all the ways in which, during his lifetime, he was aligned with the progress and innovation of the Royal Society, he was firmly grounded in older models of erudition. His respect for the 'Ancients' as well as the 'Moderns' is repeatedly born out in his art and antiquarian interests as well as his scholarly patronage. It is our mistake to try to divorce his 'scientific' pursuits from his 'cultural' pursuits. At the same time, for instance, that Mead was overseeing the *Myotomia reformata* project, he was also working to shore up support for Samuel Buckley's critical edition of Jacques-Auguste de Thou, itself a crucial text for understanding the sixteenth century. Not only did Mead help defray publication costs, he also purchased the source materials, assembled by the Jacobite Thoams Carte during his exile in France.

For Mead, an older humanist model of learning was in no way antithetical to contemporary 'scientific' thought. His coupling of mathematics and classical languages as the touchstones of the physician's education bears out the continuity. And so in the end, one of the lessons worth noting from Mead's involvement with the *Myotomia reformata* is the degree to which early modern anatomy broadly conceived not only pointed to new knowledge and thus new conceptions of what it means to be human, to inhabit a body, to interact with other bodies – it could also serve to anchor the body in entirely traditional conceptions of knowledge, or at least the *rhetoric* of traditional conceptions of knowledge. In practice, an enormous distance separated Mead from the Renaissance, and indeed Mead was himself immensely proud to be identified with the recent advances we associate with the Royal Society, and yet conceptually, Mead repeatedly stressed not a break from the past – be it the Renaissance or even Antiquity – but continuity. The body and anatomical knowledge were perhaps especially well-suited for such an outlook. In some ways, the very idea of patronizing a new edition of an older text underscores the fluidity between Mead's 'cultural' and 'scientific' interests. For him, both depended upon an antiquarian sensibility in which knowledge – and not simply historical knowledge – could be found in the past, even if those propositions were still subject to present discoveries and advancements.

In closing, a few observations on the relationship between images and texts as they relate to Cowper and Mead are perhaps useful. With each of these men, we have remarkable examples of an earlier publication being substantially revised to serve new ends. Cowper's reworking of Lairesse's illustrations effectively appropriated an anatomical treatise initially attributed to Bidloo. By contrast, Mead breathed new life into Cowper's *Myotomia reformata*, ensuring that an unremarkable book destined to be forgotten (bear in mind that the first edition was an octavo with just ten plates), is still prized as one of Cowper's great accomplishments. However, if Cowper's authorship was preserved, the second edition of the *Myotomia reformata* was nonetheless given a new use, a new voice, as Cowper's mechanistic orientation was reformulated in explicitly Newtonian terms thanks to Pemberton's introduction and the larger Newtonian context of the 1724 publication. With both *The Anatomy of Humane Bodies* and the *Myotomia reformata* there was a fairly fluid relationship between a given scientific proposition and the illustrations used to support it. In one case, the images are consistent and the text is changed; in the other case, the text persists and is newly framed with a new format, new images and a new introductory apparatus. Throughout early modern science it is easy enough to point out examples indicating the importance of images. These two cases, however, suggest that the relationship between those claims and those images was perhaps more flexible, adaptable,and varied than we sometimes acknowledge.

It perhaps explains why an anatomist like Cowper was himself interested in learning to make images. He studied drawing with the virtuosi of St Luke, an important informal predecessor to the Royal Academy. And his protégée, Cheselden, likewise learned to draw, working with the St Martin's Lane Academy, including perhaps supplying anatomical lessons for the group. That Cheselden himself produced a general anatomy – dedicated to Mead – and also a more focused text on the bones of animals makes perfect sense.

The artistic impact of the *Myotomia reformata* itself is difficult to gauge. Cowper had initially envisioned it serving artists' needs, and such thinking is consistent with Mead's patronage of contemporary artists as well, though in the end those sections were never completed.[44] Still, one explicit instance of the text's ties to the Georgian art world is notable. Hogarth, in plate 1 of *The Analysis of Beauty* (1753), includes a leg from the second edition of Cowper's treatise and references the book in the body of his text.[45] For all that was exceptional about Hogarth, I imagine in consulting the *Myotomia reformata* he was not especially unique.

As for the duo of Mead and Cheselden, both men attended not only Pope but also Newton in his final illness, with Mead sitting by the giant of British natural philosophy as he died. In the end, Newton's intellectual impact on physiology mattered little for the man himself. The rhetoric and culture of Newtonian medicine, however, mattered a great deal.

## Acknowledgements

Research for this article was supported by a summer grant from the National Endowment for the Humanities in connection with a larger project on Anglo-Dutch relations in the arts and natural sciences. I am grateful, too, for feedback I received from presenting an earlier version of the paper at the Huntington Library in September 2011 for the symposium, 'The Origins of Science as a Visual Pursuit: The Early Royal Society', organized by Sachiko Kusukawa and Alexander Marr.

# 12 ART AND MEDICINE: CREATIVE COMPLICITY BETWEEN ARTISTIC REPRESENTATION AND RESEARCH

Filippo Pierpaolo Marino

S'intese degli ignudi più modernamente che fatto non avevano gl'altri maestri innanzi a lui; e scorticò molti uomini per vedere la notomia lor sotto

[He] understood naked bodies in a way that was more modern than his predecessors; and [he] flayed many men in order to discover their internal anatomy.

What Antonio Vasari wrote on Antonio del Pollaiolo's *Ercole e Anteo* (*c.* 1475), tempera on panel, Galleria degli Uffizi, Florence, bears witness to sweeping changes in the artistic representation of the human body at the end of the fifteenth century. This shift mainly concerned the image's construction, which was based not only on merely external observation, but also on the awareness of the internal organization of the body, which is made of muscles, along with specialized organs and bones. Starting with this crucial cultural moment, specifically from Masaccio's and Donatello's artistic experiences in representing the human body's internal systems, this essay diachronically examines the production of important wax modellers, active in the city of Bologna around the eighteenth century. A close look at some artists that worked for the 'Accademia delle Scienze', such as Ercole Lelli (1702–66), Giovanni Manzolini (1700–55) and Anna Morandi (1716–74), shows how this new approach to the study of the human body mutually affected both art and medicine, paving the way for a more comprehensive and detailed understanding of anatomic systems. A special mention is of course devoted to their forerunner, Gaetano Giulio Zumbo (1656–1701). By adopting a fresh perspective that compares the disciplines of art and medicine, the present investigation on anatomic systems tries to fill an embarrassing gap in the body of criticism.

## The Body's Reconstruction

During the late Middle Ages the medical illustration and its anatomical iconography hardly managed to free themselves from an oversimplified, schematic approach in the representation of the body and its internal systems. In order to promote not only a modern relationship between art and medicine, but also an evolution of the anatomical depiction from the medieval canon cast in a Galenic mould, it was essential to adopt a new method of studying the body that went beyond the visible surface. Already from the end of the thirteenth century the contribution of the Bolognese School was decisive,[1] especially with the works of Bartolomeo da Varignana[2] (*c.* 1260–1321), Henri de Mondeville[3] (1260–*c.* 1320), and Mondino de' Liuzzi[4] (*c.* 1270–1326). These studies turned out to be of pivotal importance for the emergence of the observation of anatomy on corpses and for the application of a scientific method that went beyond the simple theoretical disquisitions borrowed from Greek texts of Galen, Hippocrates and Avicenna. Nonetheless, despite these innovations, the influence of the Alexandrian canon of *Funfbilderserie*[5] and the frog-like anatomical structure[6] were still visible in different anatomical illustrations, accompanying many treaties until the fifteenth century.

In 1491 the brothers Giovanni and Gregorio De Gregori da Forlì, typographers in Venice, published the first edition of the *Fasciculus medicinae*. This work incorporates six illustrations,[7] a series of short treatises and *Consilium*[8] by Pietro da Tossignano (*c.* 1364–1401). Although it has always been considered the prototype of an innovation within the tradition of medical illustration, it is worth noting that this volume's figures are based on a series of pathological drawings and diagrams of Germanic origin dated from the late fourteenth century.[9]

The second edition, written in 1494, in vernacular and entitled *Fasiculo de medicina*, is enriched with Mondino's *Anothomia* and new illustrations.[10] Here it is possible to notice some changes at a stylistic level and in the anatomic depiction. Artists who were interested in xylographs and illustrative prints at the end of the fifteenth century[11] – particularly medical – already recognized the importance of the study of anatomy for the body's representation, staging this metamorphosis in their paintings. It is important to remember that artists struggled to overcome medieval traditions by studying anatomy and by drawing inspiration from the works of Mondino de' Liuzzi. Attracted by the idea of *nosce te ipsum*,[12] they tore the veil that covered the human figure in Byzantine art once and for all, fiercely concentrating their attention on the body and its structure. Thus they definitively abandoned the idea of the body as a mere puppet.

Another important event that led to a new understanding of the body took place in Florence at the beginning of the fourteenth century when artists began attending apothecaries. They came into contact with physicians who, inspired by the Bolognese masters, practised anatomy on the bodies of the deceased, using the same materials employed by painters and sculptors to preserve anatomical preparations (from decomposition). The common interest for this kind of body investigation pushed painters to officially request, already in 1303, to be admitted to the union of physicians and apothecaries. This was a fruitful collaboration, which finally lead Florentine artists to establish, in the middle of that century, the so-called Company of San Luca, a society that encouraged exchanges between artists and physicians who, as a result of their profession, had easier, although secret, access to corpses. With a revolutionary impulse, both artists and anatomists discussed the osteological, arterial, venous and myological systems, hence developing a modern knowledge of surgery and the structure of the human figure. As Mario Bucci claims, at the dawn of the Renaissance 'we are discovering, or rediscovering, a treasure which was stolen from humanity since ... paganism, feared throughout the Middle Ages as an anathema: the human body'.[13]

Although anatomical drawings were still treated with a schematic approach, or tied to old prototypes, in the 1420s an amazing opus was frescoed in the Basilica of Santa Maria Novella: *Trinità*.[14] Besides mentioning the skilful use of perspective, the clever positioning of the point-of-view and the mature spatial relationship between the figures, this fresco is relevant in the context of the present study because of the image placed at the bottom of the composition. Below the altar, supported by four columns, is a skeleton reclining on a sarcophagus, accompanied by an epigraph: 'I am what you are, as I am you will be.' The work as a whole does not seem to convey any new meaning, if compared to medieval religious representations, which were loaded with chimerical horror. However, in that portion of the *Trinità*, Masaccio (1401–28) has totally transformed the prerogative of the image: the skeleton does not display macabre deformities, but rather appears to be a faithful representation of the skeletal system, contemporaneously seen from the perspectives of a naturalist, a scientist and an artist. Based on the accuracy of the bones' shapes and interconnection, it seems evident that the artist painted the skeleton rigorously from real life.

Masaccio's experience was contemporary to that of another great, if not the most important innovator, Donatello (1386–1466). While looking back to the past, Donatello gave the body a surprising definition that extended beyond a simple study of real life. During the process of restoring some of Donatello's works, Bruno Bearzi[15] shed light on the methods and techniques exploited by the Florentine artist, some of which previously only could be supposed. Donatello shaped his characters in bronze using gypsum models, portraying nude figures with meticulous anatomic detail. Subsequently, he would wrap his models in resistant cloth covered with a thick layer of wax. The addition of these materials would give the figure not only the illusion of a more realistic drapery, but it would also stress the physicality of the body.

It seems clear that the artist viewed the human figure as an important architecture which should be studied and balanced, besides being adorned. In fact, he went far beyond the simple distinction between the body and its covering in the anatomic construction of the sculpture; the concept is well described by Pliny the Elder in his *Naturalis historia*: 'Articulis membra distinxit. Venas protulit: praeterque in veste rugas et sinus invenit.'[16]

To take one example, the 'naked' figure of the bronze Christ[17] clearly displays the subcutaneous structure of muscles and tendons, as well as the veins of the arms, legs and feet. Hence, it can be asserted that Donatello, albeit secretly, might have witnessed, if not actively participated in, a corpse dissection. The transfiguration of Christ's body is not an idealized figure; instead, it demonstrates the artist's interest in the subject as pulsating material for taxonomy and classification, not to mention its dramatic attitude.

In this sense, his *Giuditta* seems to be an even more surprising work.[18] Here it is possible to find Donatello's fundamental principles as an artist and scientist, skilfully hidden beneath the metal surface. The sculptural group is magnificently balanced, despite the complexity arising from the two figures' disposition in separate levels: that of Judith, upright and dominant, and that of Holofernes, imprisoned below and venting his last breath before being overwhelmed by the winner's blade. The female statue is constructed using the above-mentioned technique.

The second statue is of even greater interest: the faint limbs of the defeated Holofernes give him a premature shade of death. It is in this figure that Donatello has delicately tied up his thorough experience of the body's dissection with supreme art. In this respect, Bruno Bearzi wisely observes:

> certain aspects, such as the too realistic nude legs of Holofernes, give the feeling that they are made out of real casts. They show a reproduction of limbs belonging to an adult man, with feet ruined by exhausting jobs ... These legs ... were created and fused separately, and inserted in the group later, fixed by using a visible metal addition.[19]

Thus it is likely that the artist modelled Holofernes's legs in a cast directly obtained from the limbs of a corpse. This nearly surgical graft poignantly recalls Beato Angelico's (c. 1393–1455) *Il Miracolo della Gamba Nera*,[20] depicted in a panel belonging to the San Marco's altar-piece.[21] Here the Saints Cosmas and Damian, protectors of medicine, replace the protagonist's leg, which was suffering from gangrene, with the healthy leg of a dead man. Nonetheless, whereas in Beato Angelico's painting the anatomic detail was exploited simply in terms of narration, in Donatello's masterpiece it acts as a subtext of the work of art. The sculptural groups hereafter epitomize new important meanings, becoming the emblem of the quest for the integration of surgery, dissection and art.

The original experiences of these fifteenth-century artists, creators of a modern way of representing the body, lead to a complete transformation and evolution of the anatomic depiction, which became increasingly detailed in the definition of the body's internal structure and its systems. Thanks to Antonio del Pollaiuolo (1432–98), artistic figures evolved by assuming also the form of proper anatomic treatises.

A still more explicit recourse to anatomy can be identified in Andrea del Verrocchio (1435–88). Indeed, his works are characterized by a remarkable taste for cruelty, as A. Busignani[22] has underscored. His repeated use of anatomic preparations, testified in Vasari's writings,[23] paved the way to an entirely fresh scientific employment of the old ceroplastics tradition. At the dawn of humanism this technique was already connected with the body's representation, among the artisan class as well as within a liturgical and funeral context. Despite this, Verrocchio succeeded in freeing the activity from the limitation of representing images and busts that aim exclusively at producing *ex-votos*.[24] These offerings convey macabre feelings, their main function being a symbolic representation of disease. Ultimately, this idea was surpassed when these works were placed in a purely artistic and scientific environment, instead of living in the limited (and limiting) religious space.

A first, remarkable example of the use of wax to reproduce the body's morphology in a modern manner can be observed in the renowned *Scorticato*,[25] realized by Ludovico Cardi, also known as 'Cigoli' (1559–1613), in collaboration with the Flemish anatomist Teodoro Maierng. In fact, the *Scorticato* poignantly witnesses Cardi's scrupulous attention to the scientific reproduction of the body in his artistic works, drawing inspiration from the anatomical studies carried out by Pollaiolo, Verrocchio and Leonardo as well as from his friendship with Galileo. This technique led to a vividly harmonious blend between art and science, thanks to the work of a Sicilian artist and abbot, Gaetano Giulio Zumbo.

## Zumbo's Art: The Anatomy of Corruption

Differently from Florentine artists and sculptors of the fifteenth century, Zumbo chose wax as the unique and fundamental material for his artistic career, a decision that could be regarded as 'ambivalence'. On the one hand, he was the creator of 'small theatres', which he used to display the body; on the other, he was an artist-scientist who exploited this method to research human anatomy. It is important to underscore the fact that in both these areas a precise study of the body performed a central role.

Despite the substantial lack of criticism on this artist and his production, likely due to the paucity of works attributed to him,[26] the significance of Zumbo's work should be considered revolutionary. His interest in the scientific aspects of artistic representation increased during his Florentine period.[27] In fact, the first part of his production is marked by a focus on the anatomy of the rotting body, decomposing and corrupted by diseases and death, from which it is possible to evince a surprisingly intense scientific objectivity. This intent can be identified in works such as *Il Trionfo del Tempo*, *La Peste*, *Il Sepolcro* or *Vanità della Gloria Umana* and in *Il Morbo Gallico*. Almost certainly these pieces were completed in Florence for Cosimo III and for the Gran Principe Ferdinando, minus the second, which can be attributed to the period spent in Naples.

The terrible realism portrayed in these figures, also described by the brothers Edmond and Jules De Goncourt,[28] was distant from the sadic cruelty that mirrored an 'unhappy epoch', to use Paolo Giansiracusa's words;[29] additionally, De Sade, besides exalting their qualities, defined *La Peste* as a group of 'tremendous reality'.[30] Interestingly, R. W. Lightbown has argued 'the terrifying realism with which Zumbo was able to present the body's corruption after death must be attributed to his anatomical studies, and to the frequentation of surgical lectures'.[31]

All the opinions expressed by these eminent artists and critics are epitomized in the *Trionfo del Tempo*. The scene of this 'small theatre', set in a cave, presents a number of bodies, each rotting in varying degrees. The details and colours of the bodies gradually foreground the flesh's caducity, slowly decomposing. To the right rests the yellowish – greenish body of a woman who died not long before; on her left Zumbo placed a male body, rendered in brownish, earthen colours. Notwithstanding the process of dismemberment, it is still possible to grasp an anatomic line. At the centre of the composition lies an almost completely putrefied body, which shows, despite its decaying condition, the internal structure, similar to a flayed man. Finally, at the bottom of the composition one can see a skeleton, which can be regarded as the last stage of decomposition. This gathering of corpses, which, significantly, begins with dead babies, is dominated by the personification of Time: the vivid exactness of its limbs strikingly contrasting the putrefied, rotten state of the other characters. Here, the message of life succumbing to death is functional to an anatomic representation. Both the anonymous author of *Mémoires de Trévoux*[32] and R. W. Lightbown agree that Zumbo

> may well have studied anatomy in Rome, where dissection was practised by the surgeon Bernardino Genga (1620–1690), whose collection of anatomical drawings from the life and from the antique statues, prepared in collaboration with Charles Errard (*c.* 1606–1689), director of the French Academy in Rome from 1660 to 1689, was published at Rome in 1691.[33]

Together with the figure of Time, the scene is dominated by the theme of decomposition, which is underlined by the presence of animals, mainly rats that seem to enter the bodies. This small detail fascinatingly recalls the oeuvre of a scientist, contemporaneous to Zumbo, active in the same court: Francesco Redi (1626–97). Redi played an important role in the second half of the seventeenth century with his book *Esperienze Intorno alla Generazione degli Insetti* (1665), in which he criticizes some theories of the time, erroneously based on old-fashioned doctrines such as the spontaneous generation of maggots in rotting bodies. By using an experimental scientific approach, Redi had the courage not only to confute explicative theories, but also, and most importantly, to add a fresh perspective on the study of the phenomenon itself by affirming its universality, at that time called *ex semine* or *ex ovo*. Bernardi aptly described his experiments:

> Redi prepared eight containers filled with different kinds of meat; he left four of them uncovered, and carefully sealed the other four. The result was unequivocal: only the first samples, on which flies could lay their eggs, originated maggots that, at a later stage, developed, becoming flies identical to the previous ones. Instead, the flesh in the sealed containers became putrid and decomposed too, but didn't give birth to any form of life.[34]

Along with its theoretical value, Redi's research represents a vital achievement in the medical field, since it made it easier to understand the infection process that lies at the base of contagious diseases. In all probability, the artist showed signs of interest in Redi's work, not only for the reason that his assumptions sparked off an intense debate starting from 1665, but also because Zumbo expressed in art what a physician had scientifically researched and demonstrated.

Due to his increasing interest in scientific matters, Zumbo decided to abandon Florence, heading to Bologna, where he spent a short but intense period in the most significant centre for European anatomy. Afterwards, Zumbo moved to Genova, where he started a fruitful collaboration with the French physician Guillaume Desnoues (*c.* 1650–*c.* 1735), professor of anatomy and surgery. Desnoues held public lectures, in which he used anatomic preparations as explicative, didactic material. These preparations, obtained through injections of alcohol and wax, were frail and they deteriorated after a short period of time.

Their cooperation gave birth to an artwork produced in two versions, now lost: the waxes of a pregnant woman, dead because of the impossibility of expelling the foetus's head, which was too big. This experience is meaningful for Zumbo. Drawing inspiration from this sculpture, he decided to reconstruct a marvellous anatomic head,[35] modelled on a female skull. Its vibrant realism and faithful beauty can be rightly regarded as the purest, most balanced synthesis between the artist's poetics and his deep anatomic knowledge of the human body and its internal systems. He managed to reproduce the skull's horizontal section as well as the brain's vertical one, displaying a detailed and precise representation of the salivary glands, the orifice of the parotid duct, the thyroid and the tracheal rings. Along with his meticulous interest for anatomic detail, Zumbo did not forget to highlight its ongoing process of decomposition, an element that has always been relevant in his production. From the feeling that shines through this half-flayed face, this work appears as the first, complete union of art and medicine.

## The Birth of 'Istituto delle Scienze' and the Osteological and Myological Investigation of Ercole Lelli

During the same years of Zumbo's activity, the city of Bologna witnessed the birth of the 'Accademias'. The rigid mentality that dominated the university at the end of the seventeenth century constituted a serious obstacle for the researcher who wished to study the natural world, thereby adopting a new, creative glance. Reacting against the substantial impossibility of innovative research, the cleverest academics organized alternative groups, promoting the growth of different associations.

In 1691 these individuals founded the Academy of Philosophers (Accademia dei Filosofi), one of the most relevant sites for science in Bologna. Also known as the Academy of the Restless (Accademia degli Inquieti), this institution symbolized the spirit's propensity to endless movement. The contribution of Luigi Ferdinando Marsili (1658–1730) was fundamental: in exchange for the vast literary and scientific patrimony he had accumulated during his trips, he erected an impressive building for a modern institute, which, starting from 1711, would be called the Institute of Sciences and Arts (Istituto delle Scienze e delle Arti).

During its first years, the institute was devoted to the teaching and researching of astronomy, experimental physics, chemistry, military architecture, natural history and mechanics. Interestingly, a special emphasis was put on the study of surgery and anatomy. Thanks to the augmented interest in this latter group, a collection of medical objects and materials was started in Palazzo Poggi. A first nucleus consisted of dried anatomic preparations ('a secco') made by Anton Maria Valsalva (1666–1723), who also authored the book *Tractatus de aure humana* (1704). Because of this institution's recognition of the value of anatomic knowledge as a support for theory, the production of such items increased.

In this regard, it is important to highlight the fundamental role of Ercole Lelli. Whereas Zumbo's work managed to render scientific detail precisely through a personal realism characterized by iconographic echoes and a taste for craftsmanship, the artistic career of the Bolognese wax modeller Lelli originated from drawing as well as from his love for truth, reality and the beauty of the body. It should be remembered that these attributes were closely linked to neoclassical aesthetics.

Already from the beginning of his activity, Lelli proved to be particularly keen at the discovery of structures and secret mechanisms of the human machine. During his apprenticeship he studied and personally experimented with the art of injecting wax in the blood vessels of the skull's intricate region. Michele Medici recalls:

> in the hospital of Santa Maria della Morte ... he injected wax in a man's head with such talent that this head seemed alive, having recovered an healthy glow; the injected wax could even be seen in the eyes' vessels.[36]

On the basis of his extensive knowledge of the human body Lelli manufactured two flayed men for the Archiginnasio[37] anatomic theatre. These statues can be regarded as an elevated, methodological achievement as well as proof of his mature anatomic investigation.[38] Lelli became increasingly interested in the morphologic study of the human body, with a particular focus on its most internal systems. It is in this context that he realized two wax model reproductions of kidneys:[39] the first pair healthy, and the second a 'horseshoe-shaped' ('a ferro di cavallo') pair (see Figure 12.1). Both would become part of the institute collection of preparations in the 1730s.

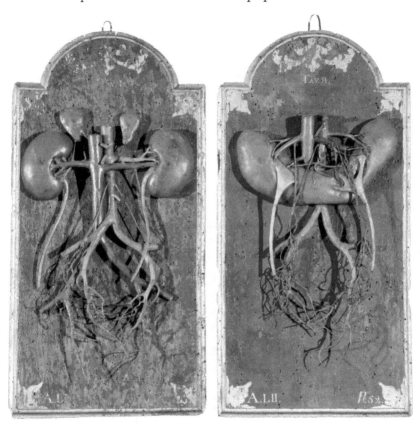

Figure 12.1: Ercole Lelli, 'Normal Kidney' and 'Horseshoe Kidney' (*c.* 1737); reproduced with permission of the Museo di Palazzo Poggi, University of Bologna, Italy.

These works appear to have been innovative, not only in their three-dimensional representation of an internal portion, which is in turn part of a bigger system, but mainly because they invited a comparison between a healthy and an ill apparatus (useful for a didactic purpose). The depiction of these two organs in all their smallest parts, such as their arterial and venous vessels, marked a turning point in the history of medicine, since it made it possible to avoid the use of corpses for medical training. Cadavers were not sufficiently available for a city that was fervently keen on this kind of study. Notably, Cardinal Prospero Lambertini showed such a real appreciation of these artefacts that, when he was elected Pope (changing his name in Benedetto XIV) in 1740, he commissioned Ercole Lelli to produce a series of wax models that would form the core for a museum of human anatomy and anthropometry (internal and external) in the Istituto delle Scienze.[40]

This moment can be considered as a milestone in the history of scientific representation. For the first time an artist was giving a detailed and precise image of the human body through its deconstruction into vital systems, thus creating a sort of a textual map. Beginning with a naked man and a woman, these statues displayed in six flayed bodies a progressive resolution, gradually moving from the superficial systems (namely, the myological) to the most internal ones, and finally arriving at the skeletal structure (see Figure 12.2). Additionally, a series of panels represented each of the small portions of the body, which could be studied separately by virtue of their function. Among these one can find the larynx, pharynx, eyes, ears and parts of the genitals. In order to produce all these objects, Lelli availed himself to the collaboration of several other artists, such as the surgeon Boari and the wax modeller Domenico Piò. Most importantly, he worked with Giovanni Manzolini.[41] Eight years later, Lelli managed to finish his protean project,[42] realizing one of the highest artistic achievements in the field of the human body's scientific documentation. It must be added that, due to his extensive experience, Lelli played a pivotal role during the following years, becoming a point of inspiration for the medical community.

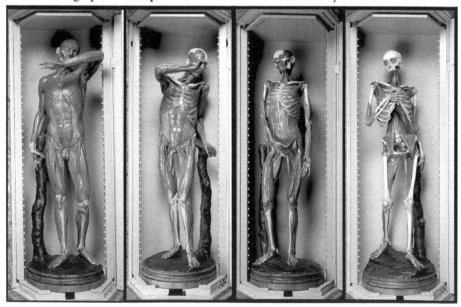

Figure 12.2: Ercole Lelli, 'Fleyed-Men' (*c.* 1750); reproduced with permission of the Museo di Palazzo Poggi, University of Bologna, Italy.

## Giovanni Manzolini and Anna Morandi: Scientific Observers, Knowledge Mediators

As discussed above, Giovanni Manzolini took part in Ercole Lelli's ambitious project. Unfortunately, due to a furious quarrel, Manzolini had to abandon the studio. This event paved the way for the construction of a laboratory at his home, where he worked with his wife, Anna Morandi, on anatomical preparations. It should be noted that Manzolini tried to avoid the moods and suggestions coming from contemporary art. Instead, he concentrated his efforts on the investigation of the most complex parts of the body, which could be seen only through a careful microscopic analysis. With regard to this aspect of his work, he was more an anatomist than an artist. His interest is evident in, for instance, the wax *Study of the Ear*[43] (see Figure 12.3). This work was created in collaboration with Morandi, as Miriam Focaccia suggests.[44] Nonetheless, a large number of critics insist on attributing it solely to his wife.

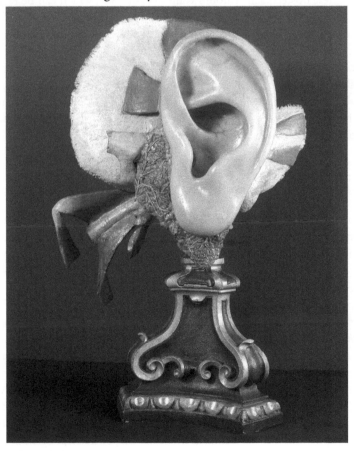

Figure 12.3: Giovanni Manzolini and Anna Morandi, *Study of the Ear* (mid-1700s); reproduced with permission of the Museo di Palazzo Poggi, University of Bologna, Italy.

Manzolini's 'Study of the Ear' was generated by scrupulous research on the auditory system, as witnessed by two letters written by the artist himself to the Istituto delle Scienze in 1750[45] and in 1751.[46] In these writings he discusses two relevant medical themes: the ears' anatomy and congenital deaf-mutism. In the first letter, besides formulating new theories on the properties and peculiarities of the vestibular nerve, Manzolini critically evaluates the veracity of certain assumptions about this system, which had been expressed in the *Tractatus de aure humana* by Valsalva. Interestingly, the artist found some imperfections in the illustrations; for this reason, he wrote a detailed report on the errors, completing it with precise references to the drawings. In the second letter, thanks to the anatomic analysis performed on the head of a deaf man, and to his intuition, Manzolini managed to discover the causes of this pathology, which originate in an anomaly of the cochlea structure.

It is important to emphasize that Manzolini's career is connected to his wife's activity. The pair realized together a series of waxes on panels commissioned by the Bolognese obstetrician Antonio Galli[47] (1708–82), which can be regarded as a model, by virtue of their completeness. Similar to a three-dimensional atlas, these twenty waxes depicted the morphological process of the womb's metamorphosis in the different stages of pregnancy.

Whereas Manzolini's works illustrated and deepened the contemporary medical knowledge, Morandi's production went rather beyond that point. After her husband's death, Anna Morandi kept working on ceroplastics and anatomy, becoming an avant-garde figure in the European context. She embodied the synthesis of theoretical knowledge and technical ability. As Galvani wrote,

> It should be taken into account that Manzolini's wife was the first one who joined two extremely dissimilar, difficult arts, namely Sculpture and Anatomy, so suitable (not to say indispensable) for such works, She combined them so well that she succeeded in both.[48]

Her fame crossed national borders, resulting in invitations to work in other institutes and academies in London and Saint Petersburg. In spite of this, Morandi chose not to leave her city, Bologna. As an answer to these invitations, she sent boxes containing some of her anatomic preparations together with books and writings. Morandi so distinguished herself, with regard to writings, that she accompanied her works of art with her own didactic texts, which clarified all of their aspects. Moreover, she put signs on her waxes that made the correspondences between the object and the text easier to recognize.

Morandi greatly contributed also to the development of modern surgery, thanks to her comprehensive knowledge of the human body, gained only after having analysed a large number of corpses. As Gabriella Berti Logan reports, the young Germano Azzoguidi (1740–1814), who would author the volume *Observationes ad uteri constructionem pertinentes*, interrogated Morandi on the presence of venous appendixes in the womb, as per Jean Astruc's description in *Traité des maladies des femmes*.[49] By giving a negative answer, she removed all his doubts.

Before Ercole Lelli, artists tried to generate a faithful representation of the human body starting with a more or less careful observation of its internal parts. Differently from them, as Rebecca Messbarger writes, Anna Morandi, 'offers a new rendering of the fabric of human bodies that envisions each organ in terms of its vital function within the context of a dynamic, interdependent physiological whole'.[50] This new approach is evident in two works: *Wax Hands*[51] (see Figure 12.4) and *Wax Muscles of the Eyeball, Muscle of the Superior Eyelid, Optic Nerve*[52] (see Figure 12.5). The first confronted, with high lyricism, an extremely complex problem: the issue of perception in relation to the nervous system. The second opus tries to describe visually these entangled connections. Starting from the internal morphology of the eye, the wax displays the veins, nerves and muscles of the eye in a succession that is functional to Morandi's explanation of the organ. Moreover, this *mise en scène* underscores the importance of the single elements and their reciprocal interconnections. Morandi was a mature wax modeller, but this practice also led her to become a brilliant scientist. Indeed, her skilled ability to synthesize art and medicine is witnessed not only by her artistic masterpieces, notably *Wax Muscles of the Eyeball, Muscle of the Superior Eyelid, Optic Nerve*, but also by her discovery that the lower oblique muscle of the eye did not stop in the nasal apophysis, as it was thought, but terminated in the lachrymal sac. This finding was made possible primarily through her faithful artistic research. Three years after her death, the Istituto delle Scienze bought her anatomic preparations, together with her scientific library.

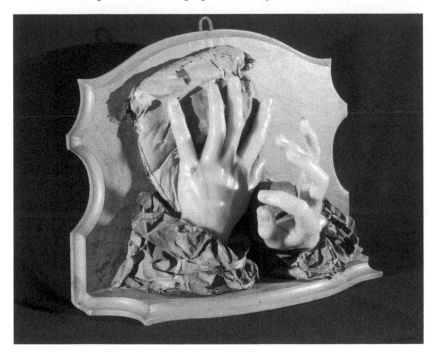

**Figure 12.4: Anna Morandi, *Wax Hands* (mid-1700s); reproduced with permission of the Museo di Palazzo Poggi, University of Bologna, Italy.**

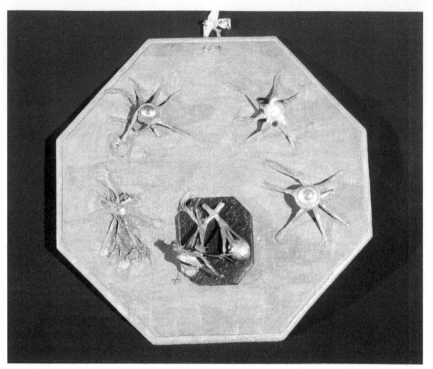

**Figure 12.5: Anna Morandi, *Wax Muscles of the Eyeball, Muscle of the Superior Eyelid, Optic Nerve* (mid-1700s); reproduced with permission of the Museo di Palazzo Poggi, University of Bologna, Italy.**

## Conclusions

The present critical analysis has highlighted the pivotal role played by the creative complicity between art and medicine in the definition of a modern concept of system. By means of the careful study and precise cataloguing of the human body, both artists and physicians have gradually gained a more comprehensive knowledge of its hidden structures. More specifically, the shift from a bi-dimensional kind of representation to purely anatomical objects expressed a mature approach articulating the idea of the human body as a unity consisting of different, interacting systems that are part of a complex architecture.

Thus it can be argued that the evolution of artistic thought, both in its theory and practice, became an essential tool in reproducing a complete mapping of the body. Notably, the practices that attracted artists and physicians proved to be fruitful for both disciplines: in the artistic field, for instance, the flat and approximate depiction of the human body was substituted by a rich and life-like rendering. The work of art tried not only to portray anatomic details, but it also made an effort to understand the underlying processes that make the human machine work, without forgetting its lyric prerogative. In turn, this innovative experience and attitude towards the subject was fundamental for the progress of medical studies, an issue that has been poorly studied.

Nonetheless, it can be asserted that it is in the production of wax modellers that the complex tangle of relationships harmoniously sublimates. Hence, the ambiguous fascination with their oeuvre: these bodies function as mirrors reflecting in a *mimetic* way their alive counterparts, resulting in a more realistic depiction of corporality, which can amaze or horrify the audience. Ambivalence seems to be a chief feature of the works of art belonging to this epoch: indeed, by escaping the purely representational, artistic context they gave birth to a realism of enormous scientific value.

Conventionally a great passion for art, which fuses with the laic and moral quest for knowledge, is thought to be the synthesis of the illuminist ideal. Significantly, these masterpieces seem to be expressing the same essence. In the words of Barbara Maria Stafford, they built a solid bridge over the 'untraversable abyss ... between the practical visual and the theoretical textual'.[53]

# 13 THE INTERNAL ENVIRONMENT: CLAUDE BERNARD'S CONCEPT AND ITS REPRESENTATION IN *FANTASTIC VOYAGE*

Jérôme Goffette and Jonathan Simon

'We stand in the middle of infinity between outer and inner space.'
– Richard Fleischer (dir), *Fantastic Voyage* (1966)

What does it mean to represent the interior of the human body? Recent scandals around exhibitions of 'real' dissected human bodies, such as Gunther von Hagens's notorious Body Worlds exhibition and the recent closure of a similar type of anatomical exhibition, 'Our Body – à corps ouvert' by a French court in 2009, have served to keep this question alive. And yet the interior of the body has been represented in the cinema practically from the beginning of narrative films. Horror films and war films regularly expose the interior of the body for its shock value. Indeed, with increasingly sophisticated special effects now available to film directors, the interior of the body is exposed with a realism designed to turn the stomach of the most hardened spectator. However, this is not the only context in which the body's interior has been represented in fiction. The interior of the body can also be explored in more artistic and scientific ways, with such representations often playing on the wonder or even the miracle of the human 'machine' both to engage the audience and to convey a message about the significance of life. Yet even if one adopts this more positive attitude to the interior of the body, there are many different ways to do so, and new scientific discoveries have served to add to this panoply. Thus, the range of visions of the interior of the human body is not the same today as it was in the past, and the relevant transformations of the vision of the body have been multiple and spread across time and geographical space. Here, we want to consider one particular development around the concept of the internal environment introduced by Claude Bernard in the nineteenth century. We will then see how this concept of the internal environment was mobilized in the twentieth century in the now classic Hollywood film *Fantastic Voyage*, which depicts humans exploring the inside of the human body in a miniaturized submarine.

Before turning to Claude Bernard, it is important to underline the ambivalence of the human body as on the one hand attractive and enticing and on the other violent and revolting. In his analysis of the imaginary, Gilbert Durand points to these two possibilities and argues that while both are present in European culture, it is increasingly the negative 'infernal' aspects that dominate.

In the first place, it is the sombre aspect of the archetypal figures of fear that wins out over the 'soft' image of the interior. '[The body's orifices] are the doors into this miniature infernal labyrinth that is constituted by the shadowy, bloody interior of the body.'[1] Thus, we can interpret the history of such representations as a struggle between these two visions of the interior of the body; the soft yielding body, warm and rounded, the body we encounter every day, versus the terrifying, bloody, infernal body which was for so long the dominant vision of the body whose integrity was compromised. Traditionally, the opening of a body would inevitably be followed by death; and the opening was often seen as the path for the soul or life to escape. A triple obstacle blocked the way to the interior of the body: the sensory obstacle of the obscurity of an unlit space; the affective obstacle constituted by the fear of the infernal vision of this forbidden space; and the symbolic obstacle of death itself and the agony of the dying. Indeed, the rise of exact anatomy in the Renaissance only overcame the first obstacle, the darkness of the interior. The best known icon of this anatomical enlightenment was Andreas Vesalius's (1514–64) *De humani corporis fabrica*, published in 1543. The classical anatomical representations found in the book show the body stripped down layer by layer, from muscle to bone. The symbolism of the gallows and the penitence of the dead keep the representations in the register of the fear of death, and the vision of a 'soft' interior remains entirely absent.

Later, the development of the microscope would lead to another transformation in the perception and representation of the interior of the body. While the plates of Robert Hooke's *Micrographia* (1665) graphically evoked a fantastic invisible living world hidden within the visible world, they did not touch on the human body. Nevertheless, the observation of red corpuscles by Jan Swammerdam and the drawings of spermatozoids by Antoni van Leeuwenhoek opened up an interior that was no longer one of suffering and horror but an image of wonder at the unexpected composition of vital fluids that had hitherto been regarded as homogeneous and simple. The microscopic analysis of blood and sperm was tangential to the anatomical tradition for understanding the nature of the human body, as it operated on samples removed from the body and so no longer involved any direct exploration of a human body. Of course, this approach shares certain elements with the physiology of Magendie and Bernard, which sought to integrate an understanding of living processes in a science of the functioning of the animal and human body.

Claude Bernard's concept of the internal environment (*milieu intérieur*) is a particularly significant innovation in the scientific conception of the human body and notably its interior. While the term was first presented to the public in 1865, Mirko Grmek in his study of Bernard's papers found that the idea was already present in his notebooks as early as 1851. The idea of the living organism as characterized by a distinct internal environment maintained against the challenges of an inanimate external environment is today so banal that it is hard to imagine how hard it would have been for Bernard and his contemporaries to accept. Here, we want to explain why this idea seemed so foreign to Bernard's contemporaries, but also to trace the path of its diffusion and acceptance by the scientific world and the wider public. To treat the second issue, we will consider not only the history of science but also the role science fiction might have played in this transition, considering the work of Maurice Renard, but with a particular focus on Richard Fleischer's *Fantastic Voyage* and to a lesser extent *Blood Music*, a more recent film on the theme by Greg Bear.

## Claude Bernard: The Internal Environment as Conceptual Revolution

After not having published for six years, Bernard released his best-known book, *An Introduction to the Study of Experimental Medicine* in 1865, and it was here that the phrase 'milieu intérieur' appeared for the first time in print. The French word 'milieu' French is not easy to translate, as is evidenced by the fact that the word has been integrated into English in a number of contexts, mostly relating to human society. Here, we use the phrase 'internal environment' to translate 'milieu intérieur'. As mentioned above, the idea of the internal environment had been present in Bernard's personal notes as early as 1851.[2] Over the course of these fourteen years the idea became increasingly central to Bernard's thinking, and became a veritable paradigm for experimental medicine.

> Ancient science was able to conceive only the outer environment; but to establish the science of experimental biology, we must also conceive an inner environment ... Only by passing into the inner, can the influence of the outer environment reach us ... Now, here is the true physiological environment; this it is which physiologists and physicians should study and know, for by its means they can act on the histological units which are the only effective agents in vital phenomena ... The organism is merely a living machine so constructed that, on the one hand, the outer environment is in free communication with the inner organic environment, and, on the other hand, the organic units have protective functions, to place in reserve the materials of life and uninterruptedly to maintain the humidity, warmth and other conditions essential to vital activity ... In a word, vital phenomena are the result of contact between the organic units of the body with the inner physiological environment; this is the pivot of all experimental medicine.[3]

Indeed, this new paradigm of the inner environment modified our way of seeing the living body in a number of ways.

## Miniaturization

First, in order to understand Bernard's approach we need to make the move from the macroscopic to the microscopic. The introduction of the microscope, notably those equipped with high-quality optical systems in the nineteenth century, changed the scale of observational perception. This was not a theoretical transformation, but a perceptual shift linked to the daily practice of microscopic analysis in the field of histology. Using the microscope involved loosening the tie to macroscopic vision, and adopting a projective capacity that allowed the researcher to inhabit a different world; but one whose difference was constituted by a difference in scale rather than place. Nevertheless, what is most surprising in Bernard is not so much the possibility of using a microscopic, but the use he makes of the perceptual perspective: 'If we could be a blood corpuscle, we would see the properties of each tissue with respect to the environment of the blood, but we are not at this point.'[4]

The phrase 'If we could be a blood corpuscle' illustrates perfectly the boldness of the imaginative work being done by Bernard in this book, as we can see him projecting himself into this alternative world. The problems he confronts are both perceptual and figurative; he is attempting to stand back from his proper perspective and place himself in the position of a living cell. Indeed, naturalists and physiologists that were his contemporaries were unreceptive to this way of thinking, and, as Grmek points out, it was only after 1885, and more particularly in the twentieth century that his ideas would take hold. In a note from 1867 that has been published by Grmek, Bernard wrote that, 'In the life sciences we need to create a science of the internal environment which would be the true experimental physiology. Here, we would be in the organism as we are in the world.'[5]

Bernard explained the incomprehension of his contemporaries in terms of the difficulty experienced by naturalists when asked to change their perspectives. He argued that they were so used to comparing species either still existent or extinct that they were not capable of passing from outside to a perspective from within. The triumph of perspective in Renaissance painting, placing the viewing subject at the centre of the construction of an image, is here undermined by a projection into the object that is being represented. Bernard posits an analogical displacement of perspective: 'We would be in the organism as we are in the world'; the physiologist's view of the internal environment should be like our view of the world around us.

## Embedded Perspectives

The perceptual and cognitive difficulties confronted by Bernard's contemporaries are amplified by a *mise en abîme* in his deployment of the concept of environment.

> [T]he lowest animal has its own organic environment; infusoria have an environment belonging to them, in this sense that they are more permeated than is a fish with the water in which he swim. In the organic environments of the higher animals, the histological units are like veritable infusoria, that is to say, they are provided an environment proper to themselves which is not the general organic environment. Thus a corpuscle of blood is permeated with a fluid different from the serum in which it floats.[6]

Thus, Bernard mobilizes an approach that is reminiscent of Leibniz's monads, with a radical perspectivalism in which every living thing is a world unto itself.[7] For Bernard, it is not a question of the world being contained in every constitutive part, but rather that each element of the living world lives in its own specific world. Like Kepler's vision of the embedded spheres of the solar system, the internal environments of the body's constituent parts exist embedded one within one another. Thus the internal environment should not be thought of as the circulatory system, the lymph system or a collection of organs that function together or separately, but rather as a physiological concept. The important thing is to consider the environment or environments in terms of the object under consideration in relation to the specific context in which it is located and all this at the appropriate scale.

## The Physiological Vision and Life

In his published work, Bernard often repeated his desire to use his idea of the internal environment as a key concept on which to found a discipline of physiology as the science of life. Here is just one example of this argument:

> To establish the science of experimental biology, we must also conceive an inner environment ... The general cosmic environment is common to living and to inorganic bodies; but the inner environment created by an organism is specific to each living being. However, this is the true physiological environment ... where one finds the only effective agents in vital phenomena.[8]

This 'biological science', a science of the living body and of living phenomena needs to escape from the common-sense view of the body from the exterior, all the more so because from this perspective it is possible to mistake inanimate objects for living beings and vice versa. In order to enter into this new science, the scientist needs to enter into the more intimate features of life located within the 'organic environment'. This approach represents a substantial rupture from the work of the anatomists, whether through dissection or the preparation of illustrative anatomical specimens. The vision of living bodies as they are in life requires rethinking what to look at and how.

## Life in an Aquatic Seascape

One of the consequences of Bernard's way of thinking is to transform the imagery associated with living organisms. The injunction to see living beings from within rather than from without, in order to understand how they function, means that the scientist should no longer be observing an object, but rather contemplating a landscape. In the case of the human body, the internal environment should, in particular, be represented by an aquatic landscape or seascape. Indeed, Bernard is clearly aware that it is the marine or the aquatic that constitutes the appropriate reference for this work.

> We are like those men who measure the state of the air in order to carry out experiments on fish in the water. Our tissues are not subject to the influence of the air any more than are fish. Our tissues are aquatic just like fish. They die when they are exposed to the air. If we could be a blood corpuscle, we would see how the properties of all the tissues exist in relation to blood as a medium.[9]

The second half of the nineteenth century was the time when large aquaria started to be built to complement the collections of killed specimens (whether dried or immersed in alcohol) in natural history. The first public aquarium in Europe was opened in London's Regent's Park in 1853. In 1870, Jules Verne published what is probably the most famous undersea novel ever, *20,000 Leagues Under the Sea*, in which the mysterious captain Nemo has numerous exciting adventures in the uncharted depths of the oceans thanks to his futuristic submarine, the *Nautilus*. The nineteenth century saw the ocean take form as more than just a dangerous expanse of water. After conquering its surface, the exploration of the hidden depths opened up a vast new space to the world's imagination. Indeed, the HMS *Beagle* on which Charles Darwin voyaged around the world in the 1850s was charged precisely with fathoming the depths of the coast of South America.

## Blood, Regulation and Distribution

Another change in perspective ushered in by Bernard's concept of the internal environment involves the integration of physiological complexity. The vision of this environment is divided between unity and disparity between the homogeneous and the heterogeneous. While blood appears to the naked eye as a homogeneous red fluid, it was already known to be composite (red blood cells separate from the liquid serum when blood is left to stand), but by asking the researcher to put himself in the position of a red blood cell Bernard took a step further in the miniaturization of the perspective. However, following the development of physiology, and notably techniques for chemical dosing, blood was discovered to be more than just a solution of red blood cells in serum.

Techniques for the measurement of glucose content, levels of toxins and other chemicals multiplied the diversity of the blood's constituents.

Finally, we need to consider the role played by Bernard's conception of homeostasis in this vision of the interior of the body. Important functions of blood include the regulation of the body and the distribution of vital materials like nutrients and oxygen. Blood is actively involved in regulating the living cells that compose the body, and coordinating their interaction with other cells and with the exterior world. Thus the internal environment can also be seen as a buffer between the outside world and the smallest components of the body, ensuring a viable context for maintaining the functions of life at the micro level in the context of an organism that evolves in a more or less hostile environment.

## *The Internal Environment as the Product of a Living Organism*

This last point leads us to an important, but far from obvious aspect of Bernard's approach. Unlike the external environment, which is independent of the organism itself, the internal environment is a product of this same organism.

> The internal environment, which is a true product of the organism, preserves the necessary relations of exchange and equilibrium with the external cosmic environment; but in proportion as the organism grows more perfect; the organic environment becomes specialized and more and more isolated, as it were, from the surrounding environment.[10]

Thus, we are dealing with an environment produced by the organism itself, an internal environment arising out of just such an internal environment. Accustomed as we are to thinking of living organisms in terms of their independence from the world, Bernard obliges us to think of the body in terms of dependence. In case of the constitutive cells being damaged the whole environment suffers and the body is put at risk. The internal environment emphasizes the interdependence between the entities composing the body and the medium in which they exist. Another way of thinking about this is to think of the internal environment as an 'intimate' environment. Indeed, Bernard uses this kind of terminology in his *Introduction to Experimental Medicine*, where he talks of 'intimate particles' as well as intimate environment.[11] The use of this kind of vocabulary offers a positive 'soft' image of the body in contrast to the bloody one of the dissection table and its accompanying anatomic plates. This suggests that we should place Bernard's physiology on the positive side of Gilbert Durand's dichotomy as championing a different kind of scientific imagery from the medical tradition of the time.

## The *Fantastic Voyage*

Bernard's theory of the internal environment represented such a radical break with medical visions of the living organism that it only managed to establish its place well after the death of its author. According to Mirko Grmek, the change of paradigm associated with this view only started at the end of the nineteenth century, despite the early interest exhibited by the American psychologist William James.[12] It is not our aim in this essay to explore the integration of this view into scientific culture, but rather to look at its effects on the wider social and cultural contexts of the twentieth century.

The first half of the twentieth century witnessed the ascension of cinema, with many successful literary narratives being adapted for the big screen. In the popular genre of horror films, the representations of the body remained quite traditional. Mary Shelley's *Frankenstein* (1818) and Robert Louis Stevenson's *The Strange Case of Dr Jekyll and Mr Hyde* (1886) were two classic novels in this genre that were not only made into films but also served as the inspiration for many others. These films featured dead and dismembered bodies with all the horror and shock of the popular images of the dissection table. Such gory representations (although before the development of special effects, more would pass by suggestion than by images of the body itself) were only made more vivid by famous murder cases from the nineteenth century, such as the story of Burke and Hare or Jack the Ripper.

Generally, in the early cinema as in the literature that informed it, the body is limited to its superficial appearance and its interior becomes an ill-defined ectoplasm, as in H. G. Wells's story *The Invisible Man* (1897). A modern anthropological study of popular conceptions of the body suggests that the vision of its interior remains unclear, with the subjects of the investigation admitting as much themselves. Thus the investigation identified not only areas of straightforward ignorance, with respect to the body, but echoes of humoural theory as well.[13] The early decades of the twentieth century did see the publication of a few texts that attempted to present a 'realist' vision of the interior of the body, like Maurice Renard's *L'homme truqué* (1921) with its insistence on the electrical phenomena of the human body. Nevertheless, the dominant vision of the body remained external or superficial (with the interior serving as evidence of violent intrusion) and macroscopic (with the organs being the finest detail to be considered).

Richard Fleischer's *Fantastic Voyage* from 1966 marks a turning point in the representation of the human body in film following the conceptual path prefigured in the writings of Claude Bernard. Before making *Fantastic Voyage*, Fleischer had already made around twenty films, including an adaptation of Jules Verne's *20 000 Leagues Under the Sea* and an historical epic *Barabbas* (1961). Although a well-established film-maker, Fleischer was probably agreeably surprised by the success of this film, which enjoyed box office success around the world followed by numerous television broadcasts. Isaac Asimov wrote a novel based on the film, and, in 1968–9, ABC showed a television series based on the film consisting of seventeen half-hour episodes. The concept, even more than the film itself, seems to have constituted a kind of 'best-seller' of the 1960s. In light of its wide diffusion, it is very possible that the film had an influence on popular representations of the body. What is important for our argument here is that this voyage into the human body offered a *mise en scène* of the vision of the body's interior proposed a century earlier by Bernard, trying to show what we would see 'if we could be a blood corpuscle'.[14]

In the analysis of the film that follows, we attempt both to explore its relationship to Bernard's idea of the 'internal environment' and to draw attention to other elements of the film that might make us think otherwise. The first part consists in a 'classic' epistemological analysis with a comparative exploration of the conceptual elements in the film and in the work of Bernard. The second part of the analysis will turn around the symbolic imaginary of the work. Here, we will leave issues concerning the literary form of the work aside to focus on the symbolic elements of the film. To summarize our approach, a semantic exploration of both the conceptual and the imaginary aspects of *Fantastic Voyage* will be presented. While the essential conceptual background for understanding the representation of the human body in the film has been examined, we have yet to broach the issue of the symbolic imaginary, and so propose a few lines of introduction to the subject.

Modern Western philosophy has dismissed the imaginary as unworthy of attention for much of its history. For a long time, the imaginary was evoked only as the counterpoint to conceptual clarity or reason, regarded as the domain of the chaotic and the irrational to be avoided at all costs. It was only in the twentieth century that the idea of the organization of the imaginary started to be developed, notably thanks to the work of Mircea Eliade (1996), Gaston Bachelard and Gilbert Durand. In his exploration of dreams and poetry, Bachelard pointed to the common elements and privileged forms of the imaginary that underwrite a shared fabric of dreams. Durand developed the idea of the anthropological structures of the imaginary, which would serve as the title for his leading publication.[15] Adopting this approach, we want to explore Fleischer's film by referring to the imaginary symbols that he deploys, relying for their interpretation on the dictionaries of symbols of Gertrude Jobes, Eduardo Cirlot and, above all, Jean Chevalier and Alain Gheerbrant.[16] This technique will allow us to highlight not only the fictional alterations of the physiological vision as it is brought to the screen, but also to recognize the places in which the film uses a process of symbolic emphasis to make certain elements visually comprehensible. As this was not a scientific film, but was aimed at a general public, concepts considered too foreign for a non-specialist audience required the emphasis of a special *mise en scène*. Indeed, the imaginary can help people to understand difficult concepts, offering a translation into other more comprehensible registers, and it is not always the case, as suggested by the Italian proverb *Traduttore, traditore*, that a translation necessarily betrays the content.

What for Claude Bernard and his disciples was a scientific representation, required an abstract schema to be translated for the film – an appropriate land-scape (or seascape) for an adventure narrative. Evidently, in order to provide the necessary escapism expected of a fantasy fiction, emphasis had to be placed on the spectacular wherever possible. The opening of the film provides the fictional background for the voyage through the body in the context of a high-stakes political thriller. In the context of the Cold War, a team is asked to take a minia-ture submarine into the body of a top scientist. They are to destroy a blood clot and thus save the man's life so that he can provide the Americans with the vital sensitive information that only he knows. Rather than considering this central story or the subplots and interpersonal intrigue that develop around it, here we wish to focus exclusively on the sets, special effects and dialogues that are used to dramatize the discovery of the interior of a human body.

## *The Change in Scale*

The first special effects associated with the voyage inside the body involve the change of scale experienced directly by the team charged with the mission. The men and woman board the submarine, *Proteus*, which is then reduced to the size of a cell in order to pass through the blood stream undetected. The minia-turization process occurs in two steps, each one representing a thousand-fold reduction, which helps the director to make this change in scale more vivid. After the first miniaturization the submarine is reduced from metres to millime-tres, a transformation illustrated by the gigantic faces of the technicians looking in from outside. The second phase of the miniaturization involves a new prop, the giant syringe. The submarine is placed in the liquid in the syringe and the whole object is shrunk down, bringing the submarine down to a few microm-eters, the size of red blood cells. Using these special effects, Fleischer brings Bernard's project of assuming the place of the red blood cell to the screen, pro-viding the premise for the visualization of the internal environment from this perspective. This 'fantastic' miniaturization process, which is presented as being without limits, is interrupted at the scale of the human blood cell. The choice of stopping at the scale of the blood cells makes it easier for the viewer to relate to the subsequent adventure in the body, and the fact that the reduction takes place continuously helps render the transformation comprehensible. Further-more, to provide a framework of suspense, the miniaturization effect is limited in time. To close this sequence, we see the contents of the syringe injected into the carotid artery of the comatose scientist and, thus, thanks to the construction of the miniaturization sequence and the suggestion that the microscopic submarine is in the syringe, the link has been made between the protagonists and the blood stream.

The realism of this opening sequence is complemented by a mobilization of the imaginary, with a visual evocation of a poetics of space. We are transported into a miniature world, or, to use one of Gaston Bachelard's paradoxical expressions, we are carried into an 'intimate immensity'.[17] This phrase should remind us of the commentary that Bachelard made concerning Jules Supervielle's poetic phrase: 'Delicate inhabitants of the forests that are ourselves'.[18] This 'forest' is a metaphor for the self, as a deep, dark place, but also an intimate space for its inhabitants. Thus the figure of speech pulls in both directions at once, towards an intimacy of the self and an immensity of un- or under-explored space. While the relevant chapter in Bachelard's *The Poetics of Space* turns around the small hidden treasure in the context of the miniature, what interests us with respect to *Fantastic Voyage* is the dialectic between the intimate and the vastness of the interior space evoked by the film. Thus, the film's approach breaks with the traditional isomorphism to be found in films that relate the macro to the microcosm. We are not plunged into a world that is just like ours; part of the appeal of the film is precisely an exoticism based on an anisomorphism. The submarine is plunged into a 'forest' or a 'labyrinth' that differs from those found on earth. The décor, the actors and even the sounds all belong to a foreign microworld. An observer reduced to the micrometer, as Bernard had imagined it, is lost in the world that is in a sense his most familiar environment. This is not the world of Lilliput where everything is like our real world but in miniature; the scientific imagination replaces the default anthropomorphism of popular literature. In the end this microscopic tourism of the body's interior is presented as a visit to the most exotic world possible.

## *The Aquatic Universe*

The first difference between this internal environment and our normal vision of the body is the aquatic nature of the medium of the blood stream. This point is already prefigured in the form of the vessel used by the team, a submarine rather than a road vehicle. The aquatic nature of the environment is underlined a number of times in the dialogues between the actors.

| | |
|---|---|
| Pr Duval: | 'An ocean of life!' (sec. 00h38m30s) |
| Captain Owens: | 'We're in some sort of current!' (during the passage through the arterio-venous fistula, which Owens refers to as a 'Whirlpool') (sec. 00h40m00s) |
| Grant: | 'It looks like the sea at dawn.'(sec. 01h06m40s) |
| Grant: | 'Skipper, we're picking up seaweed or whatever that is.' |

Dr Michaels:    'Reticular fibres, we ought to be clear of them soon.'
(sec. 01h09m20s)

Thus, we find ourselves in a great seascape, just as in Verne's *20 000 Leagues Under the Sea*. This environment was not limited to fiction either, as Jacques Cousteau had already enjoyed considerable success with his underwater documentaries, and notably with his film *The Silent World* (*Le Monde du silence*) from 1956, which won the Palme d'Or at Cannes. Cousteau also developed his own small submarine, the *SP-350*, which bears a certain resemblance to the *Proteus*. Thus, the submarine references of the film – captain, diving gear, seaweed, etc. – were already familiar, although this does not detract from the novelty of the transposition of this cast from under the ocean into the interior of a human body.

Of course, the passage from the earth's atmosphere to an aquatic medium evokes a rich web of symbolic associations. The most obvious is water as a symbol of life. Professor Duval (the brain surgeon charged with removing the blood clot in the victim's brain) refers to the serum in which the blood cells float as 'an ocean of life'. This phrase does not make sense as a scientific claim but does refer to a rich vein of symbolism, as explored by Mircea Eliade, among others. For Eliade, water is not only a cosmic symbol of life and a potent remedy because 'life, vigour and eternity reside in water'[19] but also a rich source of phantasmagorical figures 'dragons, snakes, snails, dolphins, fish, etc. are water's emblems' hidden in the depths of the ocean, they are infused with the sacred force of the abyss'.[20]

Professor Duval's exclamation clearly plays on such connotations: the ecstatic recognition of the abundance of life within life. The serum, the medium in question, is itself a physiological product, another proof of the creative power of life within a living being. Rather than a scientific trope of disenchantment and objectivity, the science is presented in a dreamlike style, with numerous statements of awe and reverie. At the moment the submarine is first introduced into Chenes's bloodstream, Harry Kleiner's film script explicitly evokes both sides of this dichotomy, with Grant, Duval and Duval's assistant, Cora Peterson, 'enthralled', while Michaels, the team's medical scientist (who would later prove to be a treacherous saboteur) retains an objective distance.

> Grant and Cora, strapped in their seats, look on enthralled at the sheer beauty of the dancing wonder-world visible through the windows. Duval appears equally moved. Michaels observes with more clinical detachment.[21]

While water is a symbol for life, it is also a medium that can generate levity, where otherwise heavy objects can float weightlessly, suspended in space. The human body can float in just this way; submerged in water we are relieved from the daily effort of holding ourselves upright. Gilbert Durand reads this property in an allegorical way, arguing that immersion in water signals the suspension of human existential fears by taking away, however temporarily, the fear of falling and the constant effort involved in our postural reflexes.[22] The argument is not one of a regression to the foetal stage of life or the desire for a uterine cocoon, but rather the idea of an intermediary situation between the struggle to hold oneself upright and the transcendent dream of flight.[23]

Indeed, the situation is reminiscent of the first analyses Durand made of the nocturnal regime of the image. These analyses start with a descent, a voyage towards the depths of the chthonian world. He then goes on to underline the image of embedding, of an image of the 'within' associated with Lilliputian dreams or images of ichthyomorphic vessels.[24] Durand includes the story of Jonah and the whale in this type of imagery, with Jonah floating in the whale who is in turn floating in the ocean. The situation of the *Proteus* and its crew in *Fantastic Voyage* shares many of these distinctive elements: miniaturization, a logic of embedding (humans within a human), the omnipresent water, as well as the labyrinthine or cavernous aspects of the story.

## Labyrinth and Arborescence

There is a particular feature of the world of *Fantastic Voyage* that sets it apart from other undersea dramas like *20 000 Leagues Under the Sea*. Under the sea, water stretches off in all directions, while in the circulatory system liquid is canalized into the vessels. Indeed, blood flows through a circulatory system in the networks of arteries and veins and the lymphatic system. The body viewed from the interior, adopting the perspective of a subject a few micrometers in size, is a labyrinth, which, from a certain distance can be seen as having a double dendritic form, evoking an anthropomorphic tree or a dendritic labyrinth, as suggested by Durand.[25] The labyrinthine structure with a localized target, a clot in the brain that the crew is supposed to destroy using a special laser gun, implies a logistics for guiding the *Proteus* through the body. Thus, in the military style control room, there is a huge map of the body's circulatory system with a glowing light that traces the submarines path towards the target. The ambience is similar to images of space flights from the same period, but also recalls control rooms from the Second World War that tracked the air battles of the time. The plan is to take a direct path from the carotid artery to the site of the clot by passing into the appropriate vessels of the brain. Having destroyed the clot, the submarine will be recuperated via the jugular vein, and all this within the sixty-minute limit to the miniaturization.

Unfortunately for the mission, but fortunately for the tension of the plot, right from the beginning the original plan comes undone due to the unforeseen presence of an arterio-venous fistula, through which the submarine is drawn directly into the venous system heading for the heart. Rather than aborting, the team decides to go around the circulatory system, through the heart and lungs to attain their target. More than a typical anatomy lesson, this detour raises numerous points of physiology. For example, they have to stop the patient's heart for the submarine to pass through unharmed – more tension, but also a chance to see the interior of the heart.

Inside the labyrinth the situation and trajectory of the submarine become of capital importance as they seek their target within the complex geography of the human circulatory system. Thanks to the fantasy technology of 'stereotaxic imaging', the crew possess a collection of detailed maps, and, at the same time, they are followed by the military control team. This schema of a voyage of initiation through a maze or labyrinth is rich in connotations, with no shortage of myths involving the passage through a labyrinth to find a sacred or personal treasure.[26] This symbolism of the labyrinth is thus superimposed on the rich symbolism of circulation itself, beyond the vision of the arterial and venous systems as versions of the tree of life.[27] There is also the image of the circulation as an ouroborous, the alchemical figure of the snake that eats its own tail. In the context of this profusion of connotations, the symbolic risks taking over the narrative from the scientific discourse. Nevertheless, the screenplay of *Fantastic Voyage* avoids entering into a reflection at this level by keeping the scientific discourse to the fore, sometimes even adopting a pedagogical style.

## Blood as a Composite Medium

The lessons on human microscopic physiology are triggered by a series of encounters with interesting or intriguing objects or phenomena throughout the voyage. Evidently this representation is in the style of the period – 1966 – and at times appears more kitsch than realistic to a viewer more than forty years later; but we also have to remember that it is a fiction film and not a documentary. On the journey, the submarine comes across red blood cells (presented as quite ethereal, closer to the projection of an object rather than a solid cell), epithelial cells, lung cells (like large nylon balloons), the reticular fibres of the ganglions, cells of Hensen (which trap Cora Peterson at one point), antibodies and the enchanting (or enchanted) spectacle of the sparks of electricity within the neuronal cells in the brain. At the end, the white blood cells make their dramatic entry to destroy Michaels, the traitor trapped within the growing *Proteus*.

Thus the scenario juggles two registers. On the one hand, we are in the physiological world proposed as a methodological ideal by Bernard, at the level where the crew of the Proteus can clearly distinguish the composite nature of the blood as an internal environment, providing an opening onto multiple observations of microscopic functions. On the other hand, the symbolic is always close to the surface, and is constantly mobilized to engage the audience in a different way. We can illustrate this point by two such examples of a symbolic turn in the *mise en scène*, although we could multiply these moments in the film. The first example is the case of the antibodies that attack Cora Peterson as she starts to grow to antigenic size. This attack of the antibodies is not very realistic, as they are represented like high-speed planes speeding through the blood directly towards their target. Nevertheless, this representation works well as the symbolic level, since these antibodies recognize the external intruder in an apparently intuitive manner and, like guard dogs, do not waste any time hunting it down. The second example where the symbolic triumphs over the quest for any realism is even more obvious, and this is the sparking between the neurones in the brain. Although there has never been any evidence for any illumination in the brain, let alone sparks of electricity, the symbolism is rich in terms of both the power and the nature of the human brain.[28] Light is a classic symbol for thought, with the rise of computing and the 'electrical brain' after the Second World War making sparks an obvious choice for representing the dynamism of human consciousness. This use of sparks serves several symbolic functions at once; representing modernity, science and technology, as well as providing a link with the modern spectacle of high-voltage electrical phenomena.

## Chemistry

In our review of the sciences represented in *Fantastic Voyage*, we want to finish by looking at chemistry and its place in the physiology of the internal environment. A good illustration of the presence of this chemistry is provided en route to the alveoli of the lung: after having damaged an air tank, the *Proteus* takes advantage of its passage through the lungs to refill with air. Here, the crew can observe the oxygenation of the red blood corpuscles up close, as they turn, in the film at least, from blue to red, a choice of colours that we discuss below. The explanation is given to the public first via an exchange between scientist and profane in the submarine, and is then taken to a higher level of reflection by a debate between scientists.

| | |
|---|---|
| Dr Michaels: | 'We're entering a capillary. Try to stay in the middle.' |
| Cap. Owens: | 'The wall's transparent.' |
| Dr Michaels: | 'It's less than one ten-thousandth of an inch thick. And porous.' |
| Cara Peterson: | 'Doctor, just think of it: we're the first ones to actually see it happen.' |
| Dr Duval: | 'The Living Process!' |
| Mr Grant: | 'Mind letting me in on what's going on out there?' |
| Dr Michaels: | 'Oh, it's just a simple exchange, Mr Grant. Corpuscles releasing carbon dioxide in return for oxygen coming through on the other side.' |
| Grant: | 'Don't tell me they're refuelling!' |

| C. Peterson: | 'Oxygenation!' |
| Dr Duval: | 'We've known it exists even though we never saw it [...] But to actually see one of the miracles of the universe: the engineering of the cycle of a breath' |
| Dr Michaels: | 'Well, I wouldn't call it a miracle. Just an exchange of gases. The end-product of five hundred million years of evolution.' |
| Dr Duval: | 'You can't believe all that is accidental? That there isn't a creative intelligence at work?' |
| | (sec. 00h52m30s) |

The chemistry of life is represented on one hand as being 'just an exchange of gases', and, on the other as being 'one of the miracles of the universe'. The conversation closes with an overture to a well-worn debate between evolutionism and creationism that has been repeated on many occasions across the twentieth century. The accompanying visual effects illustrate this discussion as never before, with the team looking on, fascinated, as the erythrocytes change before their eyes from a pale blue to a warm pink-red colour. Here, the film has rejected a literal rendition of the colours of oxygenated and de-oxygenated haemoglobin in favour of more evocative colours, notably the 'colder' colour blue, which 'represents subconsciousness opposed to red which represent consciousness. In therapeutics sedatives often are blue in color, alluding to the color's ability to sooth the spirit.'[29] While red, or at least pink, is the colour of vitality and renewal: 'Symbolic of joy and youth. Associated with the number five, a mystic number for healing.'[30]

While the whole crew can appreciate the beauty of this spectacle of regeneration, the question of its ultimate significance divides the two scientists. Dr Michaels sees it as a physiological cycle of oxygenation produced by the blind action of natural selection. Dr Duval, in contrast talks of the 'cycle of breath' and imputes its beauty to a creative intelligence. Indeed, by using the term 'breath' Duval is tapping into a rich symbolic terrain, as is suggested by Gertrude Jobes's dictionary, in which '"Breath": Creator deity, divine and immortal element in man, life force, soul, spirit.'[31]

While the context of the Cold War favours the American Christian imputation of religious significance against the materialism of the Soviet Union (Dr Michaels is ultimately revealed to be an enemy agent and saboteur), the film avoids explicitly arguing for one side or other of the debate. The oxygenation of the blood cells is left to stand as both a scientific phenomenon and a wondrous spectacle.

## *Fantastic Voyage as a Pedagogical Project*

As the name of the film suggests, *Fantastic Voyage* plays on the marvellous aspects of the representation of the interior of the human body, but it is nevertheless bound to a scientific vision of this internal environment. Thus, the narrative never appeals to supernatural or magical phenomena to drive the plot; and the film attempts within the bounds explored above to retain a realist approach, making it clearly a film in the 'science fiction' genre rather than that of 'science fantasy'. With its special effects and voyage-through-the-body narrative this popular film offers an interesting, if not highly accurate, vision of the interior environment of human that comes quite close, in principle at least, to the ideas of Claude Bernard.

The spectacular *mise en scène* serves to erase many of the difficulties associated with presenting this vision from within. While the idea of placing oneself in the situation of a blood cell was difficult and even destabilizing for Bernard's contemporaries, it becomes self-evident in the context of the film's narrative, even though this environment is represented as quite exotic. Thus, *Fantastic Voyage* serves as a pedagogical tool, helping to overcome at least two 'epistemological obstacles' identified by Gaston Bachelard: the obstacle of naïve experience and the obstacle of substantivalism. The naive conception of the body is resistant to the idea of the body as an aquatic labyrinthine environment, because our earliest conception of the body is as solid and as unified or unitary rather than as liquid and ramified. Nevertheless, the film succeeds in plausibly representing this interior, however difficult the subsequent work of reconciling this image with our naive impressions of the human body might be. The substantivalist obstacle is somewhat more complex: 'What is occult is enclosed. By analysing the references to the occult, we can characterise what we might term the myth of the interior, and then the deeper myth of the intimate.'[32]

It is clear that one of the effects of the film is, by opening the interior of the body up to the audience, to undermine the occult nature of the body, the body as an integral, impenetrable unity possessing a hidden and potentially supernatural interior. Nevertheless, the film does not thereby achieve what Bachelard suggests will happen, that is to say the elimination of all mythical resonances, but rather the film transforms the symbolism associated with the interior of the body. The voyage of the *Proteus* introduces its own mythical narrative, adopting the role of Jason's ship the *Argo*, but on a quest/voyage in the interior of the body. Indeed this reinscription of the scientific information in the narrative form of a thriller represents a pedagogical move, enabling the transmission of knowledge about the body through the use of an appropriate form. The tale or story, with its tense plot and the spectacular turns of events provides an appropriate fictional vehicle for the presentation of the internal environment. And so in order to transmit the scientific messages that come with adopting the microscopic perspective recommended a century earlier by Bernard, the film plays on a range of symbolic imagery that mobilizes implicit semantic relationships. We know that we are in the brain precisely because of the sparks of intelligence. It makes sense to us that the antibodies should single out intruders that behave differently from the body itself.

Nevertheless, *Fantastic Voyage* is not simply a work of popularization that 'dumbs down' the scientific message it is transmitting. The film itself contributed a positive construction of the body's interior for scientists and the lay public alike. The physiological vision of the body, so foreign to Bernard's contemporaries, was solidly in place by 1966, both in the biological sciences and in the cultural vision of the human body. But this knowledge and recognition of the nature of the interior remained largely theoretical, notably in a period with little or no three-dimensional medical imagery. If there was not necessarily a need, there was certainly a place for a scientific representation of this space that could serve as a new symbolic reference. Indeed, while courses in anatomy or human biology could provide a forum for teaching the accumulated wealth of scientific information about human physiology at the microscopic level, in order to engage a general public you need an appropriate narrative, in this case the narrative of a thriller-adventure. The film offered a new mytheme with new archetypes, but ones that, as we have shown, were easy to appropriate as they were anchored in a network of familiar associations both narrative and symbolic. The film no doubt owes its success to this readily acceptable combination of the symbolic with a spectacular and fantastic *mise en scène* of the interior of the body, to form a meaningful overall 'vision' of the adventure.

Our aim here is not to argue that *Fantastic Voyage* constitutes a 'great' or exceptionally visionary film. There are many awkward moments, both in terms of its narrative and the symbolism as well as a host of scientific inaccuracies, even accepting the rather implausible presuppositions that underwrite the plot. The lack of any real development of the characters and the kitsch aesthetic of the film have contributed to its status as a cult B-movie, but it has nevertheless, we believe, played an important role in establishing the interior environment in modern Western culture. The film was accompanied by a novel of the same name commissioned from Isaac Asimov (1966), which was a precursor for later nano-biotechnological science fiction stories from the 1980s, in particular, Greg Bear's *Blood Music* (1983).

## Conclusions

What can we say about *Fantastic Voyage*? It seems justifiable to argue that following the success of this 1966 film, the interior of the human body had a vision in terms of Bernard's interior environment. While the film portrayal was maybe overly exotic, it nevertheless successfully broke with the morbid, gory spectacle of the body common to horror films, marking the entry of a positive register for depicting this intimate interior space in films. The aquatic 'landscape' presented in the film offers a complex vision of the interior of the body viewed from the microscopic perspective. Labyrinthine and populated by foreign objects, this image is partly determined by a desire for realism and partly by the exigencies of Hollywood spectacle. In this context, it is interesting to note that the recent collectors' edition of the DVD of *Fantastic Voyage* does not feature the classic image of Dr Duval aiming his laser gun at the blood clot in the brain, but a large open eye looking at us out of the box. While this is the eye from which the survivors of the *Proteus* are rescued at the end of the film, it also represents our own view of ourselves, with the metamorphosis of this gaze being, in a sense, the essential subject of the film.

A second important point is how this vision of the body is informed not only by empirical scientific information but also by the artistic exigencies of the *mise en scène*, making it a work of both science and fiction. Furthermore, it is not a rigid or static representation of the body, but a dynamic one shaped by the film's tense plot, but this is a narrative that leaves space for a number of attempts to explore the human resonances of the adventure within the body. Thus, this film combines the scientific and the marvellous as proposed by M. Renard a century ago,[33] presenting both the science of the human body under construction and echoing the mystery of a more traditional enchanted vision of the human body.

To close, we would like to return to our opening presentation of the opposition between two visions of the interior of the body; the soft appealing body and the dark, bleeding body (Durand), or, in other terms, the lived body versus the dissected body. It is clear that *Fantastic Voyage*, in contrast to the wealth of horror movies that play on the feeling of revulsion provoked by the violent entry into or opening of the body, represents a vision closer to the soft appealing body, experienced by its miniaturized visitors as a wondrous machine. Nevertheless, this vision of the body lacks the subjective experience that constitutes an essential part of our embodied life. More recent narratives that follow the same orientation opened up by *Fantastic Voyage*, such as Greg Bear's *Blood Music*, take the time to explore and represent the sensitive and active dimensions of the subject as well.

# NOTES

## Landers, 'Introduction'

1. E. Tyson, *The Anatomy of a Pygmy Compared with that of a Monkey, an Ape, and a Man* (London: Printed for T. Osborne, 1751), p. A 2r.
2. Ibid., p. 2.
3. Ibid.
4. L. Goldmann, *Towards a Sociology of the Novel*, trans. A. Sheridan (London: Tavistock Publications, 1975), pp. 8–9.
5. W. Mayrl, 'Introduction', in *Cultural Creation in Modern Society* (Saint Louis, MI: Telos Press, 1976), pp. 1–27, on p. 13.

## 1 Landers, 'Early Modern Dissection as a Physical Model of Organization'

1. K. F. Russell, *British Anatomy: 1525–1800* (Winchester: St Paul Bibliographies, 1987), p xxi.
2. C. Singer, *A Short History of Anatomy from the Greeks to Harvey* (New York: Dover Publications, Inc., 1957), p. 171.
3. Russell, *British Anatomy*, p. xxiii.
4. For an extended discussion, see A. Carlino, *Books of the Body: Anatomical Ritual and Renaissance Learning*, trans. J. Tedeschi and A. C. Tedeschi (Chicago, IL: Chicago University Press, 1999), pp. 156–70.
5. Ibid., p. 127.
6. A. Vesalius, *On the Fabric of the Human Body*, trans. W. F. Richardson, 5 vols (San Francisco, CA: Norman Publishing, 1998), vol. 1, p. li.
7. Richardson translates *ratio* as 'regimen' (ibid., p. xlviii). *Ratio* also means system, or theory. To display the ambiguity of the word, I have chosen to translate *ratio* as 'doctrine', in order to highlight the importance of comprehensive systems in medical theory. Vesalius says elsewhere uses the phrase '*medendi rationem*' to describe the doctrines that govern the separate but related processes of diagnosis, prognosis and therapeutics. Though Richardson's use of the word 'regimen' implies a similar idea, I believe it fails to communicate the importance and broad acceptance of medical *theory* as a basis for praxis. N.B. – *Manus opera* refers to surgery, but also the treatment of fractures – basically all types of work performed by the hands.
8. Vesalius, *On the Fabric of the Human Body*, vol. 1, p. li.

9.   Carlino, *Books of the Body*, p. 11.
10.  Vesalius, *On the Fabric of the Human Body*, vol. 1, p. li.
11.  Ibid., vol. 1, p. liv.
12.  Carpi's edition of Mondino's *Anothomia* has numerous illustrations to accompany the text; however, Vesalius's engravings represent a much higher level of detail and accuracy.
13.  Vesalius, *On the Fabric of the Human Body*, vol. 1, pp. l–li. The original Latin reads: 'Cæterùm peruersissima hæc curationis instrumentorum ad uarios artifices diductio, adhuc multò execrabilius naufragium, aclongè atrociorem cladem præcipuæ naturalis philosophiæ parti intulit, cui quum hominis historiam complectatur, firmissimum[que] totius medicæ artis fundamentum, ac constitutionis initium iure habenda sit, Hippocrates & Plato tantum tribuerunt, ut illi inter medicinæ partes, primas esse adscribendas non dubitarint. Hæc nanque cùm prius à medicis unicè excoleretur, ipsi[que] in hac adipiscenda omnes neruos intenderent, tum demum miserè collabi cœpit, quum ipsi manuum munus ad alios reijcientes, Anatomen perdiderunt' (Vesalius, *De humani Corporis fabrica Libri Septem* (Basliae: Ex officina Ioannis Oporini, 1543), 2v–3r).
14.  Vesalius, *On the Fabric of the Human Body*, vol. 1, p. l–li.
15.  N. G. Siraisi, 'Vesalius and the Reading of Galen's Teleology', *Renaissance Quarterly*, 50:1 (1997), pp. 1–37, on p. 3.
16.  E. L. Eisenstein, *The Printing Revolution in Early Modern Europe* (New York: Cambridge University Press, 2005), p. 23.
17.  E. Wickersheimer (ed.), *Anatomies de Mondion dei Luzzi et de Guido de Vigevano* (Genève: Slatkine Reprints, 1977), pp. 51, 53, 57.
18.  Eisenstein, *The Printing Revolution*, p. 70.
19.  R. Collison, *Encyclopaedias: Their History Throughout the Ages* (New York: Hafner Publishing Company, 1964), p. 21.
20.  Carlino, *Books of the Body*, p. 40.
21.  Eisenstein, *The Printing Revolution*, p. 48.
22.  Carlino, *Books of the Body*, p. 40.
23.  Russell, *British Anatomy*, p. xix.
24.  H. Cushing, *A Bio-Bibliography of Andreas Vesalius* (Hamden, CT: Archon Books, 1962), p. 120.
25.  Ibid., pp. 124–5.
26.  Russell, *British Anatomy*, p. xxii.
27.  Although the smaller images make cross-referencing easier, much of the detail of the original illustrations is lost.
28.  He mentions the benefits of studying anatomy in the fifth chapter, and then proceeds to give various philosophical, theological and artistic reasons for having knowledge of the human form. Crooke does not become 'scientific' in his approach until the fifteenth chapter.
29.  Jonathan Sawday appears to be the only scholar to consider Crooke's contribution beyond a mere mention. See J. Sawday, *The Body Emblazoned: Dissection and the Human Body in Renaissance Culture* (New York: Routeledge, 1995)
30.  B. Smith, 'Premodern Sexualities', *PMLA*, 115:3 (2000), pp. 318–29, on p. 322.
31.  R. Sugg, *Murder after Death: Literature and Anatomy in Early Modern England* (Ithaca, NY: Cornell University Press, 2007), p. 113.
32.  C. D. O'Malley, 'The Fielding H. Garrison Lecture: Helkiah Crooke, M.D., F.R.C.P., 1576–1648', *Bulletin of the History of Medicine*, 42:1 (1968), pp. 1–18, on p. 11.

33. H. Crooke, *Mikrokosmografia: A Description of the Body of Man* (London: Printed by William Jaggard, 1615), pp. 26–7.
34. Ibid., p. 26.
35. Ibid., p. 27.
36. Ibid.
37. Ibid., p. 28.
38. Ibid., p. 27.
39. Ibid., p. 28.
40. R. A. Fox, *The Tangled Chain: The Structure of Disorder in the Anatomy of Melancholy* (Berkeley, CA: University of California Press, 1976), p. 27.
41. Ibid., pp. 22, 24.
42. Ibid., p. 28.
43. Ibid.
44. Ibid, p. 21.
45. Ibid, pp. 27–8.
46. R. Burton, *The Anatomy of Melancholy*, ed. H. Jackson (New York: New York Review Books, 2001), p. 126.
47. H. Ridley, *The Anatomy of the Brain* (London: Printed for Sam. Smith and Benj. Walford, 1695), p. 32.
48. W. J. Ong, *Ramus, Method, and the Decay of Dialogue* (Cambridge, MA: Harvard University Press, 1983), p. 76.
49. I find it likely that Crooke is using the term *cleave* in its double-sense, meaning both to separate and to adhere (see *OED*). If so, the verb works perfectly to demonstrate the point I am trying to make about systematic organization, which allows both for division and coherence on the basis of proximal and functional relationships.

## 2 Witherbee, '"Who Will Not Force a Mad Man to be Let Blood?": Circulation and Trade in the Early Eighteenth Century'

1. W. Petty, 'Preface', in *Political Arithmetick* (London, 1690).
2. W. Killigrew, *A Proposal, Shewing How this Nation may be Vast Gainers by All the Sums of Money, Given to the Crown, without Lessening the Prerogative* (London, 1663), pp. 9–10.
3. Ibid., p. 9.
4. A number of these pamphlets were published in a collection from Goldsmith's Library of Economic Literature. Far more can be found through the *Early English Books Online Database* from Gale Publishing. See *Bank of England: Selected Tracts 1694–1804. Goldsmiths' Library of Economic Literature*, University of London (London: Gregg International Publishers Ltd., 1968), pp. 103–5. See also R. Roberts and D. Kynaston (eds), *The Bank of England: Money, Power and Influence 1694–1994* (Oxford: Clarendon, 1995), and Sir J. Clapham, *The Bank of England: A History* (Cambridge: Cambridge University Press, 1944).
5. W. Harvey, *Exercitatio Anatomica de Motu Cordis et Sanguinis in Animalibus*, trans. C. D. Leake (Springfield, IL: Charles C. Thomas, 1970), p. 3.
6. R. French, *William Harvey's Natural Philosophy* (Cambridge: Cambridge University Press, 1994), p. 102.
7. Ibid., pp. 1–3.
8. Harvey, *Exercitatio Anatomica de Motu*, p. 3.
9. Ibid., pp. 106, 104.
10. French, *Harvey's Natural Philosophy*, p. 3.

11. Ibid., p. 68.
12. Ibid.
13. Ibid., p. 330.
14. Harvey, *Exercitatio Anatomica de Motu*, p. 74.
15. B. Rotman, *Mathematics as Sign: Writing, Imagining, Counting* (Stanford, CA: Stanford University Press, 2000), p. 51.
16. Ibid., pp. 51–2.
17. Ibid.
18. Ibid., p. 52.
19. Ibid., p. 24.
20. Ibid., p. 41.
21. Ibid., p. 51.
22. W. Paterson, *A Brief Account of the Intended Bank of England* (London: Randal Taylor, 1694), p. 1.
23. Ibid., p. 3.
24. Ibid., pp. 13–14.
25. Ibid., p. 14.
26. T. Aspromourgos, *On the Origins of Classical Economics: Distribution and Value from William Petty to Adam Smith* (London: Routledge, 1996), p. 124.
27. See M. Poovey, *A History of the Modern Fact: Problems of Knowledge in the Sciences of Wealth and Society* (Chicago, IL: Chicago University Press, 1998).
28. See P. Brantlinger, *Fictions of State: Culture and Credit in Britain, 1694–1994* (Ithaca, NY: Cornell University Press, 1996), and J. Thompson, *Models of Value: Eighteenth-Century Political Economy and the Novel* (Durham, NC: Duke University Press, 1996).

## 3 Cope, 'Earth's Intelligent Body: Subterranean Systems and the Circulation of Knowledge, or, The Radius Subtending Circumnavigation'

1. *Legal Planet: The Environmental Law and Policy Blog* [of Berkeley Law and UCLA Law], at http://legalplanet.wordpress.com/2010/04/28/redwashing/ [accessed 16 January 2012].
2. T. Robinson, *The Anatomy of the Earth* (London: Printed for J. Newman, 1694), pp. 1–2.
3. Ibid., p. 6.
4. Ibid., pp. 10–11.
5. T. Robinson, *New Observations on the Natural History of this World of Matter, and this World of Life: In Two Parts. Being a Philosophical Discourse, Grounded upon the Mosaick System of the Creation, and the Flood. To which are added Some Thoughts concerning Paradise, the Conflagration of the World, and a Treatise of Meteorology: With Occasional Remarks upon some late Theories, Conferences, and Essays* (London, 1696), pp. 31–2.
6. T. Robinson, *A Vindication of the* Philosophical *and* Theological *Exposition of the Mosaick System of the Creation. With Moral Inferences and Conclusions* (London, 1709), pp. 6–7.
7. Robinson, *New Observations*, pp. 6–9.
8. The mock-heroic contrast between the majesty of Moses's account and the silliness of the Bantry miners' superstitions illustrates the tendency in anatomical writing to default

into travel journalism. When an anatomist lacks the tools to penetrate into the interior of a system (in this case, to visit the trolls who allegedly live within the earth), the default strategy is the covering of more territory on the surface. A case study in the intersection of travel and anatomical writing can be found in R. R. Cawley, 'Burton, Bacon, and Sandys', *Modern Language Notes*, 56:4 (1941), pp. 271–3.

9.  Robinson, *The Anatomy of the Earth*, pp. 20–1.
10. Robinson, *New Observations*, pp. 59–60.
11. Robinson, *A Vindication*, pp. 15–16.
12. Robinson, *New Observations*, p. 66.
13. Robinson, *The Anatomy of the Earth*, pp. 13, 18–19, 67.
14. See M. Escholt, *Geologica Norvegica* (London, 1663).
15. See E. Warren, *A Defense of the Discourse concerning the Earth Before the Flood. Being a Full Reply to a Late Answer to Exceptions made against the Theory of the Earth: Wherein those Exceptions are Vindicated and Reinforced: And Objections against the New Hypothesis of the Deluge, Answered* (London, 1691).
16. For a summary of the literature responding to the 1692 Port Royal, Jamaica earthquakes, see L. Gragg, 'The Port Royal Earthquake', *History Today*, 50:9 (September 2000), pp. 28–34.

## 4 Spicci, '"After an Unwonted Manner": Anatomy and Poetical Organization in Early Modern England'

1.  R. Copland, *The Questyonary of Cyrurgyens, with the Formulary of Lytell Guydo in Cyrurgie, with the Spectacles of Cyrurgyens Newly Added, with the Fourth Boke of the Terapeutyke, or Methode Curatyfe of Claude Galyen* (London: Printed by Robert Wyer for Henry Dabbe and Rycharde Banckes, 1542), unpaginated.
2.  S. Gosson, *The Schoole of Abuse* (London: Southgate, 1868), p. 38.
3.  D. P. Thomas, 'Thomas Vicary and the Anatomy of Man's Body', *Medical History* 50:2 (2006), pp. 235–46, on p. 237.
4.  Between 1545, the year of publication of the anonymous *The Anathomy of the Inwarde Partes of Man*, and 1633, the year of Fletcher's *The Purple Island*, more than seventy texts entitled 'Anatomy of ...' were printed in England. Only 25 per cent of them have a strict medical vocation; the remaining 75 per cent are non-medical texts that deal with many different subjects, such as religion, satire, moral philosophy, and literature. For further details see M. Spicci, *The Purple Island (1633) di Phineas Fletcher: un'anatomia. Corpo e ibridazioni discorsive nell'Inghilterra elisabettiana* (Catania: Ed.it, 2009).
5.  T. Rogers, *A Philosophicall Discourse, entitled, The Anatomy of the Minde* (London: J[ohn] C[harlewood], 1576), unpaginated.
6.  J. Woolton, *A New Anatomie of Whole Man* (London: Thomas Purfoote, 1576), unpaginated.
7.  J. Sawday, *The Body Emblazoned. Dissection and the Human Body in Renaissance Culture* (London: Routledge, 1995), p. 73.
8.  G. K. Hunter, *John Lyly: The Humanist and the Courtier* (London: Routledge & Kegan Paul, 1962), p. 50.
9.  R. Underwood, *A New Anatomie* (London: Printed for Willian Jones, 1605).
10. Ibid., p. 1.
11. Ibid.

12. Ibid., p. 2.
13. Ibid.
14. Ibid., p. 3.
15. Ibid., p. 4.
16. A. B. Langdale, *Phineas Fletcher: Man of Letters, Science and Divinity* (New York: Octagon Books, 1968), p. 52.
17. The quotations from Fletcher's poem are taken from F. S. Boas (ed.). *The Poetical Works of Giles and Phineas Fletcher* (Cambridge: Cambridge University Press, 1908–9).
18. E. Benlowes, 'On the Excellent Moral Poem, entitled the *Isle of Man*', in Boas (ed.), *The Poetical Works of Giles and Phineas Fletcher*, p. 5.
19. Ibid.
20. Ibid.
21. D. Featley, 'To the Reader', in Boas (ed.), *The Poetical Works of Giles and Phineas Fletcher*, p. 4.
22. Ibid.
23. L. Roberts, 'To the Unknown Mr. P. F. Upon Survay of his Isle of Man', in Boas (ed.), *The Poetical Works of Giles and Phineas Fletcher*, p. 9.
24. Ibid.
25. P. Fletcher, *The Purple Island*, I.34.3.
26. Ibid., I.34.2.
27. Ibid., I.34.7.
28. P. C. Hoffer, *Sensory Worlds in Early America* (Baltimore, MD and London: Johns Hopkins University Press, 2006), p. 41.
29. Roberts, 'To the Unknown', p. 9.
30. W. Franklin, *Discoverers, Explorers, Settlers. The Diligent Writers of Early America* (Chicago, IL and London: University of Chicago Press, 1979), p. 22.
31. Ibid., p. 23.
32. Fletcher, *The Purple Island*, V.2.1.
33. N. Cobb, *Prospero's Island: The Secret Alchemy at the Heart of 'The Tempest'* (London: Coventure, 1982), p. 32.
34. G. U. De Sousa, 'Alien Habitats in *The Tempest*', in P. M. Murphy (ed.), *The Tempest. Critical Essays* (New York and London: Routledge, 2001), p. 449.
35. Fletcher, *The Purple Island*, I.34.6.
36. Hoffer, *Sensory Worlds*, p. 45.
37. Fletcher, *The Purple Island*, I.43.6.
38. E. Hooper-Greenhill, *Museums and the Shaping of Knowledge* (London and New York: Routledge, 1992), p. 91.
39. J. Donne, *Sermons* (Berkley and Los Angeles, CA: University of California Press, 1953), p. 67.
40. Fletcher, *The Purple Island*, I.48.1–4.
41. G. Havers (ed.), *A General Collection of Discourses of the Virtuosi of France* (London: Thomas Dring & John Starkey, 1673), unpaginated.
42. Fletcher, *The Purple Island*, I.39.3.
43. Ibid., V.5.2.
44. Ibid., I.33.5.
45. Ibid., I.45.1.
46. Ibid., IV.16.3.
47. Ibid., IV.16.4–7.

48. Ibid., V.4.3.
49. Ibid., V.11.2.
50. Ibid., V.11.5.
51. Ibid., V.30.6.
52. Ibid., V.33.1.
53. Ibid., V.33.4.
54. Ibid., V.14.2.
55. Ibid., V.16.3–4.
56. Ibid., V.16.6.
57. Ibid., V.18.3.
58. Ibid., II.22.2.
59. Ibid., II.27.1–2.
60. Ibid., II.27.7.
61. Ibid., II.9.5.
62. Ibid., II.33.5–7.
63. Hoffer, *Sensory Worlds*, p. 4.
64. Fletcher, *The Purple Island*, II.9.3.
65. Ibid., II.10.6–7.
66. Ibid., II.12.7.
67. Ibid., II.12.6.
68. Ibid., III.8.1–3.
69. Ibid., II.17.1.
70. Ibid., II.17.4–7.
71. Ibid., II.8.1–7.
72. Sawday, *The Body Emblazoned*, pp. 27–8.
73. Fletcher, *The Purple Island*, I.38.1.
74. Ibid., I.34.6.
75. J. Hart, *Columbus, Shakespeare, and the Interpretation of the New World* (New York: Palgrave, 2003), p.
76. T. Healy, 'Sound Physic: Phineas Fletcher's "The Purple Island" and the Poetry of Purgation', in *Renaissance Studies*, 5 (1991), pp. 341–52, on p. 345.
77. Fletcher, *The Purple Island*, II.14.2–7.
78. Ibid., II.15.1–6.
79. Ibid., II.15.4n.
80. Ibid., III.5.5–7.
81. Ibid., IV.4.2.
82. Ibid., IV.4.4–7.
83. Ibid., IV.10.2–3.
84. Ibid., IV.11.3–4.
85. Ibid., IV.14.1–2.
86. Ibid., IV.15.2–7.
87. Ibid., IV.15.1.
88. Ibid., IV.18.3–7.
89. Ibid., I.45.1.
90. J. C. Davies, *Utopia and the Ideal Society. A Study of English Utopian Writing, 1516–1700* (Cambridge: Cambridge University Press, 1981), p. 19.
91. Fletcher, *The Purple Island*, I.36.1–2.
92. Ibid., I.26.3–4.

93.  Ibid., I.38.6–7.
94.  Ibid., I.26.7.
95.  Ibid., I.34.2.
96.  Ibid., I.28.
97.  Ibid., I.44.5.
98.  Featley, 'To the Reader', p. 4.
99.  Fletcher, *The Purple Island*, I.34.2–7.

## 5 Parker, 'Subtle Bodies: The Limits of Categories in Girolamo Cardano's *De Subtilitate*'

1.   G. Cardano, *The First Book of Jerome Cardan's De Subtilitate*, trans. M. Cass (William-sport, PA: Bayard Press, 1934), p. 75. 'Propositum nostri negotii in hoc Opere est, de Subtilitate tractare. Est autem subtilitas ratio quaedam, qua sensibilia à sensibus, intelligibilia ab intellectu, difficilè comphreahenduntur.' H. Cardanus, *Opera Omnia*, ed. C. Spon, 10 vols (Lyons: Huguetan & Ravaud, 1663), vol. 3, p. 357.
2.   Aristotle, *Parts of Animals*, trans. J. G. Lennox (Oxford: Clarendon Press, 2001), p. 2 (639b3–5).
3.   Ibid., p. 2 (654b10–20).
4.   A. Gotthelf and J. G. Lennox (eds), *Philosophical Issues in Aristotle's Biology* (Cambridge: Cambridge University Press, 1987). The volume *Philosophical Issues in Aristotle's Biology* provides a varied and extensive investigation into the particular relationships between Aristotle's proto-scientific writings and his metaphysical claims. G. E. R. Lloyd has convincingly argued that Aristotle was not the paragon of systematic thought that he is often represented as being. See *Aristotelian Explorations* (Cambridge: Cambridge University Press, 1996). Aristotle's work was, however, received both as an argument for systematic thought and as a model of such thinking.
5.   Aristotelian philosophy also influenced the early Hellenistic physicians before Galen. See H. von Staden, 'Teleology and Mechanism: Aristotelian Biology and Early Hellenistic Medicine', in W. Kullmann and S. Föllinger (eds), *Aristotelische Biologie: Intentionen, Methoden, Ergebnisse* (Stuttgart: Franz Steiner Verlag, 1997), pp. 183–208.
6.   Galen, *Selected Works*, trans. and ed. P. N. Singer. (Oxford: Oxford University Press, 1997), p. 30. On Galen's use of classification, see I. Johnston, *Galen on Diseases and Symptoms* (Cambridge: Cambridge University Press, 2006), pp. 21–125, as well as R. Siegel, *Galen's System of Physiology and Medicine* (Basel: S. Karger, 1968). On some links between Galen's philosophy and Aristotle in early modern medicine, see A. Wear, *Knowledge and Practice in English Medicine, 1550–1680* (Cambridge: Cambridge University Press, 2000), p. 131.
7.   Galen, *Selected Works*, p. 34.
8.   Ibid.
9.   A. Falcon, 'Commentators on Aristotle', in E. N. Zalta (ed.), *The Stanford Encyclopedia of Philosophy*, at http://plato.stanford.edu/archives/fall2009/entries/aristotle-commentators/ [accessed 30 September 2011].
10.  Aristotle, *Parts of Animals*, p. 2 (645b15–16).
11.  Andrea Carlino provides a compelling history of the changes in anatomical teaching before and after Vesalius. The style described by Cardano, where the authoritative text holds more importance than the cadaver being dissected, is known as the 'quodlibertar-

ian model', which Carlino discusses in detail in his first chapter. See A. Cardano, *Books of the Body: Anatomical Ritual and Renaissance Learning*, trans. J. Tedeschi and A. Tedeschi (Chicago, IL: University of Chicago Press, 1999). For an account that is specific to the changing attitudes towards Galen in medicine more generally, see O. Temkin, *Galenism: Rise and Decline of a Medical Philosophy* (Ithaca, NY: Cornell University Press, 1973).

12.  G. Cardano, *The Book of My Life*, ed. A. Grafton, trans. J. Stoner (New York: New York Review of Books, 2002), p. 45. The entire anecdote, summarized in the excerpt quoted above, is recounted thus in Cardano's original: 'Alterum Bononiae cum Fracantiano primo professore in praxi Medicae artis: cum venisset in contentionem de meatu fellis ad ventriculum, & recitasset Graecè coram tota Academia (dissectio enim Anatomica exercebatur) dixi *deficit où* tum ille non profectò, cum ego quietius affirmarem, exclamant discipuli, mittatur pro Codice: mittit ille laetus, statim affertur, legit, invenit ut dixeram ad unguem, si luit, obstupuit, admirabatur, sed magis etiam discipuli, qui eo me per vim traxerant, ex illa die, adeò congressum meum fugiebat, ut monuerìt famulos, ut me venientem ostenderent, atque ita devitabat ne in via occurreret. Cumque semel per dolum assidenti Anatomiae superinduxissent, aufugit, & togae implicitus pronus cecidit, ex quo omnes qui aderant obstupebant, & ipse paulo post discessit, cum esset conductus ad plures annos.' Cardanus, *Opera Omnia*, vol. 1, p.10.

13.  Cardano, *The Book of My Life*, p. 58. 'Itaque cum plurimi apertè primùm sperantes me arguere posse, quod aberrassem, corpora dissecuissent, ut Senatoris Ursi, Doctoris Peregrini, Georgii Ghisileri: In quo illud visum est admirabile praedixisse me morbum fore in iecore, cum urinae essent optimae?' H. Cardanus, *Opera Omnia*, vol. 1, p. 33.

14.  A captivating account of this autopsy is provided in N. Siraisi, *The Clock and the Mirror: Girolamo Cardano and Renaissance Medicine* (Princeton, NJ: Princeton University Press, 1997), pp. 116–17.

15.  Cardano, *The Book of My Life*, p. 16. The anecdote is included in his chapter, 'Vitae ab initio usque ad praesentem diem (finem scilicet Octobris, an. 1575.) enarratio brevis.' He recounts the story thus: 'Sed post aestatem redii ad profitendi munus, & sequenti anno instante Andrea Vesaelio viro clarissimo, & amico nostro, oblata est conditio D. ccc. Coronatorum in singulos annos à Rege Daniae, quam recipere nolui cùm etiam victus impensam suppeditaret, non solum ob regionis intemperiem, sed quod alio sacrorum modo consuevissent: ut vel ibi malè acceptus futurus essem, vel patriam legem meam maiorúmque relinquere coactus.' Cardanus, *Opera Omnia*, vol. 1, p. 4. This event is also described in terms of Vesalius's biography in C. D. O'Mally, *Andreas Vesalius of Brussels, 1514–1564* (Berkeley, CA: University Press of California, 1964), p. 234.

16.  Cardano, *The Book of My Life*, p. 58. 'Ex Professoribus Franciscum Vicomercatum Mediolanensem Philosophum, & suspexi Andream Vesalium in Anatomica arte primarium.' Cardanus, *Opera Omnia*, vol. 1, p. 12.

17.  H. Cardanus, *De exemplis centum geniturarum*. In *Opera Omnia*, vol. 5. p. 500. For a discussion of this horoscope, see Siraisi, *The Clock and the Mirror*, p. 107ff. For a translation of the full text of Cardano's horoscope for Vesalius, see H. Cushing, *A Bio-Bibliography of Andreas Vesalius* (Hamden, CT: Archon Books, 1962).

18.  'I am quite certain ... that he himself [Galen] had never cut open a human body and furthermore that, deceived by his apes (although he did chance upon two human skeletons) he frequently and quite wrongly finds fault with the ancient physicians who actually did their training by dissecting human material.' A. Vesalius, *On the Fabric of the Human Body. Book I: Bones and Cartilages*, trans. W. F. Richardson and J. B. Carman (San Francisco, CA: Norman Publishing, 1998), pp. lii–liv. The original reads, 'nobis

modò ex renata dissectionis arte, diligentique Galeni librorum praelectione, & in plerisque locis eorundem non poenitenda restitutione constet, nun quam ipsum resecuisse corpus humanum: at verò fuis deceptum simiis (licet duo ipsi arida hominum cadavera occurrerint) crebro ueteres medicos in hominum confectionibus se exercentes immeritò arguere.' A. Vesalius, *De humani corporis fabrica*. (Basil: Oporinus, 1543), p. 3.

19. Nutton cites Abd-al Latif al-Baghdadi (d. 1231), whose osteological research constitutes the major exception. V. Nutton, 'Introduction', to *Andreae Vesalii, De Humani Corporis Fabrica*, ed. D. Garrison and M. Hast, at http://vesalius.northwestern.edu/flash.html [accessed 1 October 2011].

20. For a history of this group of anatomists, see N. Siraisi, *Taddeo Alderotti and His Pupils: Two Generations of Italian Medical Learning* (Princeton, NJ: Princeton University Press, 1981).

21. Vesalius, *On the Fabric of the Human Body. Book I: Bones and Cartilages*, p. lii. Vesalius, *De humani corporis fabrica*, p. 3.

22. Galen, *On the Usefulness of the Parts of the Body*, trans. M. T. May (Ithaca, NY: Cornell University Press, 1968), p. 457.

23. Galen, *Usefulness of the Parts of the Body*, p. 460.

24. Vesalius, *On the Fabric of the Human Body. Book I: Bones and Cartilages*, p. 46. The chapter is titled, 'Capitis structurae ratio, quotque, eiusdem figurae.' The passage on Galen reads: 'Humanum caput oculorum gratia efformari, cancrorum, scarabeorum, & quorundam quae capite destituuntur animalium oculos manifestò commonstrare, Galenus docuit. His fiquidem oculi super processus praelongos locantur, neque imi, quemadmodum os, nasus, & aures in pectore ipisis conduntur. Oculos enim alta eguisse sede, attestantur hostium incursus latronumque speculatores, qui muros, montes & altas turres eodem usu ascendunt, quo nautae navium antemnas, terram ocyus, quàm qui subsunt in navi, conspecturi.' Vesalius, *De humani corporis fabrica*, p. 18.

25. There is some evidence that Vesalius was not flattered by this imitation. See Cushing, *A Bio-Bibliography of Andreas Vesalius*. He proposes that Vesalius's reference to a 'Paris offender' who stole his anatomical drawings might be a reference to Estienne. The family Estienne was also known as Stephanus, a famous family of printers, which for three generations had rivalled the Aldine press in Venice. Cushing points out that Vesalius had spoken slightingly of Parisian anatomists and printers by the name Stephanus.

26. C. Estienne, *La dissection des parties du corps humain divisee en trois livres, faictz par Charles Estienne docteur en Medecine: avec les figures & declaration des incisions, composees par Estienne de la Riviere Chirurgien* (Paris: Simon de Colines, 1546), from the Huntington LACMA collection, no. 621850, p. 2 (my translation). The French reads: 'A nous, entre aultres choses, a semble meilleure la contemplation de l'homme: duquel le singulier artifice & ouvraige, nous donne a congnoistre lincredible puissance de nostre Dieu immortel.'

27. Chapter 11, '*De hominis necessitate et forma*' and chapter 12, '*De hominis, natura et temperamento*' treat man's purpose on earth and his 'form' or appearance, then human nature and temperament. These chapters make up the middle portion of the twenty-one-book volume.

28. Cardano is now most famous as a mathematician because he published a formula for finding the roots of a cubic equation. Yet his wide range of interests is reflected in the different critical and biographical works published about him in the last century. Markus Fierz's biography touches on many of Cardano's interests, focusing especially on his identity as a physician, natural philosopher and interpreter of dreams. See M. Fierz, *Girolamo Cardano: 1501–1576 Physician, Natural Philosopher, Mathematician, Astrologer, and Interpreter of Dreams*, trans. H. Niman (Boston, MA: Birkhäuser, 1983). Anthony

Grafton has written about Cardano's work in astrology in A. Grafton, *Cardano's Cosmos: The Worlds and Works of a Renaissance Astrologer* (Cambridge, MA: Harvard University Press, 1999). Ore Øystein speaks to Cardano's fascination with gambling in O. Øystein, *Cardano the Gambling Scholar* (Princeton, NJ: Princeton University Press, 1953). As mentioned above, Nancy Siraisi's perceptive work focuses on his medical writings. Ian Maclean's careful scholarship explores many aspects of Cardano's oeuvre, focusing especially on his place in Renaissance thought as an interpreter of Aristotelian psychology and natural philosophy in I. Maclean, 'Cardano's Eclectic Psychology and its Critique by Julius Caesar Scaliger', *Vivarium* 46 (2008), pp. 392–417. See also, I. Maclean, 'Cardano and his Publishers, 1534–1663', in *Girolamo Cardano: Philosoph, Naturforscher, Arzt.*, ed. E. Kessler (Wiesbaden: Harrassowitz Verlag, 1994), pp. 314–16.

29. The passage on the bones of the skull reads: 'Sed ut ad hominis revertar compositionem, os capitis è pluribus frustis constare necesse fuit, ut tutius esset: nam parte fracta non est neccesse totum vitiari, ut venae, arteriaque ingredi commodiùs possent, egredique excrementa fuliginosa. Suturis tenuissimis partes eius iunxit, ut firmius continerentur, ut calor cerebri non evanesceret, ut frigori aditus minus pateret, ut firmius membranae illis haererent: & quanquam suturae tenues essent, ossa tamen non parum crassa sunt.' Cardanus, *Opera Omnia*, vol. 3, p. 559. Cardano often uses *subtilitas* and *tenuis* interchangeably, though *subtilitas* refers more frequently to abstractions, while *tenuis* tends to be used in discussions that refer to more exclusively physical qualities, as in this description of the fine sutures joining the bones of the skull.

30. The skull's ability to release waste matter was especially important for the early modern conception of the humoural body. Drawn mostly from Galen, humoural theory understood disease as a result of imbalance within the body or the putrefaction of a particular humour. A remedy restored balance by evacuating the humour that was causing the problem. Within this framework, the sutures of the skull provided a natural evacuation for the body, since noxious humours could be released through them to prevent a potentially dangerous imbalance. For a clear summary of humoural theory and the early modern challenges to its dominance in medical treatment, see H. J. Cook, 'Medicine', in L. Daston and K. Park (eds), *The Cambridge History of Science: Volume 3, Early Modern Science* (New York: Cambridge University Press, 2006), pp. 407–34.

31. Vesalius, *On the Fabric of the Human Body*, p. 61. The chapter is titled, 'De octo capitis ossibus, & suturis haec committentibus.' The passage reads, 'sed conducebat ex multis ossibus ipsam compingi, ut si quando percussa rumpatur, ipsius rupturae in totam calvariam veluti per fictile vas, non procedant, sed destineantur, & in illus sedibus cessent, in quibus ipsum quoque os suturis terminatum definit.' Vesalius, *De fabrica*, p. 26.

32. 'A ce que si quelque coup se bailloit sur la teste, ledict tez ne se sendist comme ung pot d'ung coste jusques a l'aultre: ou en plusieurs pieces.' Estienne, *La dissection des parties du corps humain*, p. 16.

33. Vesalius, *On the Fabric of the Human Body. Book I: Bones and Cartilages*, p. 60. 'Verum quum caput tectum quoddam domus calidae referat, fumida vaporosaque subiectarum partium recrementa, quaecunque sursum conscendunt, excipiens, atque huius gratia copiosiore evacuatione caput ipsum egeat, galeam cerebro inductam non omni ex parte solidam, sed cavernosam, futurisque intertextam sagax rerum Parens efformavit, non quidem spongiae modo tenuibus inaequalibusque foraminibus, velut quibusdam cavernulis, utrinque os perforans.' Vesalius, *De fabrica*, p. 26.

34. Estienne, *La dissection des parties du corps humain*, p. 14. The French reads: 'Telle conjunction de plusieurs os ensemble a este aussy necessaire pour donner passaige aux Vapeurs du cerveau.'

35. L. Daston and K. Park, *Wonders and the Order of Nature: 1150–1750* (New York: Zone Books, 1998), p.167.

## 6 Davis, 'Mirroring, Anatomy, Transparency: The Collective Body and the Co-opted Individual in Spenser, Hobbes and Bunyan'

1.  References are to E. Spenser, *The Faerie Queen*, ed. A. C. Hamilton (London: Longman, 2001). The present discussion does not take in canto 10, an embedded narrative of mythic British and elfin history, the second of which pertains to Guyon.

2.  See L. Barkan, *Nature's Work of Art: The Human Body as Image of the World* (New Haven, CT and London: Yale University Press, 1975), and M. Kemp, 'Temples of the Body and Temples of the Cosmos', in B. Braigrie (ed.), *Picturing Knowledge: Historical and Philosophical Problems Concerning the Use of Art in Science* (Toronto: University of Toronto Press, 1996), pp. 40–85.

3.  See H. Grabes, *The Mutable Glass: Mirror-Imagery in Titles and Texts of the Middle Ages and English Renaissance*, trans. G. Collier (Cambridge: Cambridge University Press, 1982).

4.  E. R. Curtius, *European Literature and the Latin Middle Ages*, trans. W. R. Trask (London: Routledge and Kegan Paul, 1953), p. 326.

5.  The Castle of Anima episode in Passus 9 of the B-Text of *Piers Plowman* is, as is generally recognized, a particularly important intertext for Spenser's Alma episode. 'Alma' is, as Walter R. Davis explains, 'both a poetical contraction of ... Latin and Italian *anima*, whose meaning evolved from 'breath' to 'the vital principle' to 'the soul', and the feminine form of Latin *almus* ['that which nourishes'; 'fair, beautiful, gracious'], as in the common phrase *alma mater*' (24). A. C. Hamilton points out that 'Alma' can also signify 'a maiden' (from Hebrew *almah*), and that Langland's Anima is also named 'Life'; see Spenser, *The Faerie Queene*, 9.18n.

6.  Spenser, *The Faerie Queen*, II.9.11.

7.  Ibid., IV.9.2.

8.  Ibid., II.9.22.

9.  I have argued that the stanza's transcendent mathematics *is*, as presented, inherently incommensurable with surrounding statements in the poem and that, here as elsewhere, Spenser insists on the reciprocal irreducibility of significant symbolic systems; see N. Davis, *Stories of Chaos: Reason and its Displacement in Early Modern English Narrative* (Aldershot: Ashgate, 1999), p. 79. No one is going to find this stanza's hidden truth: its truth is on the surface, making for speculative openness.

10. See P. Archambault, 'The Analogy of the "Body" in Renaissance Political Literature', *Bibliothèque d'Humanisme et Renaissance*, 29 (1967), pp. 21–53.

11. See also Spenser, *The Faerie Queen*, II.21.45.

12. The *psychomachia* has its fullest known English realization in the morality play of *c.* 1400 known as *The Castle of Perseverance*. The adventures of its central figure, Humanum Genus, span crucial battles fought within the soul, as virtues and vices lock in combat, and over the fate of the human soul, as for example when Humanum Genus leaves the safety of the play's symbolic castle under the persuasion of Covetousness. The basic

motifs of the *psychomachia* are established in Prudentius's later fourth-century poem of that name.

13. Spenser, *The Faerie Queene*, II.9.16.
14. Ibid., II.9.24.
15. W. J. Ong, *Orality and Literacy: The Technologizing of the Word* (London and New York: Methuen, 1982), p. 133.
16. Spenser, *The Faerie Queene*, II.12.1.
17. Ibid., II.9.1.
18. Ibid., II.9.36–44.
19. For the relation to architectural treatises, see P. Long, 'Objects of Art/Objects of Nature', in P. Smith and P. Findlen (eds), *Merchants and Marvels: Commerce, Science, and Art in Early Modern Europe* (New York and London: Routledge, 2002), pp. 74–9, and for positive roles given to machine analogy in the era's moral thinking, see J. Wolfe, *Humanism, Machinery, and Renaissance Literature* (Cambridge: Cambridge University Press, 2004).
20. Here it is useful to compare the passage with its closest contemporary intertext, the citadel-body of Du Bartas's *Divine Weeks* (first week, sixth day, ll. 401–944; pp. 269–95). Du Bartas's account, which more closely resembles the paintings of Arcimboldo, is an ingenious, multi-focussed description of organic form as artefact, whereas Spenser's primary concern is with the working interconnectedness of the whole.
21. Spenser, *The Faerie Queen*, II.9.23.
22. Ibid., II.9.27–33.
23. Ibid., II.9.13.
24. Ibid., II.9.33–44.
25. Ibid., II.9.44–60.
26. Ibid., II.9.26.
27. See ibid. II.9.24n.
28. Ibid. II.716–6. For further discussion of the Spenserian narrative exemplar as an automated and automating life-form, see N. Davis, 'Nature, Desire and Automata in Bower of Bliss', in W. Hyman (ed.), *The Automaton in Renaissance Literature* (Aldershot: Ashgate, 2011).
29. See the work's preface, pp. xlix–lii, and Long, 'Objects of Art/Objects of Nature', pp. 76, 79.
30. This is one of the poem's several non-inclusive definitions of its understanding readership; the teachings of the egalitarian giant in book 5, for example, are said to be of interest only to 'fooles, women, and boyes', who as represented in the passage turn into a 'lawless multitude' (2.30, 52) when Artegall and Talus destroy him.
31. The central combat, for example, directly recalls that of Hercules and Antaeus.
32. Spenser, *The Faerie Queen*, II.11.39–40.
33. For the vivid conjunction in Hobbes of sensationalist psychology and a strong interest in crowd control, see P. Springborg, 'Hobbes and Historiography: Why the Future, he Says, Does Not Exist', in G. A. J. Rogers and T. Sorell, *Hobbes and History* (London and New York: Routledge, 2000).
34. T. Hobbes, *Leviathan or, The Matter, Forme and Power of A Common-Wealth Ecclesiasticall and Civill*, ed. C. B. Macpherson (Harmondsworth: Penguin, 1968), p. 379. Hobbes goes on to state with unfathomable sarcasm that if ordinary people can learn to accept the officially promulgated doctrine of the Eucharist, 'which is against Reason' (p. 379), they will certainly learn to accept his entirely rational doctrine of the sovereign state.
35. Ibid., p. 81.

36. J. Tralau, 'Leviathan, the Beast of Myth', in P. Springborg (ed.), *The Cambridge Companion to Hobbes's Leviathan* (Cambridge: Cambridge University Press, 2007), pp. 61–81, on p. 62.

37. Hobbes, *Leviathan*, p. 227.

38. I concur with Horst Bredekamp's view that the frontispiece to the first edition 'constitutes one of the most profound visual renderings of political theory ever produced', and with his high estimation of 'its capacity to address elements of political thought [which are] bizarre or even offensive to the modern reader', H. Bredekamp, 'Thomas Hobbes's Visual Strategies', in Springborg (ed.), *The Cambridge Companion to Hobbes's Leviathan*, pp. 29–60, on pp. 30, 33. Among Bredekamp's conclusions are that it was designed in Paris by the engraver Abraham Bosse with the collaboration of Hobbes's (see p. 30).

39. The image is reproduced in ibid., p. 41.

40. Ibid., p. 40.

41. See Landau's comments on the radical 'otherness' and rational irreducibility of Leviathan as invented monster with strong mythic overtones.

42. Cf. the image of the sleeping Bunyan, accompanied by one of the book's scenes *qua* dream, which appears as frontispiece to the third edition of *The Pilgrim's Progress*, a text which had already gained a considerable reputation.

43. J. Bunyan, *The Holy War* (1682), ed. R. Sharrock and J. F. Forrest (Oxford: Clarendon Press, 1980), p. 5.

44. Ong, *Orality and Literacy*, pp. 132–5.

45. For an examination of relations between authority and authorship in Bunyan, see T. Spargo, *The Writing of John Bunyan* (Aldershot: Ashgate, 1997).

46. Bunyan, *The Holy War*, pp. 51–2.

47. Ibid., p. 184. See also the text's treatment of narrative time, one of whose periods of demarcation seems to correspond to a phase of Bunyan's own spiritual development as described in *Grace Abounding*. See the comments of the editors, p. xxxii.

48. The traditional, unitary image of the soul is most in evidence in the representation of the victorious Emanuel's arrival in the town, his privileged treatment of it and the celebrations which ensue, pp. 106–16, 135–50. A climactic passage characterizes Mansoul most distinctly as feminine: 'Now did Mansoul's cup run over, now did her Conduits run sweet wine, now did she eat the finest of the wheat, and drink milk and hony of the rock! Now she said, how great is his goodness! For since I found favour in his eyes, how honourable have I been!', p. 149.

49. Bunyan, *The Holy War*, p. 144.

50. Ibid., p. 204.

51. Cf. the distinction made by Charles Taylor between *shared* (Intersubjective) *meanings* and *common meanings* (affirmed by a group in active sharing). See C. Taylor, *Philosophical Papers 2* (Cambridge: Cambridge Unievrsity Press, 1985), p. 39.

## 7 Untea, 'From Human to Political Body and Soul: Materialism and Mortalism in the Political Theory of Thomas Hobbes'

1. K. Bootle Atie, 'Re-membering the Body Politic: Hobbes and the Construction of Civic Immortality', *ELH*, 75:3 (2008), pp. 497–530, on pp. 497–8. Cf. E. Kantorowicz, *The King's Two Bodies: A Study in Medieval Political Theology* (Princeton, NJ: Princeton Univ. Press, 1997), p. 409.

2. Bootle Atie, 'Re-membering the Body Politic', p. 496.
3. Ibid., p. 498.
4. L. I. Bredvold, 'Dryden, Hobbes and the Royal Society,' *Modern Philology*, 25:4 (1928), pp. 417–38, on p. 419.
5. R. Descartes, *Meditations on First Philosophy* (1641), trans. D. A. Cress (Indianapolis: IndianaHacket, 1993), p. 420.
6. Ibid., pp. 419–20.
7. Bredvold, 'Dryden, Hobbes and the Royal Society', pp. 420–1.
8. Ibid., pp. 420, 423.
9. Ibid., p. 420.
10. T. Hobbes, *Leviathan, or the Matter, Form, and Power of a Commonwealth, Ecclesiastical and Civil* (1651; London: John Bohn, 1839), p. 85.
11. Ibid., pp. 443–4.
12. N. H. Henry, 'Milton and Hobbes: Mortalism and the Intermediate State,' *Studies in Philology*, 48:2 (1951), pp. 234–49, on pp. 236, 239.
13. Ibid., pp. 237–9.
14. Ibid., p. 442.
15. Ibid., p. 443.
16. Brevold, 'Dryden, Hobbes and the Royal Society', p. 424.
17. Ibid., pp. 422–4.
18. S. Frost, *Lessons from a Materialist Thinker: Hobbesian Reflections on Ethics and Politics* (Stanford, CA: Stanford University Press, 2008), p. 71.
19. Ibid., p. 72.
20. Ibid., pp. 71–2. J. Bramhall, *A Defence of True Liberty from Antecedent and Extrinsicall Necessity* (1655), ed. G. A. J. Rogers (London: Routledge/Thoemmes Press, 1996), p. 79.
21. Frost, *Lessons from a Materialist Thinker*, p. 33.
22. Ibid.
23. T. Sorell, 'Hobbes's Scheme of the Sciences', in T. Sorell (ed.), *The Cambridge Companion to Hobbes* (Cambridge: Cambridge Univ. Press, 1996), pp. 45–62, on p. 53.
24. T. Hobbes, *On the Citizen* (1642), trans. R. Tuck and M. Silverthorne (Cambridge: Cambridge University Press, 2003), pp. 4–5.
25. T. Hobbes, *The Elements of Law Natural and Politic: Human Nature; De Corpore Politico* (1640), ed. J. C. A. Gaskin (Oxford: Oxford University Press, 1999), p. 19.
26. Ibid., p. 20; emphasis added.
27. T. Hobbes, *Elementorum philosophiae; sectio prima: de corpore* (Londini: Andrea Crook, 1655), A 3. Cf. D. M. Jesseph, 'Galileo, Hobbes and the Book of Nature,' *Perspectives on Science*, 12:2 (2004), pp. 191–211, on p. 199.
28. Jesseph, 'Galileo, Hobbes and the Book of Nature', p. 202.
29. Ibid.
30. Ibid., p. 207.
31. Ibid., p. 201. Hobbes, *Leviathan*, p. 3.
32. Jesseph, 'Galileo, Hobbes and the Book of Nature', pp. 201, 208.
33. Ibid., pp. 202, 208.
34. Descartes, *Meditations on First Philosophy*, Objection IV, p. 105.
35. Hobbes, *Leviathan*, p. 2.
36. Ibid., p. 42.
37. Frost, *Lessons from a Materialist Thinker*, p. 69.
38. Hobbes, *Leviathan*, p. 13.

39. Ibid., pp. 47–8.
40. Ibid., p. 14.
41. Ibid., p. 47.
42. Bernard Gert considers that, because of the possibility of altruistic behaviour for Hobbesian individuals, Hobbes's psychology should not be called egoistical, but pessimistic. This interpretation is based on the assumption that, according to psychological egoism 'men never act in order to benefit others'. In the light of the text quoted above from chapter 6, Hobbes's 'compassion' is not purely altruistic, but rather it is an involuntary egoistical feeling. B. Gert, 'Hobbes and Psychological Egoism', *Journal of the History of Ideas*, 28:4 (1967), pp. 503–20, on p. 505.
43. Hobbes, *Leviathan*, ch. 11, p. 86.
44. Ibid., p. 119.
45. L. T. Sarasohn, 'Motion and Morality: Pierre Gassendi, Thomas Hobbes and the Mechanical World-View', *Journal of the History of Ideas*, 46:3 (1985), pp. 363–79, on p. 365.
46. S. Frost, 'Faking It: Hobbes's Thinking-Bodies and the Ethics of Dissimulation', *Political Theory*, 29:1 (2001), pp. 30–57, on p. 34. J. Hampton, *Hobbes and the Social Contract Tradition* (Cambridge: Cambridge University Press, 1999), p. 13.
47. Hobbes, *Leviathan*, p. xi.
48. T. H. Miller, 'The Uniqueness of Leviathan: Authorizing Poets, Philosophers and Sovereigns', in T. Sorell and L. Foisneau (eds), *Leviathan after 350 Years* (Oxford: Clarendon Press, 2004), pp. 75–105, on pp. 98–9.
49. Hobbes, *Leviathan*, p. xi.
50. S. H. Daniel, 'Civility and Sociability: Hobbes on Man and Citizen', *Journal of the History of Philosophy*, 18:2 (1980), pp. 209–15, on p. 210.
51. Hobbes, *Leviathan*, pp. 24–5; p. 36; pp. 102–3; p. 139.
52. Ibid., p. xi.
53. Ibid., pp. xi–xii; emphasis added.
54. Hobbes, *De Cive*, I, 7, p. 27.
55. Ibid., I, 7, p. 27.
56. Hobbes, *Leviathan*, p. 139.
57. Ibid., p. x.
58. Ibid., p. 138.
59. Ibid., p. ix.
60. Ibid., p. 87.
61. Ibid., p. 89.
62. Ibid., p. 307.
63. Ibid., p. 32; p. 113.
64. Ibid., p. 153.
65. Ibid., p. 321.
66. Ibid., pp. 199–200.
67. Ibid., p. 239.
68. Ibid., p. 147.
69. Sorel, 'Hobbes's Scheme of the Sciences', p. 58.
70. Hobbes, *Leviathan*, p. ix.
71. J. Mitchell, 'Hobbes and the Equality of All under One,' *Political Theory*, 21:1 (1993), pp. 78–100, on p. 82.
72. R. S., Woolhouse, *The Empiricists* (Oxford: Oxford University Press, 1988), p. 30.

73. Hobbes, *Leviathan*, p. 56.
74. Ibid.
75. Ibid.
76. Ibid., p. 114.
77. Ibid., p. 95.
78. Ibid., p. 312.
79. Ibid., p. ix.
80. Ibid., p. 158.
81. Ibid., pp. 308–9.
82. Ibid., pp. 319–20.
83. Brevold, 'Dryden, Hobbes and the Royal Society', p. 419.
84. Hobbes, *Leviathan*, p. 319
85. Ibid., p. 320.
86. Ibid., p. 321.
87. Ibid., p. 437.
88. Ibid., p. 574.
89. Ibid., p. 317.
90. Ibid., p. 321.
91. Ibid., pp. 315–16.
92. Ibid., p. 341.
93. Ibid., p. 233.
94. Ibid., p. 239.
95. Ibid., pp. 239–40.
96. Ibid., p. 665.
97. Ibid., p. 335.
98. Ibid.
99. P. Pasqualucci, 'Hobbes and the Myth of "Final War"', *Journal of the History of Ideas*, 51:4 (1990), pp. 647–57, on p. 656.
100. Hobbes, *Leviathan*, p. 113.

## 8 Ishizuka, 'Visualizing the Fibre-Woven Body: Nehemiah Grew's Plant Anatomy and the Emergence of the Fibre Body'

1. J. B. Banborough, *The Little World of Man* (London: Longman, 1952). p. 53; S. Collins, *A Systeme of Anatomy* (London, 1685), p. 3.
2. T. Gibson, *The Anatomy of Humane Bodies Epitomize*, 6th edn (London, 1703), p. ii.
3. A. G. Van Melsen, *From Atomos to Atom: The History of the Concept of Atom* (1952; New York: Harper & Brothers, 1960), pp. 41–4, 74; E. N. Emerton, *The Scientific Reinterpretation of Form* (Ithaca, NY: Cornell University Press, 1984), p. 90.
4. R. Bolye, *Selected Philosophical Paper of Robert Boyle*, ed. M. A. Stewart (Cambridge: Hackett, 1991), p. 41.
5. On Malpighi, see M. Fournier, *The Fabric of Life: Microscopy in the Seventeenth Century* (Baltimore, MD: Johns Hopkins University Press, 1996), pp. 55–60 and G. Gigglioni, 'The Machine of the Body and the Operations of the Soul in Marcello Malpighi's Anatomy', in Domenico Bertoloni Meli (ed.), *Marcello Malpighi, Anatomist and Physician* (Firenze: Olschki, 1997), pp. 149–74.
6. F. J. Cole, 'The History of Anatomical Injections', in C. Singer (ed.), *Studies in the History and Method of Science*, 2 vols (Oxford: Clarendon Press, 1921), vol. 2, pp. 285–343, on p. 287.

7. Ibid., p. 303.
8. E. G. Ruestow, 'The Rise of the Doctrine of Vascular Secretion in the Netherlands', *Journal of the History of Medicine*, 35 (1980), pp. 265–87, on p. 272.
9. Ibid., p. 271; L. Belloni, 'Marcello Marpighi and the Founding of Anatomical Microscopy', trans. T. B. Settle, in M. L. Righini Bonelli and W. R. Shea (eds), *Reason, Experiment, and Mysticism in the Scientific Revolution* (New York: Science History Publication, 1975), pp. 95–110, on p. 98; Fournier, *The Fabric of Life*, p. 129.
10. Fournier, *The Fabric of Life*, pp. 136–8, 55.
11. C. Wilson, *The Invisible World: Early Modern Philosophy and the Invention of the Microscope* (Princeton, NJ: Princeton University Press, 1995).
12. R. Hooke, *Micrographia: or Some Physiological Descriptions of Minute Bodies made by Magnifying Glasses with Observations and Inquiries Thereupon* (London, 1665), p. 138.
13. Ibid., p. 135.
14. Ibid., p. 141.
15. E. King, 'Some Considerations Concerning the Parenchymous Parts of the Body', *Philosophical Transactions*, 1 (1665–6), pp. 316–20, on pp. 316–17.
16. F. Glisson, *English Manuscripts of Francis Glisson (1): From Anatomica Hepatis (The Anatomy of the Liver), 1654*, ed. A. Cunningham (Cambridge: Wellcome Unit for the History of Medicine, 1993), p. 53.
17. N. Grew, *The Anatomy of Plants. With an Idea of a Philosophical History of Plants and Several Other Lectures Read before the Royal Society* (London, 1682), p. 19.
18. Ibid., pp. 120–1.
19. N. Grew, *Cosmologia Sacra: or, A Discourse of the Universe as it is the Creature and Kingdom of God* (London, 1701), p. 18.
20. Grew, *The Anatomy of Plants*, p. 121. Contemporaries also observed that Grew discovered the more minute fibres composing the bladders, which made up the Pith; see the editor's notes to Leeuwenhoek's letter in *Philosophical Transactions* (1676), vol. 11, pp. 653–60, on p. 660.
21. Grew, *The Anatomy of Plants*, pp. 59, 62. Other examples are 'as it were ... a Diversified Woof' (for the uniform contexture of the parenchymous part of the barque), 'Threds ... Braced together in the form of *Net-Work*' (for the texture of the barque), 'Fine and close *Needle-work*' (for the fibrous structure of the pith), 'a piece of *Linsy-Woosly Work*, or like manner other *Manufactures* in which the *Warp* and the *Woof* are of different Sorts of *Stuff*' (for the insertions in the wood) (pp. 64, 65, 77, 114).
22. Ibid., p. 77.
23. Ibid., pp. 121–2.
24. Grew, 'Epistle Dedicatory', in *The Anatomy of Plants*.
25. He also wrote the *Comparative Anatomy of Stomachs and Guts*, which is included in his *Musaeum Regalis Societalis, or A Catalogue and Description of the Natural and Artificial Rarities* (London, 1681).
26. Grew, *The Anatomy of Plants*, p. 112.
27. Ibid., p. 131. Other illustrations of the analogy between plants and animals are seen on p. 60 (transformation); p. 66 (the fibre); p. 77 (skin); p. 84 (nutrition).
28. Grew, *Cosmologia Sacra*, p. 18.
29. J. Bolam, 'The Botanical Works of Nehemiah Grew, F.R.S. (1641–1712)', in *Notes and Records of the Royal Society of London*, 26 (1971), pp. 219–31, on pp. 227–8.
30. The anatomists also often found in the micro-structures of the organs their similarity to the morphological form of the plant; branches, twigs, leaves and trees were recurrently

mentioned in anatomists' writings and shown in the illustrations, and sometimes those illustrations of animal/human anatomy weirdly resembled the micro-fibrous structures of the plant. So, Grew's choice of the study of plant anatomy for explicating the animal/ human anatomy was not fortuitous, for the inner animal/human body (the animal kingdom) was increasingly viewed as the place inhabited by the vegetable kingdom.

31. S. I. Mintz, *The Hunting of Leviathan* (1962; Bristol: Thoemmes Press, 1996).
32. Grew wrote *Cosmologia Sacra* as an antidote to Spinoza's philosophy (preface n.p.).
33. N. C. Gillespie, 'Natural History, Natural Theology, and Social Order: John Ray and the "Newtonian Ideology"', in *Journal of the History of Biology*, 20 (1987), pp. 1–49, on p. 21.
34. M. Hunter, *Science and the Shape of Orthodoxy: Intellectual Change in Late Seventeenth-Century Britain* (London: Boydell Press, 1995), p. 15.
35. Atheism, in this period, meant the belief that God does not exist or the universe perpetuates without the divine intervention; however, the term was often employed by controversialists to their opponents who they thought did not conform to orthodox theology. The heterodoxies of the period include Hobbes's materialism, Spinoza's hylozoism (matters endowed with life), and atomism. Very few professed themselves as true atheists.
36. J. Rogers, *The Matter of Revolution: Science, Poetry, & Politics in the Age of Milton* (Ithaca, NY: Cornell University Press, 1996), p. 36; S. Clucas, 'Poetic Atomism in Seventeenth-Century England: Henry More, Thomas Traherne and "Scientific Imagination"', *Renaissance Studies*, 5 (1991), pp. 327–40, on p. 335.
37. Clucas, 'Poetic Atomism', pp. 328–9.
38. Ibid., p. 333.
39. J. Keill, *The Anatomy of the Human Body Abridged* (London, 1698), p. 1.
40. G. S. Rousseau, *Nervous Acts: Essays on Literature, Culture and Sensibility* (Basingstoke: Palgrave, 2004).
41. The doctrine of 'animal spirits' is ancient, tracing back to Galenian notion of *pneuma* which is secreted in the brain and distributed throughout the body by means of hollow nerves. It retained its explanatory force even in late seventeenth century partly because of Cartesian mechanization of the body as the hydraulic machine.
42. G. Cheyne, *The English Malady; or, A Treatise of Nervous Diseases of all Kinds* (London, 1733), p. 62. For more on this, see my essay on Blake and fibre medicine, H. Ishizuka, 'Enlightening the Fibre-Woven Body: William Blake and Eighteenth-Century Fibre Medicine', *Literature and Medicine*, 25 (2006), pp. 72–92; I am preparing a paper devoted to this theme ('"Fibre Body": The Concept of the Fibre in Eighteenth-Century Medicine', *Medical History* (forthcoming)).
43. H. Boerhaave, *Dr. Boerhaave's Academic Lectures on the Theory of Physic*, 6 vols (London, 1742–6), vol. 2, p. 310.
44. T. de la Roche, *L'Amour dévoilé ou le système des sympathistes* (n.p., 1749), p. 113.

# 9 Wolfe, 'Forms of Materialist Embodiment'

1. J. O. de La Mettrie and H. Boerhaave, *Institutions de médecine de M. Hermann Boerhaave*, trans. with commentary by La Mettrie, 2nd edn, 8 vols (Paris: Huart & Cie, 1747), vol. 5, p. 111.
2. R. Boyle, *The Origin of Forms and Qualities* (1666), in R. Boyle, *The Works of Robert Boyle*, ed. T. Birch, 6 vols (London: J. and F. Rivington et al. 1772; Hildesheim: Georg

Olms, 1965), vol. 3, p. 13; R. Boyle, *Some Considerations Touching the Usefulness of Experimental Natural Philosophy* (1671), vol. 2, in Boyle, *The Works*, vol. 3, p. 427.

3.    R. Descartes, *Treatise on Man*, in *Œuvres*, ed. C. Adam and P. Tannery, 11 vols (Paris: Vrin, 1964–74), vol. 11, pp. 120, 130–1, 202.

4.    H. Boerhaave, *De usu ratiocinii mechanici in medicina*, in *Opuscula selecta Neerlandicorum de arte medica*, 19 vols (1703; Amsterdam: F. van Rossen, 1907), vol. 1, p. 146. *Boerhaave's Orations*, trans. and ed. E. Kegel-Brinkgreve and A. M. Luyendijk-Elshout. (Leiden: E. J. Brill / Leiden University Press, 1983), p. 96.

5.    J. Toland, *Letters to Serena* (London: B. Lintot, 1704; New York: Garland, 1996), letter 5, p. 192.

6.    D. Diderot, *Œuvres complètes*, ed. H. Dieckmann, J. Proust and J. Varloot, 33 planned volumes (Paris: Hermann, 1975), vol. 17, p. 128.

7.    For an early rebuttal of this view see A. Thomson, 'L'homme-machine, mythe ou métaphore?', *Dix-huitième siècle*, 20 (1988), pp. 368–76. For the case of Diderot, see C. Wolfe, 'Machine et organisme chez Diderot', *Recherches sur Diderot et l'Encyclopédie*, 26 (1999), pp. 213–31.

8.    J.-P. Dupuy, *The Mechanization of the Mind: On the Origins of Cognitive Science*, trans. M. B. DeBevoise (Princeton, NJ: Princeton University Press, 2000).

9.    Cf. E. Husserl, 'Philosophy as Rigorous Science', trans. and ed. P. McCormick and F. Elliston, in *Husserl. Shorter Works* (1910; Notre Dame: Notre Dame University Press, 1981), pp. 166–97; R. Ruyer, 'Ce qui est vivant et ce qui est mort dans le matérialisme', *Revue Philosophique*, 116:7–8 (1933), pp. 28–49; H. Jonas, *The Phenomenon of Life. Towards a Philosophical Biology* (New York: Harper & Row, 1966).

10.    J. Schiller, *La notion d'organisation dans l'histoire de la biologie* (Paris: Maloine, 1978).

11.    C. Merchant, *The Death of Nature: Women, Ecology, and the Scientific Revolution* (New York: Harper & Row, 1980); L. R. Kass, 'Appreciating the Phenomenon of Life', *Hastings Center Report*, 25:7 (1995), pp. 3–12.

12.    U. Rublack, 'Fluxes: The Early Modern Body and the Emotions', *History Workshop Journal*, 53 (2002), pp. 1–16; C. McClive, 'Menstrual Knowledge and Medical Practice in France, c. 1555–1761', in G. Howie and A. Shail (eds), *Menstruation: A Cultural History* (London: Palgrave Macmillan, 2005), pp. 76–89; L. W. Smith, 'The Body Embarrassed? Rethinking the Leaky Male Body in Eighteenth-Century England and France', *Gender and History*, 23:1 (2010), pp. 26–46.

13.    I. Hacking, 'The Cartesian Body', *BioSocieties*, 1 (2006), pp. 13–15. An entire generation of prominent Descartes scholars has rejected this reading, emphasizing instead an 'embodied Descartes'. See, for example, A. Oksenberg Rorty, 'Descartes on Thinking with the Body', in J. Cottingham (ed.), *The Cambridge Companion to Descartes* (Cambridge: Cambridge University Press, 1992), pp. 371–92; J. Sutton, 'The Body and the Brain', in S. Gaukroger, J. A. Schuster and J. Sutton (eds), *Descartes' Natural Philosophy* (London: Routledge, 2000), pp. 697–722. And, differently, D. Des Chene, *Spirits and Clocks: Machine and Organism in Descartes* (Ithaca, NY: Cornell University Press, 2001), however, this does not affect the prevalence of our concept of the 'Cartesian body' (aka Gilbert Ryle's 'ghost in the shell'), which is all that matters here.

14.    D. Haraway, 'A Cyborg Manifesto: Science, Technology, and Socialist-Feminism in the Late Twentieth Century', in *Simians, Cyborgs and Women: The Reinvention of Nature* (New York: Routledge, 1991), pp. 149–81; N. K. Hayles, 'The Life Cycle of Cyborgs: Writing the Posthuman', in M. Benjamin (ed.), *A Question of Identity: Women, Science and Literature* (New Brunswick, NJ: Rutgers University Press, 1993), pp. 152–70. Cf.

N. K. Hayles, 'Flesh and Metal: Reconfiguring the Mindbody in Virtual Environments', *Configurations*, 10 (2002), pp. 297–320.

15. J. Riskin, 'The Defecating Duck, or, The Ambiguous Origins of Artificial Life', *Critical Inquiry*, 29:4 (2003), pp. 599–633. C. T. Wolfe, 'Le mécanique face au vivant', in B. Roukhomovsky, S. Roux et al. (eds), *L'automate: modèle, machine, merveille* (Bordeaux: Presses universitaires de Bordeaux, forthcoming, 2013).

16. T. Hobbes, *Leviathan or The Matter, Forme and Power of a Commonwealth Ecclesiastical and Civil*, ed. E. Curley with Latin variants (1651; Indianapolis: Hackett, 1994), ch. 4, § 46, p. 459. T. Hobbes, *Thomas White's 'De Mundo' Examined* (1642–3), trans. H. W. Jones (London: Bradford University Press, 1997), ch. 37, § 4, p. 447.

17. F. Bacon, *Novum Organum*, bk 2, ch. 2, in F. Bacon, *The Works of Francis Bacon*, ed. J. Spedding, R. L. Ellis and D. D. Heath, 14 vols (London: Longman & Co., 1857–74), vol. 8, p. 168.

18. D. Diderot, *Éléments de physiologie*, in *Œuvres complètes*, op. cit., vol. 17, pp. 334–5.

19. La Mettrie, *Institutions de médecine de M. Hermann Boerhaave*, p. 125.

20. R. Cudworth, *The True Intellectual System of the Universe* (London: R. Royston, 1678; Hildesheim: Georg Olms, 1977), vol. 1, ch. 2, § 30, p. 135.

21. A. Furetière, *Dictionnaire universel, contenant généralement les mots français, tant vieux que modernes, et les termes des sciences et des arts*, 3 vols (The Hague: A. & R. Leers, 1727), vol. 3, s.v. 'Matérialiste'; in the earlier (1690) edition we find an entry 'Matériel' that gives a rather conformist yet telling example for the word 'material': 'composed of matter. The soul of animals is *material*, that of humans is *spiritual*.'

22. M. Merleau-Ponty, *Phenomenology of Perception*, trans. C. Smith (London: Routledge & Kegan Paul, 1962), p. 104.

23. Rublack, 'Fluxes: The Early Modern Body and the Emotions', p. 13.

24. Aside from various works in 'history of the body' that appeared at a bewildering rate during the 1980s and 1990s, in early modern studies one can mention C. W. Bynum, 'Why All the Fuss about the Body? A Medievalist's Perspective', *Critical Inquiry*, 22 (1995), pp. 1–33; T. Reiss, 'Denying the Body? Memory and the Dilemmas of History in Descartes', *Journal of the History of Idea*, 57:4 (1996), pp. 587–607; G. K. Paster, 'Nervous Tension: Networks of Blood and Spirit in the Early Modern Body', in D. Hillman and C. Mazzio (eds), *The Body in Parts* (London: Routledge, 1997), pp. 107–25; S. Pilloud and M. Louis-Courvoisier, 'The Intimate Experience of the Body in the Eighteenth-Century: Between Interiority and Exteriority', *Medical History*, 47 (2003), pp. 451–72; McClive, 'Menstrual Knowledge and Medical Practice in France'; Smith, 'The Body Embarrassed?'. In embodied cognitive science, see I. M. Young, *On Female Body Experience: 'Throwing Like a Girl' and Other Essays* (Oxford: Oxford University Press, 2005). For an interesting and original twist on their programmes, combining 'humoural materialism' with 'historical cognitive science', see J. Sutton, 'Spongy Brains and Material Memories', in S. Gaukroger, J. A. Schuster and J. Sutton (eds), *Descartes' Natural Philosophy* (London: Routledge, 2000), and J. Sutton, 'Carelessness and Inattention: Mind-Wandering and the Physiology of Fantasy from Locke to Hume', in C. T. Wolfe and O. Gal (eds), *The Body as Object and Instrument of Knowledge: Embodied Empiricism in Early Modern Science* (Dordrecht: Springer, 2010). For a recent attempt to compensate for the total absence of 'embodiment' discourse in the history of science (here, early modern life science), see C. T. Wolfe and O. Gal (eds), *The Body as Object and Instrument of Knowledge. Embodied Empiricism in Early Modern Science* (Dordrecht: Springer, 2010).

25. The example of Sanctorius (and Harvey, cf. A. Salter and C. T. Wolfe, 'Empiricism contra Experiment: Harvey, Locke and the Revisionist View of Experimental Philosophy', *Bulletin de la SHESVIE*, 16:2 (2009), pp. 113–40) shows that antireductionism needs to improve its vision of the history of modern science, particularly medicine. However, conversely, mainstream history of philosophy has much to gain by understanding 'humouralist' models of the body in early modernity (see the references in note 24, above).

26. M. Merleau-Ponty *The Structure of Behaviour*, trans. A. L. Fisher (Boston, MA: Beacon Press, 1963), p. 209.

27. Ibid., p. 154.

28. J. Sawday, *The Body Emblazoned: Dissection and the Human Body in Renaissance Culture* (London: Routledge, 1995), p. 29.

29. Thompson, 'L'homme machine, mythe ou métaphore?', p. 238.

30. Boerhaave, *De usu ratiocinii mechanici in medicina*, p. 81.

31. G. Baglivi, *The Practice of Physick*, trans. G. Sewell and J. T. Desaguliers, 2nd edn (1696; London: A. Bell et al., 1704), pp. 135–6.

32. W. Croone, *De ratione motus musculorum* (London: S. Hayes, 1664), §26, p. 15, quoted in L. G. Wilson, 'William Croone's Theory of Muscular Contraction', *Notes and Records of the Royal Society*, 16:2 (1961), pp. 158–78, on p. 161.

33. Boerhaave, *De usu ratiocinii mechanici in medicina*, p. 146; also in *Boerhaave's Orations* (1983), p. 96.

34. The *Dictionnaire de l'Académie*, in 1694, defines 'machine' as 'a set of parts or organs which form a whole, living or not, and produce determinate effects without transmitting a force externally; organism, body'; quoted in G. Cayrou, *Le français classique. Lexique de la langue du dix-septième siècle* (Paris: Didier, 1948), s.v. 'Machine', p. 530.

35. See J. Vaucanson, *An Account of the Mechanism of an Automaton or Image Playing on the German-Flute*, trans. J. T. Desaguliers (1738; London, T Parker, 1742); J. Riskin, 'The Defecating Duck, or, The Ambiguous Origins of Artificial Life', *Critical Inquiry*, 29:4 (2003), pp. 599–633, and for new analyses of Vaucanson and the status of automata in early modern Europe, B. Roukhomovsky, S. Roux, et al. (eds), *L'automate: modèle, machine, merveille* (Bordeaux: Presses universitaires de Bordeaux, forthcoming 2013).

36. T. Kaitaro, *Diderot's Holism. Philosophical Anti-Reductionism and its Medical Background* (Frankfurt: Peter Lang, 1997), ch. 3 ; D. Boury, 'Théophile de Bordeu: source et personnage du *Rêve de D'Alembert*', *Recherches sur Diderot et sur l'Encyclopédie*, 34 (2003), pp. 11–24.

37. L. de, La Caze, *Idée de l'homme physique et moral pour servir d'introduction à un traité de médecine* (Paris: Guérin & Delatour 1755), p. 2.

38. Ibid., p. 12.

39. C. T. Wolfe and M. Terada, 'The "Animal Economy" as Object and Program in Montpellier Vitalism', *Science in Context*, 21:4 (2008) pp. 537–79, in § 4.

40. J.-J. Ménuret de Chambaud, 'Œconomie Animale (Médecine)', in D. Diderot and J. D'Alembert (eds), *Encyclopédie ou Dictionnaire raisonné des arts et des métiers* (Paris: Briasson, 1765), vol. 11, pp. 360–6, on p. 364b.

41. Sutton, 'The Body and the Brain'.

42. La Mettrie, *L'Homme-Machine*, in *Œuvres philosophiques*, ed. F. Markovits, 2 vols (1751; Paris: Fayard, 1987), vol. 1, p. 67.

43. O. Temkin, *Galenism: Rise and Decline of a Medical Philosophy* (Ithaca, NY: Cornell University Press, 1973).

44. La Mettrie, *L'Homme-Machine*, vol. 1, p. 62.
45. Ibid., vol. 1, p. 91.
46. H. Fouquet, *Discours sur la clinique* (Montpellier: Izar & Ricard, an XI [1803]), pp. 16–7; he does not mean the older, Galenic idea that the study of the body's anatomy reveals to us such miracles of design that our metaphysical confidence in the existence of a God should be bolstered!
47. I do not attempt here to provide a cultural *survol* of early modern anatomy and embodiment, as in Sawday, *The Body Emblazoned* (esp. pp. 66ff on the cultural context of anatomy and Vesalius); C. Mazzio, 'The Senses Divided: Organs, Objects and Media in Early Modern England', in D. Howes (ed.), *The Empire of the Senses* (Oxford: Berg, 2005), pp. 85–105; P. Mitchell, *The Purple Island and Anatomy in Early Seventeenth-Century Literature* (Madison, NJ: Fairleigh-Dickenson University Press, 2007) (with discussion in A. Salter, 'The Early Modern Imagination has a Change of Heart: Peter Mitchell's *The Purple Island and Anatomy in Early Seventeenth-Century Literature, Philosophy, and Theology*', *Metascience*, 18 (2009), pp. 131–4).
48. Sydenham/Locke, *Anatomia* (1668) (attributed both to Sydenham and to Locke); Locke's 'version' is Locke MS, National Archives PRO 30/24/72/2 ff. 36v–37r., quoted in J. C. Walmsley, 'Sydenham and the Development of Locke's Natural Philosophy', *British Journal for the History of Philosophy*, 16:1 (2008), pp. 65–83, on p. 70 (also in K. Dewhurst, *Dr. Thomas Sydenham (1624–1689), his Life and Writings* (London: Wellcome Medical Library, 1966), pp. 85–93). For further discussion of this text see Salter and Wolfe, 'Empiricism contra Experiment' and, especially on questions of attribution, P. Anstey and J. Burrows, 'John Locke, Thomas Sydenham, and the Authorship of Two Medical Essays', *eBLJ* (British Library) 1 (2009), at http://www.bl.uk/eblj/2009articles/pdf/ebljarticle32009.pdf [accessed January 5, 2010].
49. F. Bacon, *Advancement of Learning*, ch. 2, in *The Works of Francis Bacon*, vol. 6, p. 246.
50. Bacon, *Novum Organum*, bk. 1, ch. cxxiv, in *The Works of Francis Bacon*, vol. 8, p. 156.
51. Diderot, letter to Landois, 29 June 1756, in Diderot, *Œuvres complètes*, vol. 9, p. 258; see also his early letter to Voltaire, 11 June 1749, in D. Diderot, *Correspondance*, ed. G. Roth, 9 vols (Paris: Éditions de Minuit, 1955–70), vol. 1, p. 78.
52. T. Willis, *Two Discourses Concerning the Soul of Brutes, Which is That of the Vital [Soul] of Man*, trans. S. Pordage (London: Dring, Harper and Leigh, 1683), p. 23.
53. B. Fontenelle, *Traité de la liberté de l'âme*, in *Œuvres complètes*, ed. G.-B. Depping, 3 vols (1700; Geneva: Slatkine Reprints, 1968), vol. 2, § 1–2. I translate *âme* as 'mind', since the term in this context means strictly the locus of mental properties, of which the brain is the physical substrate – and not, say, the metaphysical opposite of 'matter', or even that which survives after the death of the body; I return below to the gradual process of 'naturalization' of the soul in the later Enlightenment.
54. J. Priestley, *Hartley's Theory of the Human Mind, on the Principle of the Association of Ideas, with Essays relating to the Subject of it* (London: J. Johnson, 1775), p. xx.
55. Anon., 'Passions, s. f. pl. *(Philos. Logique, Morale.)*', in D. Diderot and J. D'Alembert (eds), *Encyclopédie ou Dictionnaire raisonné des arts et des métiers* (Paris: Briasson, 1765), vol. 12, pp. 142–6, on p. 142.
56. *Nouvelles ecclésiastiques*, 18 November 1758, p. 188, cited in F. Salaün, 'La culture matérielle et morale dans l'*Encyclopédie*', in *La matière et l'homme dans l'*Encyclopédie, ed. S. Albertan-Coppola and A.-M. Chouillet (Paris: Klincksieck, 1995), pp. 187–218, on p. 190.
57. A. Comte, *Discours sur l'esprit positif*, new edn (1844; Paris: Vrin, 1974), § 771.

58. A. Thomson, *Bodies of Thought: Science, Religion, and the Soul in the Early Enlightenment* (Oxford: Oxford University Press, 2008); C. T. Wolfe, 'A Happiness Fit for Organic Bodies: La Mettrie's Medical Epicureanism', in N. Leddy and A. Lifschitz (eds), *Epicurus in the Enlightenment* (Oxford: Voltaire Foundation, 2009), pp. 69–83.

59. La Mettrie, *L'Homme-Machine*, in *Œuvres philosophiques*, p. 286.

60. To Damilaville, November 1760, in Diderot, *Œuvres complètes*, vol. 3, p. 216.

61. *Lettre sur les sourds et muets*, in Diderot, *Correspondance*, vol. 4, pp. 15, 54.

62. Kaitaro, *Diderot's Holism. Philosophical Anti-Reductionism and its Medical Background*, and C. T. Wolfe, 'Machine et organisme chez Diderot', *Recherches sur Diderot et l'Ency-clopédie*, 26 (1999), pp. 213–31.

63. F. Engels, *Ludwig Feuerbach und der Ausgang der klassischen deutschen Philosophie*, in Marx and Engels, *Werke*, 39 vols (Berlin: Dietz Verlag, 1888/1982), vol. 21, p. 278 (translation mine); in English in K. Marx and F. Engels, *Basic Writings on Politics and Philosophy*, ed. L. S. Feuer (New York: Doubleday, 1959), p. 211.

64. G. Vassails, 'L'*Encyclopédie* et la physique', *Revue d'histoire des sciences*, 4 (1951), pp. 294–323, on p. 315.

65. Diderot and D'Alembert (eds), 'Méchanicien', in *Encyclopédie ou Dictionnaire*, vol. 10, pp. 220–2, on p. 221.

66. A. Thomson, 'Mechanistic Materialism versus Vitalistic Materialism', in *Mécanisme et vitalisme*, ed. M. Saad, special issue of *La Lettre de la Maison française d'Oxford*, 14 (2001), pp. 21–36; P. H. Reill, *Vitalizing Nature in the Enlightenment* (Berkeley, CA: University of California Press, 2005); Wolfe and Terada, 'The "Animal Economy" as Object and Program in Montpellier Vitalism'.

67. Diderot in F. Hemsterhuis, *Lettre sur l'homme et ses rapports, avec le commentaire inédit de Diderot*, ed. G. May (1772; New Haven, CT: Yale University Press / Paris: PUF, 1964), p. 277.

68. Anon., *L'Âme matérielle* [*c.* 1725–3], ed. A. Niderst (Paris: Champion, 2003), p. 174 (Lucretius, *De rerum natura* III, 327–30).

69. La Mettrie, *L'Homme-Machine*, vol. 1, p. 98.

70. P. M. Churchland, *A Neurocomputational Perspective: The Nature of Mind and the Structure of Science* (Cambridge, MA and London: MIT Press, 1989).

71. This shift in usage towards *âme* (soul) as a synonym of *esprit* (mind) became increasingly established after La Mettrie's time: many treatises on *les facultés de l'âme* from the later eighteenth century are treatises of psychology, not reflections on an immaterial, immortal soul (J. Schneewind, 'The Active Powers', in K. Haakonssen (ed.), *The Cambridge History of Eighteenth-Century Philosophy* (Cambridge: Cambridge University Press, 2005), pp. 557–607.

72. Thomson, *Bodies of Thought*, ch. 4.

73. C. Vogt, *Physiologische Briefe*, 14th edn (1847; Gießen: Rickersche Buchhandlung, 1874), vol. 13, p. 323; the original formulation is actually from P.-J. Cabanis, *Rapports du physique et du moral* (Paris: Crapart, Caille et Ravier, 1802), p. 151.

74. *Discours sur le Bonheur*, in La Mettrie, *Oeuvres philosophiques*, vol. 2, p. 262. For more on this kind of determinism see C. T. Wolfe, 'Determinism/Spinozism in the Radical Enlightenment: The Cases of Anthony Collins and Denis Diderot', *International Review of Eighteenth-Century Studies*, 1:1 (2007), pp. 37–51. That this was an *embodied* determinism is also evidenced more amusingly by juxtapositions such as those found in the libertine, clandestine work *Thérèse philosophe* (approx. 1748), in which philosophical arguments for 'Spinozistic' determinism are presented within an erotic narrative inspired

by a contemporary scandal involving a priest and a gullible young woman (Thomson, *Bodies of Thought*, p. 171).

75. In D. Diderot, *Œuvres*, vol. 1: *Philosophie*, ed. L. Versini (Paris: Laffont-'Bouquins', 1994), p. 804.

76. P. H.-T., Baron D'Holbach, *Système de la Nature ou des lois du monde physique et du monde moral* (1770), 2nd edn, ed. J. Boulad-Ayoub (1781; Paris: Fayard-'Corpus', 1990), bk 1, ch. 1; § 18 in 1990 edition.

77. Ménuret, 'Œconomie Animale (Médecine)', p. 364b.

78. Hobbes, *Leviathan*, p. 3.

79. D. Dennett, 'Eliminate the Middletoad! Comment on J.-P. Ewert's "Neuroethology of Releasing Mechanisms: Prey-Catching in Toads"', *Behavioral and Brain Sciences* 10:3 (1987), pp. 372–73, on p. 373.

80. E. Hill, 'Materialism and Monsters in the *Rêve de D'Alembert*', *Diderot Studies*, 10 (1968), pp. 67–93, on p. 90.

81. The image that the (immaterial) soul is in the (material) body like a sailor in a ship is entertained by Aristotle (*De Anima* II.i.413a5) and rejected by Descartes in the Sixth Meditation, sounding for all the world like a phenomenologist: 'Nature . . . teaches me, by these sensations of pain, hunger, thirst and so on, that I am not merely present in my body as a sailor is present in a ship, but that I am very closely joined and, as it were, intermingled with it, so that I and the body form a unit' (Descartes, *Treatise on Man*, vol. 9, p. 64 / *The Philosophical Writings of Descartes*, ed. J. Cottingham, R. Stoothoff and D. Murdoch. Cambridge: Cambridge University Press (CSM), vol. 2, p. 56).

82. D'Holbach, *Système de la Nature ou des lois du monde physique et du monde moral* (1770; 1781), bk 1, ch. 11; p. 220 in 1990 edition.

83. A. Gaultier, *Parité de la vie et de la mort. La Réponse du médecin Gaultier*, ed. O. Bloch. (1714; Paris: Universitas / Oxford: Voltaire Foundation, 1993), pp. 142, 170.

84. *Éléments de physiologie*, in Diderot, *Œuvres*, p. 1282.

85. Diderot, *Œuvres complètes*, vol. 17, pp. 237, 470.

86. Merleau-Ponty, *The Structure of Behaviour*, pp. 208–9 (trans. modified).

87. P. S. Churchland, 'Reduction and the Neurobiological Basis of Consciousness', in A. Marcel and E. Bisiach (eds), *Consciousness and Contemporary Science* (Oxford: Oxford University Press, 1988), pp. 273–304, on p. 282.

88. G. W. Leibniz, *New Essays Concerning Human Understanding*, ed. and trans. P. Remnant and J. Bennett (Cambridge: Cambridge University Press, 1982), bk 2, ch. I, § 15.

89. Descartes, *Treatise on Man*, vol. 9, p. 60.

90. D. M. Armstrong and N. Malcolm, *Consciousness and Causality. A Debate on the Nature of Mind* (Oxford: Blackwell, 1984), p. 112.

91. D'Holbach, *Le bon sens, ou idées naturelles opposées aux idées surnaturelles*, ed. J. Deprun (1770; Paris: Éditions Rationalistes, 1990) § 41, p. 30.

92. Ibid., § 46, pp. 36–7.

93. W. G. Lycan, 'What is the "Subjectivity" of the Mental?', *Philosophical Perspectives*, 4: Action Theory and the Philosophy of Mind (1990), pp. 109–30, on p. 110.

94. P. Duhem, *Le mixte et la combinaison chimique. Essai sur l'évolution d'une idée* (1902; Paris: Fayard-'Corpus', 1985), p. 50.

## 10 Ghadessi, 'Visualizing Monsters: Anatomy as a Regulatory System'

1.  A. Carlino, 'Strani corpi. Come farsi une ragione dei mostri nel XVI secolo', *Phantastische Lebensräume, Phantome und Phantasmen* (Marburg an der Lahn: Basilisken-Press, 1997).

2.  I. G. Saint-Hilaire, *Histoire générale et particulière des anomalies de l'organisation chez l'homme et les animaux, ouvrage comprenant des recherches sur les caractères, la classification, l'influence physiologique et pathologique, les rapports généraux, les lois et les causes des monstruosités, des variétés de vices de conformation, ou Traité de teratology* (Paris: J.-B. Baillière, Libraire de l'Académie Royale de Médecine, 1832).

3.  I use the term 'monster' to refer to beings, mostly humans, whose physical appearances strayed far enough from either the idealized body or the normative body as to be impossible to recuperate as 'normal', or in certain cases, 'human'. During the historical period discussed here, the term would be applied to hermaphrodites, conjoined twins, dwarves and hirsutes, among others.

4.  J. B. de C. M. Saunders and C. D. O'Malley, *The Illustrations from the Works of Andreas Vesalius of Brussels* (New York: Dover Publications, Inc., 1950).

5.  In fact, this drive is also found in artistic representations. The new academic curricula emphasizing the need for artist to master anatomical knowledge allowed them to become fluent in both visual and anatomical languages. For works on artists' burgeoning interest in anatomy in the early modern, see A. Carlino, *Books of the Body: Anatomical Ritual and Early-Modern Learning* (Chicago, IL and London: University of Chicago Press, 1999); A. Carlino, *Paper Bodies: A Catalogue of Anatomical Fugitive Sheets 1538–1687* (London: Wellcome Institute for the History of Medicine, 1999); M. Cazort, et al. (eds), *The Ingenious Machine of Nature: Four Centuries of Art and Anatomy* (Ottawa: National Gallery of Canada, 1996); J. V. Hansen and S. Porter, *The Physician's Art: Representations of Art and Medicine* (Durham, NC: Duke University Medical Center Library and Duke University Museum of Art, 1999); M. Kemp and M. Wallace, *Spectacular Bodies: The Art and Science of the Human Body from Leonardo to Now* (Berkeley, CA: University of California Press, 2000); and B. Schultz, *Art and Anatomy in Early modern Italy* (Ann Arbor, MI: UMI Research Press, 1985).

6.  R. Mandressi, *Le regard de l'anatomiste: Dissections et invention du corps en Occident* (Paris: Editions du Seuil, 2003), p. 90.

7.  R. Mandressi, 'Textes scientifiques et savoirs sur le corps à l'époque moderne', seminar, École des hautes études en sciences sociales, Paris, 22 November 2005.

8.  For the dissection of monsters I am particularly referring to Colombo's dissection of a hermaphrodite – though the other anatomically unusual bodies he dissected could fall into this same category – and to Agnolo Bronzino's participation in the dissection of conjoined twins at the Palazzo Rucellai in 1538, see Z. Hanafi, *The Monster in the Machine: Magic, Medicine, and the Marvelous in the Time of the Scientific Revolution* (Durham, NC and London: Duke University Press, 2000), pp. 18–21.

9.  For instance, in his encyclopaedic work on animals, Conrad Gesner borrowed images from earlier German sources and from biblical texts and combined them with recently-discovered animals from the new world. See C. Gesner, *Historiae animalium* (Frankfurt: H. Laurent, 1620) where the author describes a beast from the new world (title page of book 1), a unicorn (book 1, p. 689) and a salamander (book 2, p. 80).

10. L. Daston and K. Park, *Wonders and the Order of Nature 1150–1750* (New York: Zone Books, 1998), pp. 177–80.
11. See for instance G. Canguilhem, *Le normal et le pathologique* (Paris: Presses Universitaires de France, 1966).
12. Saunders and O'Malley, *The Illustrations*, p. 204. For a detailed biography of Vesalius and his numerous productions and publications, see pp. 9–40.
13. B. Schultz, *Art and Anatomy in Early-Modern Italy* (Ann Arbor, MI: UMI Research Press, 1985), p. 11.
14. Ibid., p. 13; and N. Siraisi, *Medieval and Early Early-Modern Medicine: An Introduction to Knowledge and Practice* (Chicago, IL: Chicago University Press, 1990).
15. L. Conrad, et al., *The Western Medical Tradition 800 B.C. to A.D. 1800* (Cambridge: Cambridge University Press, 1995), pp. 66–7.
16. Ibid., p. 60.
17. Most notably, Vesalius's demonstration in the winter of 1539–40 on Galen's erroneous views and descriptions of the insertion of an abdominal muscle, the shape of the liver, the motion of the head and the azygos vein. See R. French, *Dissection and Vivisection in the European Renaissance* (Aldershot: Ashgate, 1999), pp. 165–6.
18. Carlino, *Books of the Body*, p. 2.
19. Ibid., pp. 40–1.
20. For centuries, the lecturer would read Galenic texts from the chair in Latin, while the pointer directed the audience's gaze to the supposed part of the body being discussed. The only person touching the corpse was the barber-surgeon whose knowledge of the actual body was considerable, but who often did not understand the Latin words being read. Consequently, discrepancies occurred between textual descriptions and the parts of the body being dissected. For Vesalius's acquisition of actual bodies in the hope of eradicating such inconsistencies, see J. Sawday, *The Body Emblazoned: Dissection and the Human Body in Early-Modern Culture* (London and New York: Routledge, 1995), p. 195.
21. J. V. Hansen and S. Porter, *The Physician's Art: Representations of Art and Medicine* (Durham, NC: Duke University Medical Center Library and Duke University Museum of Art, 1999), p. 32
22. Carlino, *Books of the Body*, p. 43.
23. See, for instance, G. Harcourt, 'Andreas Vesalius and the Anatomy of Antique Sculpture', *Representations*, 17 (1987), pp. 28–61.
24. While Vesalius does make some comparative anatomical and visual analyses in the *De fabrica* (in his discussion on skulls, for instance), he mostly seeks to establish an ideal anatomical norm.
25. P. Findlen, *Museums, Collecting, and Scientific Culture in Early-Modern Italy* (Berkeley and Los Angeles, CA and London: University of California Press, 1994), pp. 194–208.
26. P. Boaistuau, *Histoires prodigieuses* (Paris: Robert le Mangnier, 1566). Some of the chapter titles are as follows: 'Nabuchodonosor', 'Diables qui conçoivent', 'Monstre ayant ailes & les pieds d'oyseau engendré du temps du Pape Iule second & du Roy Louys douziesme' and 'Filles collées'.
27. Boaistuau, preface following the dedication: 'Monseigneur, entre toutes les choses qui se peuvent contempler soubs la concavité des cieux, il ne se voit rien qui plus efeuille l'esprit humain, qui ravisse plus les sens, qui plus espouvente, qui engendre plus grande admiration ou terreur aux creatures, que les monstres, prodiges & abomination, sequels nous voyons les erreures de nature ou seulement preposterées, renuersées, mutilées & tronquées, mais (qui plus est) nous y decouvrons le plus souvent un secret iugement & fleau

de l'ire de Dieu, par l'object des choses qui se presentment lequel nous faict sentir la violence de sa iustice si aspre, que nous sommes contrains d'entrer en nous mesmes, frapper au marteau de nostre conscience, esplucher noz vices, & avoir en horreur nos meffaicts, specialement quand nous lisons aux histories, sacrées & prophanes, que quelquefois les Elemens on esté Heraulx, Trompettes, ministres & executeurs de la iustice de Dieu'. All translations are by the author, unless otherwise indicated.

28.  See A. Paré, *Des monstres et prodiges* (Paris: G. Buon, 1585), bk 25, preface: 'Or disent-ils que je ne devoy escrire en François, & que par ce moyen la Medecine en seroit tenue à mespris: ce qui me semble le contraire: car ce que j'en ay faict', est plustost pour la magnifier & honorer.'

29.  See Paré, *Des monstres et prodiges*, p. 1020 : 'Monstres sont des choses qui apparoissent outre le cours de Nature (&sont le plus souuent signes de quelques malheurs à advenir) comme un enfant qui naist avec un seul bras, un autre qui aura deux testes, & autres membres outre l'ordinaire. Prodiges, ce sont des choses qui viennent du tout contre Nature, comme une femme qui enfentera un serpent, ou un chien, ou autre chose tout contre Nature ... Les mutilez, ce sont aveugles, borgnes, bossus, boiteux, ou ayant six doigts a la main ou aux pieds, ou moins de cinq ou joincts ensembles, ou les bras trop courts, ou le nez trop enfoncé comme ont les camus, ou avoir les levres grosses et renversées ... ou toute autre chose contre Nature.'

30.  L. Daston and K. Park, *Wonders and the Order of Nature, 1150–1750* (New York: Zone Books, 1998), p. 146.

31.  I. Norwich, 'A Consultation between Andreas Vesalius and Ambroise Paré at the Deathbed of Henri II, King of France, 15 July 1559', *SAMJ*, 80:5 (1991), pp. 245–7.

32.  Paré, *Des monstres et prodiges*, p. 1030.

33.  N. R. Smith, 'Portentous Births and the Monstrous Imagination in Early modern Culture', in T. S. Jones and D. A Sprunger (eds), *Marvels, Monsters, and Miracles – Studies in the Medieval and Early Modern Imaginations* (Kalamazoo: Board of the Medieval Institute, 2002), p. 270.

34.  Paré, 'un être que l'on monstre', in *Des monstres et prodiges*, p 1020.

35.  Paré, 'furent portées par plusieurs villes d'Italie' and 'le peuple qui était fort ardent de voir ce nouveau spectacle de nature', in *Des monstres et prodiges*, p. 1045.

36.  F. Gaffiot, *Dictionnaire Latin-Français: Le Grand Gaffiot* (Paris: Hachette, 2000); and E. Benveniste, *Vocabulaire des institutions indo-européennes* (Paris: Edition de Minuit, 1969), vols 1 and 2.

37.  Daston and Park, *Wonders and the Order of Nature*, pp. 173–214; 175–6.

38.  F. Liceti, *De monstrorum natura, caussis et differentiis – Libri Duo, Aeneis iconibus ornate et aucti* (Padua: Paolo Frambotti, 1634), preface: monsters 'quoque unicuique alteri monstrantur'.

39.  F. Liceti, *Description anatomique des Parties de la Femme qui servent à la Generation; avec un Traité des monstres, de leur Causes, de leur Nature, & de leur differences: Et une description anatomique de la disposition surprenante de quelques Parties Externes, & Internes de Deux Enfans Nés dans la Ville de Gand Capitale des Flandres le 28 Avril 1703 &c. &c., par Mons.r Jean Palfyn, Anatomist & Chirurgien de la Ville de Gand, Desquels ouvrages on peut considerer comme une Suite de l'Accouchement des Femmes par Mons.r Mauriceau* (Leiden: Chez la Veuve Bastiaan Schouten, 1708). Interestingly, this French version pairs the cause of monsters with a treatise on female reproductive parts, thus accentuating the generative emphasis of the book. The preface to Liceti's translation includes: 'Comme donc il n'y a rien de tout ce qui vit sous le Soleil, qui cause plus de surprise & d'admiration

que les Monstres; Ce n'est pas sans raison que les hommes desirent si universellement de connoitre leur Essence.'

40. M. Foucault, *The Order of Things: An Archeology of the Human Sciences* (New York: Random House, 1994), pp. 156–7.

41. In total, Liceti gives ten different categories of monsters and explains each one by using case studies. Furthermore, Liceti's treatise is actually written in Latin and therefore borrows from the medical textual tradition.

42. R. Colombo, *De re anatomica – Libri XV* (Venice: Nicholas Bevilacqua, 1559).

43. R. J. Moes and C. D. O'Malley, 'Realdo Colombo: "On Those Things Rarely Found in Anatomy': An Annotated Translation from the *De Re Anatomica* (1559)', *Bulletin of the History of Medicine*, 34:6 (1960), p. 508. Colombo replaced Vesalius temporarily as the chair of surgery and anatomy on 19 January 1543 and permanently in 1544.

44. Carlino, *Strani corpi*, p. 143: 'during the Early modern they were perceived and understood in many different ways: monsters were prodigies and natural wonders, monsters were signs of future catastrophes, they were used for religious and political propaganda. At the same time, they started to be conceived and studied into a medical framework ... My claim is that Colombo's approach to monstrous subjects through anatomical dissections induced him to conceive their morphological 'differences' as anatomical abnormalities. This approach signifies inscribing monstrosity in pathology'. I am indebted to Andrea Carlino who very generously shared this article and discussed his research with me.

45. Colombo, *De re anatomica*, p. 268.

46. Saint-Hilaire, *Histoire générale*.

47. Ibid., vol. 1, preface, p. x: 'J'ai cherché et je crois avoir réussi à démontrer que l'ensemble de nos connaissances sur les anomalies, ou pour employer dès à présent le nom que je lui donne dans cet ouvrage, la *tératologie* ne peut plus être considérée comme une section de l'anatomie pathologique; qu'on ne saurait non plus voir en elle un simple rameau, ni de la physiologie, ni de l'anatomie philosophique, ni de l'embryogénie, ni de la zoologie; qu'elle a avec toutes ces sciences des rapports presque également intimes, sans pouvoir être confondue avec aucune d'elles; qu'elle constitue par conséquent une branche particulière, un *science* distincte, dans le sens spécial qu'on a donné à ce mot.'

48. Ibid., vol. 1, p. 1, footnote referring to the first time the author uses the term 'tératologie': 'Je n'ignore pas que je m'écarte de l'opinion de tous les anatomistes, en considérant l'ensemble des nos connaissances sur les monstruosités comme une science distincte, comme un branche spéciale de la grande science de l'organisation: mais je crois pouvoir dire que cette innovation, importante pour les progrès futurs de la théorie des anomalies, et la création d'un mot nouveau, qui en est la conséquence nécessaire, seront complètement justifiées dans la suite de cet ouvrage.'

49. Ibid., vol. 1, p. xij: 'Aussi ai-je constamment cherché à déduire des faits tératologiques, les conséquences générales et les applications qui résultent de leur étude, et n'ai-je jamais perdu de vue le but principal que je m'étais proposé en commençant cet ouvrage; celui d'arriver, par l'étude des anomalies, de leurs caractères, de leur influence sur l'organisation, de leur mode de production et de leurs lois, à la connaissance plus exacte et plus approfondie des modifications de l'ordre normal, de leur essence, de leur raison d'existence, et des principes auxquels peut se rattacher leur infinie variété.'

50. I am being purposefully broad by using the term 'representation'. Often, the inclusion of an engraving of a monster, for instance, was accompanied by a textual description of its origins and physical appearance, or a poem relating the state of this particular being. The

actual representation of a monster might thus include a visual one alone, or a visual one together with a textual one.

51. P. Findlen, *Museums, Collecting, and Scientific Culture in Early Modern Italy* (Berkeley, Los Angeles, CA and London: University of California Press, 1994), pp. 209–10; and J. V. Hansen, 'Resurrecting Death: Anatomical Art in the Cabinet of Dr. Frederick Ruysch', *Art Bulletin*, 78 (1996), pp. 663–77, on p. 667.

52. G. Olmi, 'Il collezionismo scientifico', in R. Simili (ed.), *Il teatro della natura di Ulisse Aldrovandi* (Bologna: Editrice Compositori, 2001), p. 20.

53. The translation of Aldrovandi's own description is found in Daston and Park, *Wonders and the Order of Nature*, p. 154, n. 3.

54. Findlen, *Museums*, p. 60.

55. Ibid., p. 199. Also see G. Olmi, *Ulisse Aldrovandi: Scienza e natura nel secondo cinquecento* (Trent: UNIcoop. Soc. Coop. a.r.l., 1976), and S. P. Tugnoli, *La formazione scientifica e il 'Discorso naturale' di Ulisse Aldrovandi* (Trent: UNIcoop. Soc. Coop. a.r.l., 1977).

56. See for instance, Agnolo Bronzino's portrait of Cosimo I de'Medici's dwarf Morgante (before 1553), or Lavinia Fontana's portrait of the hirsute girl Antonietta Gonsalus (1595).

57. Such documents were often engravings representing the actual collection. See Ferrante Imperato, *Dell'historia naturale* (1672); Benedetto Ceruti and Andrea Chiocco, *Musaeum Francisci Calceolari Iunioris Veronensis* (1662); Lorenzo Legati, *Museo Cospiano annesso a quello del famoso Ulisse Aldrovandi e donato alla sua patria dall'illustrissimo Signor Ferdinando Cospi* (1677); and Ulisse Aldrovandi's illustrations in *Monstrorum historia* (1642).

58. F. H. Jacobs, *The 'Living' Image in Early-Modern Art* (Cambridge: Cambridge University Press, 2004), pp. 134, 137, 153, 160, 166 (from ch. 5: 'Nosce te ipsum: Narcissus, Mirrors, and Monsters').

# 11 Hanson, 'Anatomy, Newtonian Physiology and Learned Culture: The *Myotomia Reformata* and its Context within Georgian Scholarship'

1. H. Cook, 'Good Advice and Little Medicine: The Professional Authority of Early Modern English Physicians', *Journal of British Studies*, 33:1 (1994), pp. 1–31. The crucial conditions Cook establishes for understanding the seventeenth century still largely pertained in the eighteenth century, particularly at the level of elite medical care.

2. Mead appears throughout Pope's correspondence, and the two regularly dined together. Pope characterized Cheselden as 'the most noted, and the most deserving man, in the whole profession of Chirurgery', *Corr* 4:6, quoted in P. Rogers, *The Alexander Pope Encyclopedia* (Westport, CT: Greenwood Press, 2004), p. 60.

3. W. Cowper, *Myotomia reformata, or, A New Administration of All the Muscles of Humane Bodies wherein the True Uses of the Muscles are Explained, the Errors of Former Anatomists concerning them Confuted, and Several Muscles not hitherto Taken Notice of Described: To Which are Subjoin'd a Graphical Description of the Bones, and other Anatomical Observations: Illustrated with Figures After the Life* (London: Samuel Smith and Benjamin Walford, 1694), usefully described in the essential compendium, K. B. Roberts and J. D. W. Tomlinson, *The Fabric of the Body: European Traditions of Anatomical Illustration* (Oxford: Clarendon Press, 1992), pp. 412–17.

4.  W. Cowper, 'An Account of Two Glands and their Excretory Ducts Lately Discover'd in Human Bodies', *Philosophical Transactions*, 21 (November 1699), pp. 363–9. The glands, however, were apparently first detected by the French surgeon Jean Méry in 1684; F. Beekman, 'Bidloo and Cowper, Anatomists', *Annals of Medical History*, 7 (1935), pp. 113–29 is often cited for the claim, though he relies on an anonymously authored essay, 'William Cowper, The Anatomist', *British Medical Journal*, 1 (15 January 1898), pp. 160–1.

5.  Cowper, *Myotomia reformata*, p. 228. Whether these actually exist in humans is still unclear. See, for instance, A. Batistatou, J. Panelos, A. Zioga and K. Charalabopoulos, 'Ectopic Modified Sebaceous Glands in Human Penis', *International Journal of Surgical Pathology*, 14 (2006), pp. 355–6.

6.  E. Tyson, *An Anatomy of a Chimpanzee, Orang-outang, sive homo sylvestris, or, The Anatomy of a Pygmie compared with that of a Monkey, an Ape, and a Man* (London: Bennet, 1699). Tyson and Cowper together published a paper on the generative organs of the male opossum that appeared in the *Philosophical Transactions*, 24 (1704), pp. 1565–90; see S. S. Parrish, 'The Female Opossum and the Nature of the New World', *William and Mary Quarterly*, 54 (July 1997), pp. 475–514.

7.  A full discussion is available in C. A. Hanson, *The English Virtuoso: Art, Medicine, and Antiquarianism in the Age of Empiricism* (Chicago, IL: University of Chicago Press, 2009), pp. 58–69.

8.  D. Margócsy, 'A Museum of Wonders or a Cemetery of Corpses? The Commercial Exchange of Anatomical Collections in Early Modern Netherlands', in S. Dupré and C. Lüthy (eds), *Silent Messengers: The Circulation of Material Objects of Knowledge in the Early Modern Low Countries* (Berlin: LIT Verlag, 2011), pp. 185–215 (the essay is drawn from the fourth chapter of Margócsy's doctoral thesis 'Commercial Visions: Trading with Representations of Nature in Early Modern Netherlands' (PhD dissertation, Harvard University, 2009). As he notes, details of the contract are available in I. H. van Eeghen, *De Amsterdamse boekhandel 1680–1725*, 5 vols (Amsterdam: Scheltema & Holkema, 1960–78), vol. 4, pp. 129–31. In response to Bidloo's charges, Cowper himself notes the agreement between publishers; see his *Eucharistia* (London: Samuel Smith and Benjamin Walford, 1701), p. 27, though given that Cowper also claims that Lairesse's images were initially prepared for Jan Swammerdam, historians have been appropriately skeptical. In any case, scholarship on the Bidloo–Cowper conflict has been much poorer for the omission of this crucial primary source material.

9.  See, for instance, Beekman, 'Bidloo and Cowper, Anatomists', esp. p. 127; W. A. McIntosh. 'Cowper: The Anatomist', *Canadian Medical Association Journal*, 10 (1920), pp. 938–45; and K. F. Russell, 'The Anatomical Plagiarist', *Medical Journal of Australia*, 46 (1959), pp. 249–52. Roberts and Tomlinson, in *The Fabric of the Body*, provide a useful conclusion to these approaches: 'It has been the fate of Cowper, surgeon, to be best remembered as a plagiarist, and as the anatomist whose name has been applied to the male urethral glands ... His own writings, however, show Cowper to have been intelligent, reliably informed, and, on many occasions, original', p. 412.

10. R. Knoeff, 'Moral Lessons of Perfection: A Comparison of Mennonite and Calvinist Motives in the Anatomical Atlases of Bidloo and Albinus', in O. P. Grell and A. Cunningham (eds) *Medicine and Religion in Enlightenment Europe* (Aldershot: Ashgate, 2007), pp. 121–43.

11. In addition to Robert and Tomlison, *The Fabric of the Body*, pp. 309–10, see L. van Poelgeest, 'The Stadholder-King Wiliam III and the University of Leiden', in P. Hoftijzer

and C. C. Barfoot (eds), *Fabrics and Fabrications: The Myth and Making of William and Mary* (Amsterdam: Rodopi, 1990), pp. 97–134, esp. pp. 130–4.

12. For an insightful discussion of the staffing shortages Leiden faced in the late seventeenth and early eighteenth century, see M. Ultee, 'The Politics of Professorial Appointment at Leiden, 1709', *History of Universities*, 9 (1990), pp. 167–94. Although Boerhaave studied at Leiden, he completed his MD at Harderwijk, in 1693 – an indication, for Ultee, of the 'minor part' Leiden's medical faculty played in his education, p. 173. At one point early in the decade, just before Boerhaave was hired as a lecturer, the faculty has consisted of just two medical professors (there should have been five). Boerhaave was not appointed a professor until 1709 and this amazingly in the field of botany, an area for which he was completely unqualified. For his reputation as an exemplary teacher as well as the reputation of Leiden's medical school generally, see R. Knoeff, 'Herman Boerhaave at Leiden: *Communis Europae Praeceptor*', in O. P. Grell, A. Cunningham and J. Arrizabalaga (eds), *Centres of Medical Excellence? Medical Travel and Education in Europe, 1500–1789* (Aldershot: Ashgate, 2010), pp. 269–86.

13. Margocsy, 'A Museum of Wonders or a Cemetery of Corpses?'

14. Roberts and Tomlinson, *The Fabric of the Body*, p. 415. Bernhard Albinus (1653–1721) joined the medical faculty at Leiden in 1702; his son Bernhard Siegfried (1697–1770) was appointed to the position in 1722. C. B. Albinus (1696–1752) was appointed professor of anatomy at Utrecht in 1723.

15. As an institution, the Royal Society famously avoided involvement in personal squabbles, and so its refusal to address Bidloo's claims hardly come as a surprise. I am grateful to Moti Feingold for stressing the point to me.

16. A. Guerrini, 'The Tory Newtonians: Gregory, Pitcairne, and Their Circle', *Journal of British Studies*, 25 (1986), pp. 288–311; A. Guerrini, 'Archibald Pitcairne and Newtonian Medicine', *Medical History*, 31 (1987), pp. 70–83; and A. Guerrini, 'Isaac Newton, George Cheyne, and the *Principia Medicinae*', in R. French and A. Wear (eds), *The Medical Revolution of the Seventeenth-Century* (Cambridge: Cambridge University Press, 1989), pp. 222–45.

17. My hunch is that the question of 'Cowper's plagiarism' has received so much attention from medical historians (especially physicians) precisely because Cowper's text is superior to Bidloo's and was treated accordingly in the eighteenth century. For those focusing on an 'internal' narrative of medical progress in which advances come through noble, heroic action, Cowper poses problems. That he was supported by many physicians who are highly regarded within such accounts just makes matters worse. I am suggesting that the social and political contexts are far more interesting and useful for understanding the period.

18. Mead figures prominently in chapters 4 and 5 of Hanson, *The English Virtuoso*. For Mead's biography generally, see M. Maty, *Authentic Memoirs of the Life of Richard Mead, M.D.* (London, 1755); A. Zuckerman, 'Dr Richard Mead (1674–1754): A Biographical Study' (PhD dissertation, University of Illinois, Urbana, 1965); and R. H. Meade, *In the Sunshine of Life: A Biography of Dr Richard Mead, 1673–1754* (Philadelphia, PA: Dorrance & Co., 1974).

19. R. Mead, *A Mechanical Account of Poisons in Several Essays* (London, 1702), unpaginated preface.

20. Anita Guerrini's work is crucial, in addition to sources noted earlier, see 'James Keill, George Cheyne, and Newtonian Physiology', *Journal of the History of Biology*, 18 (1985), pp. 247–66. Also, see T. Brown, 'Medicine in the Shadow of the *Principia*', *Journal of the History of Ideas*, 48 (1987), pp. 629–48. More generally, see M. Feingold, *The Newtonian Moment: Isaac Newton and the Making of Modern Culture*, exhibition catalogue (New York: Oxford University Press, 2004).

21. K. F. Russell, 'The Anatomical Library of Dr Richard Mead (1673–1754)', *Journal of the History of Medicine and Allied Sciences*, 2 (Winter 1947), pp. 97–109, esp. p. 103.

22. Mead, who would later become royal physician to George II, understood the importance of politics as well as any of his peers, but he repeatedly resisted party politics, especially when it threatened to trump professional expertise and intellectual achievement. Similarly, as Ultee makes clear with his essay on 'The Politics of Professorial Appointment at Leiden, 1709', various factors beyond one's immediate qualifications continued to shape hiring practices at Leiden as indicated by Boerhaave's appointment to a chair of botany when he was anything but a botanist. On the other hand, Boerhaave, as the well-liked 'inside candidate', presents an example directly opposite that of Bidloo. As a teacher of medical theory, Boerhaave was effective, and given that he had been promised a professorship position as one became available, his colleagues feared that he would leave if he were passed over. He was hired as a result of academic politics not state politics.

23. Mead, *A Mechanical Account of Poisons in Several Essays*, p. 98. In the two twentieth-century biographies of Mead, Arnold Zuckerman and Richard Meade both mistakenly state that Mead had previously served as anatomy lecturer for the Barbers Surgeons for six or seven years, starting in 1703; the source of the error seems to be W. Macmichael, *Lives of British Physicians* (London: John Murray, 1830), p. 158.

24. Brown, 'Medicine in the Shadow of the *Principia*', p. 631. From this opening lecture, Pitcairne offered a series of talks that Andrew Cunningham has characterized as 'a progressive, chapter by chapter, demolition of Cartesian explanations' that made room for 'what Pitcairne believed to be Newtonian ones'. See 'Sydenham versus Newton: The Edinburgh Fever Dispute of the 1690s between Andrew Brown and Archibald Pitcairn', *Medical History*, supplement (1981), pp. 71–98, on p. 89. The notable precedent for connecting astronomy (at least in terms of method), mathematics, and anatomy – as discussed below – comes from Nicolaus Steno, whose *Myology* of 1667 was inspired by Galileo.

25. A. M. Roos, 'Luminaries in Medicine: Richard Mead, James Gibbs, and Solar and Lunar Effects on the Human Body in Early Modern England', *Bulletin of the History of Medicine*, 74 (2000), pp. 433–57.

26. Brown, 'Medicine in the Shadow of the *Principia*', p. 646.

27. A. Cunningham, *The Anatomist Anatomis'd: An Experimental Discipline in Enlightenment Europe* (Aldershot: Ashgate, 2010), p. 158.

28. Ibid., p. 198.

29. Mead, *A Mechanical Account of Poisons in Several Essays*, unpaginated preface.

30. Cunningham, *The Anatomist Anatomis'd*, p. 9: 'Without some understanding of what constituted a particular past discipline it is too easy for us to project back the concerns and boundaries of modern disciplines inappropriately, and thereby multiply our misunderstandings. And example of such disciplinary misunderstanding ... is that between the old discipline of anatomy and the old discipline of physiology, where much modern writing about the history of physiology has simply got hold of the wrong past discipline!'

31. Ibid., pp. 12, 149, 156.

32. Ibid., p. 19.

33. 'Biographical Preface', in J. Wilson (ed.), *A Course of Chemistry, Divided into Twenty-four Lectures given by the Late Learned Doctor Henry Pemberton* (London: J. Nourse, 1771), quoted in I. B. Cohen, 'Pemberton's Translation of Newton's *Principia*, With Notes on Motte's Translation', *Isis*, 54 (1963), pp. 319–51, on p. 321.

34. Domenico Bertoloni Meli, 'The Collaboration between Anatomists and Mathematicians in the mid-Seventeenth Century with a Study of Images as Experiments and Galileo's Role in Steno's *Myology*', *Early Science and Medicine*, 13 (2008), pp. 665–709. Steno's explicit rationale for linking mathematics to the study of muscles is notable: 'In this dissertation I wished to show that unless myology becomes part of mathematics, the parts of a muscle cannot be distinctly designated, nor can its motion be considered adequately. And why should we not give to the muscles what astronomers give to the sky, geographers to the earth, and, to take an example from the microcosm, what writers on optics concede to the eyes?' (quoted in Meli, ' The Collaboration', p. 700).
35. Pemberton, 'Introduction', *Myotomia reformata*, pp. iv, xxxiv.
36. Crucial background for the history of the study of the muscles comes from E. Bastholm, *The History of Muscle Physiology: From the Natural Philosophers to Albrecht Von Holler* (Amsterdam: Swets & Zeitlinger, 1968). For seventeenth-century theories of muscular motion, see the fine introduction by T. Kardel for the recent publication of Johann Bernoulli's *Dissertations: On the Mechanics of Effervescence and Fermentation and On the Mechanics of the Movement of the Muscles* in *Transactions of the American Philosophical Society*, 87 (1997), pp. 1–158.
37. Kardel, *Dissertations*, pp. 1, 32.
38. P.A. Michelloti (a member, incidentally, of the Royal Society) edited the second edition, which was published in Venice. See Kardel, *Dissertations*, pp. 1, 29–32.
39. Pemberton, *Myotomia reformata,* pp. liii, lxiii, lxxiii.
40. Ibid., p. lxxvii.
41. Bernoulli, *Dissertations*, p. 103.
42. M. Sanders, 'William Cowper and His Decorated Copperplate Initials', *Anatomical Record, Part B: The New Anatomist*, 282B (2005), pp. 5–12.
43. I am especially grateful to Sachiko Kusukawa who, in noting the temporal proximity between the two texts, raised the question of how they might be related. For Boerhaave, see G. A. Lindeboom, 'Boerhaave: Author and Editor', *Bulletin of the Medical Library Association*, 62 (1974), pp. 137–48.
44. Mead states in his 'Advertisement', that Cowper's preface 'ends abruptly, and is otherwise defective, for besides the Additions, which are here made to the Preface of his former Book, he intended some others, particularly there were found in his Papers a few Sketches concerning the Usefulness of Anatomy in Painting and Statuary, but these were so imperfect, that they were not fit to be printed'.
45. W. Hogarth, *The Analysis of Beauty*, ed. R. Paulson (New Haven, CT and London: Paul Mellon Centre for British Art, 1997), pp. 53, 151.

# 12 Marino, 'Art and Medicine: Creative Complicity between Artistic Representation and Research'

1. A fundamental contribution to the development of this kind of science in Bologna was given by Guglielmo da Saliceto (1210–77), the author of *Cyrurgia* (*c.* 1275). Moreover, Taddeo degli Alderotti (1223–1303) encouraged an intensification of the study of anatomy in this city. Later on, his lessons paved the way to a generation of distinguished doctors including Bartolomeo da Varignana, Mondino de' Liuzzi and Henri de Mondeville.
2. Bartolomeo da Varignana was a lecturer of medicine in Bologna from 1293 to 1301. The paternity of one of the first autopsies has to be attributed to him, as witnessed by an offi-

cial document. In fact he was the coroner in a criminal trial in Bologna on 1 March 1302. For further reading, see L. Premuda, *Storia dell'Iconografia Anatomica* (Saronno: Ciba Edizioni, 1993), p. 47; and A. Simili, 'Considerazioni su una Perizia Medico-Legale Inedita del "300"', *Giornale di Clinica Medica*, 17 (1941), pp. 921–27.

3.   Henri de Mondeville, a student in Bologna, became a doctor and professor in Montpellier. He is the author of *Cyrurgia* (*c.* 1320). His research seems particularly innovative because of his meticulous body examinations and the numerous illustrations accompanying the text. It is worth noting that in these illustrations the typically medieval frog scheme occurs only in one table; in addition to that, the practice of representing simply the 'five' systems disappears. The most striking element consists of the depiction of the subject deprived of his skin, which is held up by sticks lying on the corpse. This image appears as a precursor in its attitude and attempt to describe anatomy; in this respect it is comparable to a figure by Gaspar Becerra in the *Historia de la Composición del Cuerpo Humano* (1556), written by Juan de Valverde. For further reading see M. Tabanelli, *Un Secolo d'Oro della Chirurgia Francese* (Forlì: Tipografia Valbonesi, 1969).

4.   Mondino de' Liuzzi is the author of *Anothomia*, completed in 1316 (without illustrations). Even if it looks more like a manual of sectorial technique than a compendium of medicine, it is the first work which approaches the study of the body and its systems in a modern way. His treatise was widely employed in order to teach surgery until 1500. For further reference see P. P. Giorgi and G. F. Pasini, *Anothomia, Mondino de'Liuzzi da Bologna* (Bologna: Istituto per la Storia dell'Università, 1992).

5.   For further reference on *Funfbilderserie* see Premuda, *Storia dell'Iconografia Anatomica*, p. 40.

6.   See for example the illustrations in the *Ashmole* MS 399, Bodleian Library of Oxford, England, with particular reference to tables 018r, 019r, 020r, 021r, 022r.

7.   The six illustrations of *Fasciculs Medicinae* are: *The Bleeding Man*, *The Pregnant Woman*, *The Man of Wounds*, *The Man of the Diseases*, *The Wheel of Urine* and *The Zodiac Man*.

8.   The full title of the treatise is: *Consilium pro Peste Evitanda* (1398). The work is part of the numerous '*consilia*' against plague which were very popular between 1300 and 1400.

9.   For further reference see the interesting critical and philological work of T. Pesenti, *Il Fasciculus Medicinae, ovvero Le Metamorfosi del Libro Umanistico* (Treviso: Antilia, 2001). Here Pesenti underscores the presence of this series in another German code, the Palatino Lat. 1325, presumably composed in late 1400, and now part of the Vatican Library Collection. Karl Sudhoff too has tracked this series down in numerous manuscripts of German origin, dating from the end of the fourteenth century. Some drawings can also be found in the code Wellcome 49 (1420), preserved in the Wellcome Library of London, in Pal. Lat. 1305 (Vatican Library) and in another manuscript held by the Bayerische library, Monaco.

10.   The new illustrations of the 1494 edition are *A Visit to a Patient Suffering from Plague*, *A University Lecture of Anatomy*, *A Consult with the Horoscope* and *Petrus de Montagnana*.

11.   Those artists that at the end of the fifteenth century were interested in this kind of activities were defined by Adam Bartsch as *peintres graveurs*. For further reading see A. Bartsch, *Le Peintre Graveur* (Nieuwkoop: Nouvelle édition, 1982).

12.   'Know yourself'. Unless otherwise stated all translations are my own.

13.   M. Bucci, *Anatomia come Arte* (Firenze: Il Fiorino, 1969), p. 72.

14.   *Trinità* (*c.* 1426), fresco, Basilica of Santa Maria Novella, Florence.

15. B. Bearzi, 'Considerazioni di Tecnica sul San Ludovico e la Giuditta di Donatello', in L. Dolcini (ed.), *Donatello e il restauro della Giuditta* (Firenze: Centro Di della Edifimi, 1988), pp. 64–6, on p. 64.

16. 'Let's distinguish the limbs from joints. Let's show the veins: unless you find folds and sinuosity in the dress', Pliny the Elder, *Naturalis Historia* (Leipzig: Teubner, 1897), b. XXXVI, par. 56.

17. I am referring to the *Crocifisso* (*c.* 1449), bronze, Basilica of Saint Anthony, Padua.

18. *Giuditta* (*c.* 1457), bronze, Palazzo Vecchio, Florence.

19. Bearzi, 'Considerazioni di Tecnica', p. 65: 'certi aspetti troppo realistici come le gambe nude di Oloferne danno la sensazione che si tratti di calchi eseguiti dal vero. Esse mostrano la riproduzione di arti appartenenti ad un uomo di età avanzata e dai piedi distorti da faticosi lavori ... Tali gambe ... sono state create e fuse a parte ed inserite per ultime nel gruppo e fissate, mediante visibile rigetto di metallo.'

20. 'The black leg's miracle'.

21. *Pala di San Marco* (*c.* 1440), tempera on panel, Museo di San Marco, Florence.

22. A. Busignani, *Verrocchio* (Firenze: Sadea Editore, 1966), p. 11.

23. 'Andrea, dunque, usò di fermare con forme così fatte le cose naturali, per poterle con più comodità tenere innanzi e imitarle, cioè mani, piedi, ginocchi, gambe braccia torsi.' ('Thus Andrea tried to fix things in these forms, so that he could comfortably take them in front of him in order to imitate them, that is hands, feet, knees, legs arms and busts.'). G. Vasari, *Le Vite de 'piu Eccellenti Pittori Scultori, e Architettori*, 3 vols (Firenze: Giunti, 1568), vol. 2, p. 485.

24. For a long time, the church of the Annunziata in Florence hosted the largest number of such figures, the oldest of which can be dated back to 1300. Of particular interest is their description made by George Eliot. For further reading see G. Eliot, *Romola* (Torino: Utet, 1969), ch. 14.

25. *The Flayed* (1600), bronze, Museo Nazionale del Bargello, Firenze.

26. The works certainly attributed to Zumbo are *The Triumph of Time, The Plague, The Tomb* or *Vanity of the Human Glory, The Gallic Disease*, the *Head* at the Florence museum Specola and the *Head* at the Muséum National d'Historie Naturelle in Paris.

27. The Florentine period is dated, as in the documents found by François Cagnetta, between 1691 and 1694. For further reference see P. Giansiracusa (ed.), *Giulio Gaetano Zumbo* (Milano: Fabbri Editori, 1988), p. 63.

28. E. e J. De Goncourt, *L'Italia di Ieri* (Milano: Pirinetti Casoni Editore, 1944), p. 123.

29. P. Giansiracusa (ed.), *Antologia degli Scritti sull'Opera di Gaetano Giulio Zumbo* (Noto: Amministrazione comunale di Siracusa, 1990), p. 25.

30. D. A. F. De Sade, *L'Histoire de Juliette* (Paris: Ed. Pauvert, 1940), p. 248.

31. R. W. Lightbown, 'Gaetano Giulio Zumbo – 1: The Florentine Period', *Burligton Magazine*, November (1964), pp. 486–96, on p. 494.

32. AA. VV., *Mémoires de Trévoux* (*Mémoires pour l'Histoire des Sciences et des Beaux-Arts*), Octobre (1707), pp. 1830–37.

33. Lightbown, 'Gaetano Giulio Zumbo', p. 489.

34. W. Bernardi, *Francesco Redi. Esperienze Intorno alla Generazione degli Insetti* (Firenze: Giunti, 1966), p. 15: 'Redi allestì una serie di otto recipienti riempiti di vari tipi di carne, di cui quattro li lasciò all'aria aperta e gli altri quattro li sigillò accuratamente. Il risultato si dimostro inequivocabile: solo i primi campioni, nei quali le mosche avevano potuto posarsi sulla carne e deporvi le loro uova, avevano dato origine a larve che poi si erano sviluppate in mosche identiche alle prime. La carne dei recipienti sigillati, invece, era

diventata anch'essa putrida e si era decomposta, ma senza dar luogo a nessuna forma di vita.'

35. The oeuvre can be admired at the 'Specola' museum in Florence. Von Haller wrote memorable pages on it in A. Von Haller, *Bibliotheca Anatomica, qua Scripta ad Anatomen et Physiologiam, Facentia a Rerum Initiis Recensetur* (Tiguri: apud Orell, Gessner, Fuessli, et socc., 1774), p. 809.

36. M. Medici, *Elogio d'Ercole Lelli* (Bologna: Tipi a S. Tommaso D'Aquino, 1856), p. 164: 'l'avere egli injettato nello Spedale di S. Maria della Morte ... una testa d'uomo così compiutamente, che parea la testa d'uomo vivente, avendo essa ripigliato il suo naturale colorito, e veggendosi dell'injettato liquore ripieni perfino i vasi capillari dell'albuginea dell'occhio.'

37. *Scorticati del Teatro Anatomico dell'Archiginnasio* (1734), lime, Teatro anatomico dell'Archiginnasio, Bologna.

38. It is thus important to have an insight on how these works have been produced: 'per la formazione delle quali notomizzò non meno di cinquanta cadaveri ... Prese il Lelli due scheletri umani, e, posti negli ideati atteggiamenti, con canapa inzuppata di cera mischiata con semola, e trementina cominciò a foggiare i vari muscoli, e ad affiggerli a' loro luoghi imitando colla più scrupolosa esattezza il vero, ed il naturale, cui avea sempre sott'occhio, e di tal guisa proseguiva fino ad opera compiuta.' – 'in order to create them he analyzed not less than fifty corpses ... Lelli took two human skeletons and, after having put them in the desired position, he forged their muscles with a mixture of hemp, wax, bran, turpentine, putting them in the right place, trying his best to imitate reality, which was always under his eyes. He worked in this way until he finished.' M. Medici, *Elogio d'Ercole Lelli*, p. 171.

39. *Rene Normale* and *Rene a Ferro di Cavallo* (*c.* 1737), wax on panel, Museo di Palazzo Poggi, Bologna.

40. 'Ercole Lelli si esibisce di formare e scolpire in cera la Miologia e l'Osteologia del corpo umano figurato, e rappresentato in diverse statue, e tavole al naturale ... Adi 5 ottobre 1742.' ('Ercole Lelli will produce and sculpt with wax the myological and osteological systems of the human body; he will represent them in different statues, as well as in panels ... Today 5 October 1742.'). M. Armaroli, *Le Cere Anatomiche Bolognesi del Settecento* (Bologna: Clueb, 1981), p. 43.

41. This cooperation did not end happily: after working for three years, Manzolini was substituted by Luigi Dardani.

42. Ercole Lelli's works are part of the collection of the Museo di Palazzo Poggi in Bologna. They have been realized between 1742 and 1751.

43. *Orecchio staccato dal Capo con relative Ghiandole e Muscoli*, wax and wood, Museo di Palazzo Poggi, Bologna.

44. M. Focaccia, *Anna Morandi Manzolini, una Donna tra Arte e Scienza* (Firenze: Olschki, 2008), table 2.

45. G. Manzolini, *Sopra l'orecchio*, Archivio dell'Antica Accademia delle Scienze, Bologna, Reg. Atti, 16 April 1750.

46. G. Manzolini, *Osservazioni Sopra le Orecchie, e le Parti Inservienti all'Articolazione della Voce Fatte in un Cadavero che Vivendo Muto e Sordo e Nativitate*, Archivio dell'Antica Accademia delle Scienze, Bologna, Reg. Atti, 4 marzo 1751.

47. For further reference see AA. VV., *Ars Obstetricia Bononiensis: Catalogo ed Inventario del Museo Ostetrico Giovan Antonio Galli* (Bologna: Clueb, 1988).

48. Luigi Galvani (1777), quoted in S. Gherardi, *Opere Edite ed Inedite di Luigi Galvani* (Bologna: Tipografia di Emidio dall'Olmo, 1841), p. 101: 'nella Manzolini inoltre questo ancor più mirabile si deve considerare, che per prima congiunse due arti tanto dissimili, tanto difficili, anche, ma del tutto adatte (per non dire indispensabili) a compiere lavori di tal genere, Scultura e Anatomia, e le congiunse in modo da eccellere in ambedue.'

49. G. Logan Berti, 'Women and the Practice and Teaching of Medicine in Bologna in Eighteenth and Early Nineteenth Centuries', *Bulletin of History of Medicine*, 77 (2003), pp. 505–35, on p. 516.

50. R. Messbarger, 'Waxing Poetic: Anna Morandi Manzolini's Anatomical Sculptures', *Configurations*, 9:1 (2001), pp. 65–97, on p. 65.

51. *Mani*, wax and fabric on panel, Museo di Palazzo Poggi, Bologna.

52. *Muscoli del Globo e dell'Occhio, Muscolo della Palpebra Superiore, Nervo Ottico*, wax on panel, Museo di Palazzo Poggi, Bologna.

53. M. B. Stafford, *Body Criticism: Imaging the Unseen in Enlightenment Art and Medicine* (Cambridge, MA and London: MIT Press, 1991), p. 53.

## 13 Goffette and Simon, 'The Internal Environment: Claude Bernard's Concept and its Representation in *Fantastic Voyage*'

1. G. Durand, *Les structures anthropologiques de l'imaginaire* (Dunot, 1960), pp. 132–3.

2. M. D. Grmek, *Le legs de Claude Bernard* (Paris: Fayard ,1997), pp. 124–5.

3. C. Bernard, *Introduction à l'étude de la médecine expérimentale* (Paris: Baillères, 1957), p. 76.

4. Ibid., p. 139; quoted in Grmek, *Le legs de Claude Bernard*, p. 139.

5. Bernard, quoted in Grmek, *Le legs de Claude Bernard*, p. 169.

6. Bernard, *Introduction*, p. 120.

7. G. W. F. V. Leibniz, *Monadology* (Prentice Hall College Div., 1965), §67.

8. Bernard, *Introduction*, p. 76.

9. Ibid., p. 153 ; quoted in Grmek, *Le legs de Claude Bernard*, p. 139.

10. Bernard, *Introduction*, p. 64.

11. Ibid., pp. 103–4.

12. See Grmek, *Le legs de Claude Bernard*, p. 168: 'Le lecteur qui feuillette aujourd'hui les revues médicales et biologiques de la deuxième moitié du XIXe siècle a toutes les raisons de s'étonner de l'accueil froid qui fut réservé à la notion bernardienne de 'milieu intérieur'. Appréciée par quelques jeunes chercheurs, tels Paul Bert (1833–1886) dans l'entourage du maître ou William James (1842–1910) de l'autre côté de l'Atlantique, cette conception n'exerça qu'une influence très restreinte sur la plupart des physiologistes de l'époque. Bien entendu, on n'ignorait ni l'idée bernardienne ni son syntagme, mais on ne savait pas trop comment s'en servir. C'est vers 1885, et surtout après 1900, que l'expression fera fortune.'

13. See C. Durif-Bruckert, *Une fabuleuse machine. Anthropologie des savoirs ordinaires sur les fonctions physiologiques* (Paris: Métailié, 1994).

14. Bernard, *Introduction*, p. 153 ; also quoted in Grmek, *Le legs de Claude Bernard*, p. 139.

15. See G. Durand, *Les structures anthropologiques de l'imaginaire. Las estructuras antropologicas del imaginario. Introduccion a la arquetipologia general.* (México: Fondo de

Cultura Economica, 2005), and G. Durand, *As estruturas antropológicas do imaginário* (Lisboa Portugal: Presença, 1989).

16. See G. Jobes, *Dictionary of Mythology, Folklore and Symbols* (New York: Scarecrow Press, 1962); J. E. Cirlot, *Dictionary of Symbols* (London: Routledge/Taylor & Francis, 1971) ; J. Chevalier and A. Gheerbrant, *Dictionnaire des symboles: Mythes, rêves, coutumes, gestes, formes, figures, couleurs, nombres* (Paris: Robert Laffont, 1997), printed in English as *Dictionary of Symbols* (London: Penguin,1997).

17. G. Bachelard, *La poétique de l'espace* (Paris: Puf, 1957), ch. 8; trans. J. R. Stilgoe as *The Poetics of Space* (Boston, MA: Beacon Press, 1992), ch. 8.

18. Ibid., p. 171.

19. M. Eliade, *Traité d'histoire des religions* (Paris ; Payot, 1949), ch. 5, § 63, p. 169.

20. Ibid., ch. 5, § 70, p. 179.

21. Harry Kleiner, final script for *Fantastic Voyage*, version from 26 February 1965, available at http://leonscripts.tripod.com/scripts/FANVOY.htm [accessed 28 November 2010]; the actors do their best to deliver (particularly Owens, the captain of the submarine) – 36 minutes, 31 seconds.

22. Durand, *Les structures anthropologiques de l'imaginaire*, introduction, pp. 46–51.

23. G. Bachelard, *L'air et les songes* (Paris : José Corti/Livre de Poche, 1943), ch. 1: 'Le rêve de vol' ; G. Bachelard, *Air and Dreams: An Essay on the Imagination of Movement* (Dallas, TX: Dallas Institute Publications, 1988).

24. Durand, *Les structures anthropologiques de l'imaginaire*, pp. 46–51, 225–47.

25. Ibid., pp. 395–9.

26. Chevalier and Gheerbrant, 'Labyrinthe' entry, in *Dictionnaire des symboles*, p. 555.

27. Cirlot, *Dictionary of Symbols*, p. 347: 'In its most general sense, the symbolism of the tree denotes the life of the cosmos: its consistence, growth, proliferation, generative and regenerative processes.' Thus we see how the symbolism of the tree resonated both with the idea of life in general and the arterio-venous system.

28. Chevalier and Gheerbrant, 'Lumière' entry, in *Dictionnaire des symboles*, pp. 584–9.

29. Jobes, *Dictionary of Mythology*, p. 228.

30. Ibid., p. 1274.

31. Ibid., p. 245.

32. G. Bachelard, *La formation de l'esprit scientifique* (1938; Paris : Puf, 1993), p. 98; translated in English as *The Formation of the Scientific Mind* (Manchester: Clinamen Press, 2001).

33. M. Renard, 'Du roman merveilleux-scientifique et de son action sur l'intelligence du progrès', *Le Spectateur* (6), in M. Renard, *Romans et contes fantastiques – Du roman merveilleux-scientifique et de son action sur l'intelligence du progrès, Le Spectateur, n° 6, octobre 1909* (Paris: Robert Laffont, 1990), pp. 1205–13.

# INDEX